NEUROPSYCHODIAGNOSIS
IN PSYCHOTHERAPY

Revised Edition

Neuropsychodiagnosis in Psychotherapy
Revised Edition

by **LEONARD SMALL, Ph.D.**

*Chief Consulting Psychologist, Altro Health and
Rehabilitation Services, New York City*

BRUNNER/MAZEL, *Publishers* • New York

Library of Congress Cataloging in Publication Data

Small, Leonard, 1913-
    Neuropsychodiagnosis in psychotherapy.

    Includes bibliographies and index.
    1. Brain—Diseases—Diagnosis. 2. Neuropsychology. 3. Psychodiagnostics.
4. Psychotherapy. I. Title. [DNLN: 1. Mental disorders—Diagnosis. 2. Psychotherapy. 3. Nervous system diseases—Diagnosis. WL141 S635a]
RC386.5.S58   616.8'0475   80-19415
ISBN 0-87630-243-6

Published by
BRUNNER/MAZEL, INC.
19 Union Square
New York, N. Y. 10003

To

VERNA

Introduction

We now recognize that many symptoms and behaviors that appear to indicate psychopathology may have part or all of their etiology in damage, disease, or dysfunction of the brain, particularly the cerebral cortex. Estimates of the failure to detect neurological disorders in "psychiatric" patients range from 3 to about 50 percent. Significant numbers of persons with brain tumors first seek the assistance of a psychiatrist (6). Psychotic symptoms most often appear conspicuous in the clinical picture in these neurological disorders and the patient is usually so diagnosed, to his detriment (3, 5, 14, 16, 18, 22, 23, 24, 25, 27). Other symptoms reported as having masked neurological disorders are hysteria (7, 9), malingering (7), depression (9, 21), anorexia nervosa (10), behavioral problems in children (17), personality "change" (24), and "mental" symptoms (26). While no similar information is available for the percentage of patients suffering neurological pathology who come to psychologists or social workers for psychotherapy, the difficulties in differential diagnosis from those starting points are obviously similar. The more severe the symptom, the greater is the danger that the possibility of some degree of physical etiology will be overlooked by both therapist and patient. Psychodynamic explanations when applicable are indispensable to treatment, but used alone without investigation they may all too readily offer a false hypothesis. Other etiologies must be carefully considered if the interview and history-taking are to be complete, an approach that in no way abandons psychogenic hypotheses, but rather extends diagnostic reasoning to include the possible physical etiologies as well.

Neurological disorders both simulate and directly produce emotional and psychological disorders. Cantwell and Baker (4) have estimated that children with true brain damage are five times more likely than the general population to suffer psychiatric disorders. Psychomotor epilepsy, observes Lawall (11), ". . . is perhaps the quintessential example of a disorder on the borderline between psychiatry and neurology." Its behavioral manifestations may include laughter, hallucinations, involuntary obscenity, assaultiveness, hypo- and hypersexuality, *déjà vu, jamais vu,* depersonalization, derealization, paranoia, changes in mood. Petit mal may result in laziness, learning disabilities, depression, withdrawal, hostility and suicidal thoughts.

Chronic brain disorders of moderate degree appear to be even more numerous among the psychotherapy population than among those treated for acute neurological conditions (8). Behavior consequences here are also frequently mistaken for psychogenic symptoms. These conditions fall into a gray zone in both diagnosis and treatment. The ambiguities are not clarified, nor is the patient helped, when the psychotherapist automatically accepts such symptoms as hallucinations and anxiety as psychogenic. These symptoms and many more may arise from other causes. The experienced diagnostician may be alerted by symptoms that have about them an organic "flavor" or "smell." Once they are known, their resemblance to more obvious organic symptoms is pronounced. Their number and variety make them a proper concern for any clinician, so that organicity may be considered and, if absent, ruled out. *Déjà vu* experiences, depersonalization, sensory distortions and hallucinations, bizarreness, concreteness or vagary of thought, even depression, severe anxiety, each of these should have its etiological contributants sorted out and weighed. Each may have a physiological or neurological cause as well as a psychogenesis, or, even more complicated, in addition to it.

"Soft" or equivocal signs do not necessarily mean that whatever cerebral disorder may be involved is of slight degree. Following cerebrovascular accidents emotional and behavioral changes may be inconspicuous, caution Benton and Joynt (2), and identifiable only by careful comparison with peers or with the patient's own preceding behavior. And Reitan (20) also warns that there may be no correlation between severity of behavioral impairment and specific deficits on neurological examination. These equivocal situations tax the psychotherapist's tolerance for uncertainty. Some may respond to their challenge with a hermetic confidence in psychogenesis. Far more effective is careful clinical appraisal of all the probabilities, coupled with willingness to postpone judgment if data are lacking.

Alerting the psychotherapist to these possibilities is a major goal of this book. Symptoms and syndromes that frequently appear in both neurological and psychological etiologies are presented in Section I, with case histories. Because the equivocal signs often elude clear-cut neurological verification, yet clinically implicate the neurological, this section begins with a discussion of the "equivocal" or "soft signs" in neurology and neuropsychology. These represent in a most striking way the phenomena we are concerned with here. This is how all these symptoms and syndromes are often best described: "equivocal," "soft," "ambiguous." The psychotherapist must recognize them and adapt his treatment procedures and goals when they are established if treatment is not to fail. Psychotherapy that ignores a patient's handicap of cerebral dysfunction fails even as psychotherapy. Brain dysfunction not only lowers the individual threshold for the emergence of emotional problems but also makes their successful treatment more difficult, and often requires a modification of psychotherapeutic procedures.

A second objective is to suggest readily available procedures with which the psychotherapist may implement his usual diagnostic inquiry in order to weigh realistically all the etiological possibilities presented by the clinical data. Section II outlines additions to the usual interviewing procedures, with a neuropsychological way of looking at the usual psychodiagnostic tests and the information they yield. Section III presents some foundation in theory and research methods from the present state of the art of neuropsychodiagnosis and the science of neuropsychology.

One might read section III on neuropsychology before the sections on syndromes and clinical applications. However, the Case of Sam should be read first. Sam's search for nearly forty years for relief from painful and perplexing symptoms epitomizes those human dilemmas to which this book is addressed. His story identifies all too clearly the possibilities for incomplete diagnosis or mis-diagnosis and its consequences. Sam's was the predicament of the patient whose failure to respond to psychotherapy elicits in the helping professional only increasing firmness in pursuit of the psychogenic rather than a search for alternatives.

The book is intended for all psychotherapists, be they social workers, psychiatrists, or psychologists. Social workers may have neither the biological background nor the psychological one that psychiatrists and psychologists respectively bring to psychotherapy. Psychologists may lack the medical background which many social workers have, as well as lack the psychiatrist's training in biological sciences. Yet psychiatrists can be biased in favor of psychological causation and hence psychological treatment; in my experience, few psychiatrists retain much neurological emphasis. Many use from their medical training largely a reliance upon psychotropic medication. Even fewer psychiatrists in my ken have been open to the consideration of alternative diagnoses when these are based only upon soft or equivocal signs. Few of today's older generation of clinical psychologists, those with whom I am identified, much value their training in psychodiagnostic testing; even fewer use it. The younger clinical psychologists I know are frequently impatient with psychodiagnosis and chomp at the bit to be practicing psychotherapy. Their training, unfortunately, has not acquainted them with the rewarding productive potential of the test instruments they learn but so often find boring. And as happened with psychiatrists, many psychologists turned away from the neurological influences upon behavior; some were never taught them in any depth. Perhaps, too, this book will prove useful to those neurologists who have not been trained in a psychological approach to neurology, the contribution of Henry Head and Hughlings Jackson.

Neuropsychodiagnosis in psychotherapy crosses professional, scientific, and technical borders. A principle of exploitation operates in effective neuropsychodiagnosis: we must use any procedure that clarifies the relationship between brain function and behavior. Each therapeutic discipline offers something to the others here; each has much to learn from the sciences of neurology and neuropsychology, and indeed much to offer these fields in return. A work of extraordinary value by Lishman (13) extensively and minutely sets out the interactions between the neurogenic and psychogenic. Its subtitle, *The Psychological Consequences of Cerebral Disorder,* reflects the need to build and cross the bridges between disciplines if we are to understand and help these patients.

Contributing to that cooperative interaction becomes a third objective of this book. Several authors have stressed the "borderland" (12) between neurology and psychiatry, or the "interface" (19), or suggested that the disciplines "integrate" (28). A symposium explored the interface between Clinical Psychology and Clinical Human Neuropsychology (1).

To a considerable degree, these efforts examine pairs of disciplines —neurology and psychiatry, clinical psychology and clinical human neuropsychology—looking for the facets of the "interface," for the obstacles to and the possibilities for relationships within each of the disciplines. These efforts deserve support, but we must remember that the "interface" is not to be found in our disciplines but in our patients. The need is that the disciplines respond both individually and jointly to the requirements at the important "interface," that contact between phenomena within a suffering human being.

In general, etiological factors in both neurologically damaged and psychiatric patients are *more or less* definitely identifiable, as is the interaction between etiological forces. This results in *more or less* ambiguity in diagnostic statements about cause and effect, *more or less* ambiguity in identifying the appropriate interventions and their probable outcomes. It is this *more or less* status in the diagnosis and treatment of both neurological and psychiatric patients that presents an interface to the disciplines, a situation that belongs not to any discipline but to the condition of the patient. This *more or less* status will at times confound the hypotheses and empirical data of the neurologist or neuropsychologist, as it will sometimes confirm the more speculative reachings of the clinical psychologist or the psychiatrist.

The disciplines meet, then, in the presence of ambiguity about the patient's diagnosis and treatment. Without such ambiguity, each of the disciplines can go its own way, happy and productive in relative isolation. Faced with ambiguity, we need each other if we are to increase the effectiveness of our responses to our patient's needs.

BIBLIOGRAPHY

1. *Benton, A. L.,* Chairman: Symposium: Interface of Clinical Psychology and Human Neuropsychology. Clinical Psychologist, 29:2, 1976.
2. *Benton, A. L.,* and *Joynt, R. J.:* Conclusions and indications for future investigative work. *In* A. L. Benton (Ed.): Behavioral Change in Cerebrovascular Disease. New York: Harper and Row, 1970.
3. *Brock, S.* and *Wiesel, B.:* Psychiatric symptoms marking the onset in cases of brain tumor. Med. Clin. North Amer., 32:759, 1948.
4. *Cantwell, D.* and *Baker, L.:* Psychiatric disorder in children with speech and language retardation. Arch. Gen. Psychiat., 34:5, 1977.
5. *Chambers, W. R.:* Neurosurgical conditions masquerading as psychiatric disorders. Amer. J. Psychiat., 112:387, 1955.
6. *Donald, A. G., et al.:* Reported anon. Frontiers of Psychiat., 1:16, 1971.
7. *Epstein, B., et al.:* Tumors of the spinal cord simulating psychiatric disorders. Dis. Nerv. Syst., 32:11, 1971.
8. *Gomez, M. R.:* Neurologic approach to specific language disability. Bull. Orton Soc., 20, 1970.
9. *Harris, J.:* Depression and hysteria as symptoms of brain tumor. Henry Ford Hosp. Med. Bull., 13, 1965.
10. *Heron, G. B.* and *Johnston, D. A.:* Hypothalamic tumor presenting as anorexia nervosa. Amer. J. Psychiat., 133:5, 1976.

11. *Lawall, J.:* Psychiatric presentation of seizure disorders. Amer. J. Psychiat., 133, 1976.
12. *Lipowski, Z. J.* and *Kiriakos, R. Z.:* Borderlands between neurology and psychiatry: Observations in a neurological hospital. Psychiat. in Med., 3:2, 1972.
13. *Lishman, W. A.:* Organic Psychiatry: The Psychological Consequences of Cerebral Disorder. London: Blackwell, 1978.
14. *McIntyre, H. D.* and *McIntyre, A.:* The problem of brain tumor in psychiatric diagnosis. Amer. J. Psychiat., 98, 1942.
15. *Malamud, N.:* Psychiatric disorder with intracranial tumors of limbic system., Arch. Neurol., 17, 1967.
16. *Misra, P. C.* and *Hay, G. G.:* Encephalitis presenting as acute schizophrenia. Brit. Med. J., 5748, 1971.
17. *Nordan, R.:* The psychiatric reactions of children with neurological problems. Child Psychiat. Human Devel., 6:4, 1976.
18. *Olin, H.* and *Weisman, A.:* Psychiatric misdiagnosis of early neurological disease., JAMA, 189:7, 1964.
19. *Rangell, L.:* Psychoanalysis and neuropsychiatry: A look at their interface. Amer. J. Psychiat., 127:2, 1970.
20. *Reitan. R. M.:* Objective behavioral assessment in diagnosis and prediction. Presentation 15. *In* A. L. Benton (Ed.): Behavioral Change in Cerebrovascular Disease. New York: Harper and Row, 1970.
21. *Remington, F. B.* and *Rubert, S. L.:* Why patients with brain tumors come to a psychiatric hospital. Amer. J. Psychiat. 119, 1962.
22. *Scott, M.:* Transitory psychotic behavior following operation for tumors of the cerebello-pontine angle. Psychiatria, Neurologia, Neurochirugia, 73:1, 1970.
23. *Simon, M.:* The diagnosis of brain tumor masked by mental symptoms. Military Surgery, 111:411, 1952.
24. *Soniat, I. L.:* Psychiatric symptoms associated with intracranial neoplasms. Amer. J. Psychiat., 108:19, 1951.
25. *Tucker, B. E.* and *Benaron, H. W.:* The immediate effects of prolonged labor with forceps delivery, precipitate labor with spontaneous delivery, and natural labor with spontaneous delivery on the child. Amer. J. Obstet. Gynec., 66, 1953.
26. *Waggoner, R. W.* and *Bagchi, B. K.:* Initial masking of organic brain changes by psychiatric symptoms: Clinical and EEG studies. Amer. J. Psychiat., 110: 904, 1954.
27. *Wilson, L. G.:* Viral encephalopathy mimicking functional psychosis. Amer. J. Psychiat., 133:2, 1976.
28. *Wilson, W. P., et al.:* Should psychiatry and neurology integrate? Amer. J. Psychiat., 128:5, 1971.

Contents

Acknowledgments

This revised edition has benefited from the comments about the first edition by knowledgeable colleagues, who called attention to errors and/or encouraged with favorable comments. Their generosity and concern are much appreciated by me.

One colleague cannot be allowed this anonymous role. With the appearance of the first edition, Aaron Smith wrote a long, constructive letter to a stranger, praising where he could, gently and firmly pointing out errors, omissions, and theoretically questionable material. There followed a steady exchange of letters about issues in neuropsychology, several meetings at different places in the country, and a rewarding week in his laboratory at the University of Michigan where I worked with neurological patients under his supervision. I am indebted to him and most grateful.

My wife Verna, as she has before, found time among her commitments to review carefully the entire manuscript. Without her expert editorial skill, the writing would be less clear, less focussed. And, as before, I am the beneficiary of her "perceptive questions and integrative insights on those walks and talks along city streets, country lanes and coastal beaches."

LEONARD SMALL

New York City
June, 1980

PROLOGUE

The Case of Sam: Diagnostic Ambiguity and the Life of a Man

"I know I have an emotional problem, but I believe I also have a physical organic illness," said Sam, age 57. He was being readmitted to a vocational rehabilitation program from which he had been discharged 12 years before, after discharge from his sixth or seventh stay in a psychiatric hospital.

Six months before, he had again sought help at a private hospital. The current report from its staff described a clinical picture that had existed almost unchanged for more than 35 years. He came to them saying, "I feel violent and suicidal." He was in treatment with a private psychiatrist, but felt that too much anger was coming out too fast. He had become increasingly depressed, isolated, and unable to work during the two preceding years. On admission to this hospital, he was unshaved and slouched; he said, "I am angry at all doctors. My head feels as if it is shrinking; my body is empty. My body and head feel separated from each other." He feared leaving the house, he was afraid that he would lose consciousness and be blown over by the wind. Otherwise, he appeared oriented, responsive, and appropriate. The hospital reported that an electroencephalogram examination with photic stimulation was normal. They did *not* report his subsequent complaint that the photic stimulation had disturbed him extremely. He was given the drug Prolixin; his rage decreased, but as it did, his depression increased. Elavil was added to his regimen and he was discharged with a diagnosis of Schizophrenia, Chronic, Undifferenti-ated, and directed back into a rehabilitation work program.

The available history on this man is enormous. Its important details are presented here as economically as possible, with the significant facts of his upbringing, the chronology of his progress in life until the psychiatric and psychological assessment in 1971 when this writer first knew him, and finally a report of his status in 1979.

No prenatal or delivery difficulties are recorded. A sickly child, he was said to have occasional convulsions for which he frequently was taken to a clinic, but no diagnosis was made. He learned from his mother that he had had double pneumonia when he was about one year old, and that the convulsions followed this illness, continuing until age six. No nightmares or behavioral disturbances were reported.

He felt that his father was distant from him during his childhood. Later, as the patient's illness developed and he had trouble finding and keeping employment, violent quarrels broke out between them. He had certain intellectual interests which his father resented, and the father persuaded him finally to leave school to take a job. How-ever, Sam did not feel that he was singled out by his father for special mistreatment; rather the father treated all the children alike. His mother was said to be energetic, popular, and sociable, with a literary interest despite little education. She was strongly willed and indus-trious. Sam did not feel close to her either.

A brother seven years older who became successful is described as cold and reserved. A sister three years older is "intelligent, courageous, flexible." A sister eight years younger is described as pretty, likable, and good natured. Another older sister died in an accident, the nature of which, as will be seen, has strong psychodynamic implications for Sam.

Sam recalled no significant sexual events in childhood. He believes that he began to masturbate when he was 10 or 11. At 16 he began to masturbate exhibitionistically before a younger neighbor who was then eight. He continued this practice, apparently with her tacit con-sent, until she married and moved away when she was 18. His mas-turbatory fantasies were always exhibitionistic, and masturbation con-tinued throughout his marriage at age 30. He generally felt more sa-tisfied by it than by intercourse. He continued to masturbate every couple of days, and with increased frequency when bothered by symptoms.

When Sam was 10 years old, his older sister was killed by a truck, her head almost severed from her body. Sam was in the crowd but did not see the body. He heard his mother screaming and recalls the episode as a nightmare in which he felt "numb." A bystander described the details to him. During the next four years he frequently dreamed that his sister was alive; these dreams were not frightening.

When he was 15, Sam himself was hit by an automobile. He recalls sailing through the air with a vivid image of his dead sister before him. Then he hit his head against a parked car and became unconscious. No sequelae were reported. Skull x-rays were normal.

Until the age of 17 he earned good grades in school, was industrious and conforming. In high school his math work was poor, his other work good. He felt himself to be an observer and was relatively isolated.

After graduation in the midst of the economic depression, he accepted his father's urging to seek employment. This was difficult: he was fearful about job applications, felt inadequate, and could not "sell himself." He took college classes at night for three terms, but gave up because there was no money. During this time he became interested in sociology and corresponded with a famous sociologist for several years. They met and Sam was urged by the scholar to study. This relationship is documented through letters which had been examined.

At 18 he suddenly experienced "jolts" shooting up his back and into his head. Thereafter he suffered severe headaches, dizziness, weakness in the legs, and a fear of collapsing. The next year he was hospitalized for psychiatric observation for one week and discharged.

When 22, he was admitted to a large city hospital for neurological observation. Electroencephalograms and pneumoencephalograms were said to have been obtained, with negative results, and he was referred to the psychiatric clinic for psychotherapy. For several months after that the "numbness" in his head progressed to convulsions. There was no loss of consciousness or continence. Gradually, the convulsions progressed from a shaking of the body and tongue to "complete paralysis." He remained at home with his parents for nine months. When the paralysis improved, he requested readmission to the public psychiatric hospital again, and was placed in a state hospital where he remained for 14 months to be discharged at about the age of 24.

Thereafter, he gave up his intellectual interests and accepted menial jobs to please his father. He kept one such job for three years, then was promoted to a clerk's job, which he also held for three years.

But at the age of 27 his symptoms exacerbated, the head symptoms particularly. He reported feelings in his head of shrinking and expanding with numbness and emptiness. He felt that his eyes travelled around to the back of his head. At this time, when 27, he began private psychotherapy three times weekly while continuing to work. At first he was hopeful, then he became discouraged; some of the motor symptoms stopped, but the head symptoms and dizziness remained and the feelings of estrangement increased. (To jump ahead, after five years this therapy was stopped by agreement.)

At 30 he married a warm, sweet woman. He told her of his symptoms; she promised to stay with him always. Two years later he took a rather responsible job. He worked well, though he was not educated to the job's technical aspects, and he was praised for his work. When 35, he collapsed on the job. His wife was then three months pregnant. He was unable to work for several months after his son was born. Resentment of his child's troubled sleep pattern and rage at the child as a competitor appeared to be central to this collapse. He resumed psychotherapy, which continued for three years with little or no change evident.

When he was 40 years old, he again collapsed, and was away from work so long that he lost the job he had held for about eight years. He became deeply depressed. He had trouble getting out of bed, suffered spells of weeping and shaking, and was preoccupied with suicidal thoughts. He tried to hurt himself but could not carry through. These efforts led to hospitalization again. The hospital described him as regressed, with suicidal ideas, fearful, complaining of dizziness and numbness in his head, feeling empty and unreal "like a ghost." He was treated with Serpasil, one of the early tranquilizers. On discharge from the hospital he was first referred to the vocational rehabilitation agency (to which he would return 16 years later at age 57). The records of this agency describe him when first applying at age 40 as intellectually intact, seemingly appropriate. They noted the long history and the symptoms, and the diagnosis suggested was Pseudoneurotic Schizophrenia. As the agency psychologist, I saw him then and commented upon the wide scatter of subtest scores of the Wechsler-Bellevue from a low of 8 on Picture Arrangement to 17 on Similarities. Attention was called to severe depersonalization, without evidence, however, of a schizophrenic process. "Powerful depressive, suicidal trends" were reported. Feelings of lack of love, of homelessness, of separation from his parents, and a sense of loss at the death of his

father were described. I commented that Sam needed distance from
people. There was a need for closeness but a fear of it; I advised that
he be permitted to adjust his own interpersonal distances. His relationship to authority was expected to be a problem, since he defended
himself against passivity wishes with rebellious anger.

As part of the rehabilitation program, he returned to psychotherapy,
and 18 months of psychiatric treatment are recorded, as synopsized
below. (The months are numbered from the start of this rehabilitation
program when he was 41 years old.)

During month one, three weeks after admission to the program, he
was said to seem worse, to be more depressed, tense, and withdrawn
than before. Depersonalization feelings were getting stronger. He was
aware of the lack of objective reality, and feared he would destroy
himself or the world. He profoundly feared loss of sanity. He had
been medicated with Dexamyl, with Doriden at night, up to this point,
but was switched to Equanil (meprobamate), an early tranquilizer.

By month three he had adjusted to a certain extent, and continued
regular attendance at the workshop.

In month nine various changes in medication from Equanil to
Dexamyl to Thorazine and back to the Equanil were recorded. He
complained of feeling like a machine, with no self, of a terrible apathy.
In month 10, he was so depressed that he was unable to keep appointments. Finally, he came, and the report notes, "he pulls his hair, tries
to pluck his eyes out, hits against furniture, bangs into walls, has
severe suicidal urges. He can no longer endure his 'dead head.'"
Equanil seemed ineffective and Thorazine was reinstated.

At this time the agency psychiatrist began to consider electric-shock
therapy because the depression was so severe and all efforts to ventilate
his hostility produced no response. Sam consented, and during months
10 and 11 he received eight electric-shock treatments. The doctor saw
improvement, but the patient felt no better. He complained that he
was becoming increasingly anxious about the treatments, and the doctors agreed to discontinue after the eighth treatment. His psychiatrist
observed him to be less agitated, better able to concentrate. Objectively, he worked more hours per day. Sam complained of feeling
"shocks" in his head.

In month 12, Same became obsessed with death, which was attributed
to the electric-shock treatments. Head symptoms and dizziness were
prominent, and the patient for the first time recalled and talked about
seizures during childhood. Much guilt about sexual experiences and

thoughts was ventilated during these sessions, and the therapeutic focus was on fear of castration as retaliation for his sin.

In month 13, his feeling that his head was shrinking and expanding and his dizziness intensified. These were discussed in relationship to anger at the therapist for presumed rejection of him. Sam did not agree that this was a cause, and spontaneously associated his head symptoms to his sister's death, and further associated the feelings of changes in head size to tumescence and detumescence of the penis.

In month 14 Sam complained bitterly of depression, and reluctantly accepted a single electric-shock treatment. Then 42, he himself expressed conviction that his symptoms have an organic basis, since psychotherapy had not helped him. The therapist began to record doubt that psychotherapy had potentiality for helping Sam. In month 15, an eminent psychiatrist called in consultation recommended that the treating psychiatrist drain off Sam's aggression toward his wife and toward a friend, repair the damage to self-esteem over his loss of the job, define the defensive separation of body and head as isolation of emotions, and strengthen the patient's ego by asking him to undertake library research on the topic "Sociology of Work." Sam was enthusiastic about the project, and the therapist was impressed by his "logical, lucid expression of his ideas." But nothing came of this venture.

In month 16, Sam complained that his concentration was deteriorating, that he was "going to hell." He reiterated the idea that he has a neurological disease, an idea the psychiatrist termed "obsessive." Interpretation focused upon the transference; Sam was told that he saw the therapist as an authority and failed in order to defy him.

In month 17, Thoradex was substituted for some of the Thorazine; at first Sam responded well, but then complained of worsening symptoms. Both Thorazine and Thoradex were discontinued, and Trilafon was prescribed, probably for its anti-emetic property. The psychotherapeutic work emphasized his defiance of his parents about going to work and his present need to be ill in order to resist them through resisting the therapist. Agitation increased, Trifalon was discontinued, and Compazine prescribed. Psychotherapeutic work continued on his need to defy by being ill. At first Sam was angry, then his depression increased. Again a consultation was held, and lobotomy was discussed as a possibility because of Sam's failure to respond to either psychotherapy or medication.

In the 18th month his depression deepened. The therapist wrote of his own feeling that the interpretive work on Sam's need to be ill had failed. The patient said in one session, *"Despite years of psychotherapy my symptoms remain a mystery to me.* I am convinced more than ever that some organic damage has been done to my brain." Hospitalization was discussed but did not become necessary. During the next year the patient gradually improved, and was able to leave the security of the agency for a good job. His improvement came during a harmonious working relationship with one of the workshop foremen with whom he had developed what was for him a unique relationship with an authority figure. Follow-up continued for one year, then the case was closed.

The agency did not see Sam again for 12 years.

In the interval Sam worked well for ten years in a responsible job. Then he developed abdominal pains. When he was 54, two surgeries were required for removal of gall bladder and stones from the duct, but there was no relief of pain. He lost 30 pounds, became unable to concentrate and the feeling of numbness in his head increased. The following year, he stopped work altogether because he could not concentrate. He returned to the vocational agency in a severe depression. He had been taking Valium; the agency psychiatrist ordered a change back to Elavil. Sam could not tolerate the workshop. He was admitted to a state hospital where the diagnosis of Involutional Melancolia, Psychotic Depression, was made. After discharge from the state hospital, he sought out-patient treatment at a private hospital in the city. This hospital suggested that he return once more to the vocational agency.

At this point, as the agency psychologist, I saw Sam again. In reporting the current findings, I reviewed the long history. My notes comment that it presents ". . . a rare combination of equivocal neurological and psychiatric symptoms, with uncertainty as to where the proper etiology rests." I then reviewed present symptomatology and tried to relate these to the test data, as follows:

"Sam reports many current symptoms that indicate a seizure disorder. He experiences blurred vision. Moving lights make him dizzy (specifically, if he is driving with someone in a car at night the oncoming and passing lights produce the dizziness). He experiences phosphenes (visual hallucinations of flashing light) on occasion. He has episodes of frequent dizziness, then long periods during which there is no dizziness. He has never lost consciousness (expect when struck by an auto when he was 15), but he has had to hold on for fear that he would fall. On occasion he experiences a sudden tilting of the environment. One of his worst experiences is when he stops walking and the ground seems to continue to move away from him. This often is accompanied by head-pressure, which he associates with the greatest degree of illness. With this comes depression, difficulty in concentrating, the dizziness increases, he feels as if he is drunk, his gait becomes unbalanced, he has the strange experience of jolts going through the back of the spine to his head, and tremors of the knees. This progresses to numbness of the head with '. . . dead emotions. I lose all my previous enthusiasm and loves and I become like a vegetable.' He experiences convulsive jerking and tingling of the legs. There are experiences of altered states of consciousness with feelings of depersonalization. No automatic behavior or blackouts are reported.

"He believes that emotional tension is a precipitating condition, particularly if he is discontent or angry with a superior person. If, for example, he feels that he is not being instructed clearly and correctly, he becomes angry and hostile and feels that if he cannot express this, he is in danger of precipitating one of these strange experiences that culminate in depression. In the past these depressions have reached a least suicidal ideation.

"It is important to comment about his reaction to medication. Valium is the only medication which he reports has seemed to help him 'sometimes.' Elavil disturbs him. Thorazine was upsetting to him and gave him some curious side effects. (Later we were to learn that Thorazine may potentiate a seizure disorder, while Dexedrine and Dexomyl have anti-convulsant properties, and in Thoradex the addition of Dexedrine may counteract the seizure-potentiating qualities of Thorazine.) One private doctor and another at a state hospital in September, 1971, prescribed Dilantin. The private doctor tried it for two months, then stopped it. Sam says Dilantin makes him restless. There is indication in the record that Dexedrine or Dexamyl was prescribed at one time but then discontinued. I am not able in this voluminous record to find the reason for its having been prescribed, nor for its termination. Compazine also was prescribed at one time as was Thoradex. When first given Thoradex, Sam was said to be enthusiastic about it, and to feel that it improved his ability to read.

"The impression is obtained from reading the extensive reports of psychiatric contacts, that for inexplicable causes, he was sometimes ac-

cessible to psychotherapy, while at other times he seemed unreachable and unresponsive.

"On contact today, Sam is a wiry, wry, intelligent man. His depression is quite clear. There is a great deal of hostility. The major result of this hostility, in addition to the depression, appears to be an obsessive-compulsive personality. He has little tolerance for imprecision in others and in himself. Because of his difficulties, a tendency toward clouded consciousness on occasion, and because of marked cognitive defects, he becomes imprecise, and his anxiety mounts.

"When I tested him nearly 16 years ago, he achieved the following subtest and overall scores on the Wechsler-Bellevue scale: Information 14, Comprehension 12, Arithmetic 10, Similarities 17, Digit Span 13, Digit Symbol 15, Picture Completion 9, Block Design 9, Picture Arrangement 8, Verbal I.Q. 124, Performance I.Q. 113, Full Scale I.Q. 120.*

"Since then there has been some decrease in functioning level in some subtests, and not in others. Information has dropped by 2 scale points to 12, and here he complains of memory difficulties, that there are some things he has forgotten: for example, the source of rubber. While he is able to operate at a high level in this area, memory difficulties interfere with items at easier level. Comprehension remains the same, Arithmetic about the same as 16 years ago. There has been a marked decrement in ability to conceptualize, with increasing concreteness and loss of capacity for abstract thinking. A good example of this is the "fly-tree" item; he says, "a tree is high up and a fly can fly high up." Digit Span remains about the same. Finger dexterities (Digit Symbol) have dropped markedly by four scale points to 11. Recognition of essential details is decreased somewhat; spatial visualization has dropped slightly by two scale points to seven.

"The best way of looking at the current intellectual assets and liabilities is to compare overall scores. These indicate that constructional and spatial tasks are not as well mastered as are verbal ones: The Performance I.Q. is 18 points lower than the Verbal. A com-

---

* Some readers may not be familiar with the scoring system of the Wechsler tests of intelligence. They are constructed as batteries of subtests. Each subtest presents a different type of problem and is scored according to the subject's responses or solutions. These, called "raw" scores, are converted into "scale scores," e.g., Information 14, which in turn are used to compute the intelligence quotients.

parison of average scale scores is helpful: verbal tasks average to 12; attention-memory tasks to 12, and perceptual-analytic ones to six.*

The prorated I.Q. for Object Assembly is 38 points lower than Information at 116.**

"Even in areas of specialization, even among seemingly intact functions, such as attention and recall of auditory material, deficits appear when the complexity of the task is increased: he can retain nine digits forward but only four in reverse. On Arithmetic, he functions quite well until the upper level of difficulty is reached, then he makes near-hits or misses, however one cares to express it. In Block Design, he has tremendous difficulty making the shift from a two by two square to a three by three square; he was puzzled and insisted there needed to be an even number of pieces. With Picture Arrangement, he could complete only the first three items successfully, but as the number of pictures in a story increased and the theme became more complicated, failures appeared, so that he only achieved a prorated I.Q. of 91. This was the case too with the assembly of familiar objects. Here he had difficulty with every item, and required nearly a minute to complete the easiest item. His perplexity was apparent: 'I got it together but it doesn't seem to fit, something seems to be wrong.'

"The Heimburger-Reitan Test and dual administration of the Bender Gestalt support the impression of impairment of perceptual-analytic, spatial visualization functions.***

"No evidence of a psychotic process is obtained. The data appear to be consistent with a diagnosis of a depressive, obsessional-compulsive personality who appears subject to seizure phenomena that have escaped detection by standard neurological means. A recent electroencephalograph is reported to be normal. Photic stimulation was employed, but it is noteworthy that no sleep recording was made.

"The patient should be under protracted neurological observation.

---

* The significance of averaging certain scale scores is discussed in Chapter 11. Briefly, some of the Wechsler tests have been found to be related to each other as to which "function" or aspect of intelligence they appear to evaluate. The groups of related subtests have been identified by statistical analysis; they are Verbal, Attention-Memory and Perceptual-Analytic. Each is called a "factor." The scale scores of the tests making up a factor may be averaged and compared with similar averages for the other factors.

** The prorated I.Q. for a single subtest of the Wechsler is obtained by presuming uniform functioning in all of the subtests, and in effect states "If scale scores for all the other subtests were the same as the scale score for this subtest, the individual's I.Q. would be the following. . . ."

*** These tests are discussed in Chapter 11.

It may be wise to repeat some of the special neurological tests because of the deterioration in intellectual and cognitive functioning in the absence of a psychosis. He appears to have highly idiosyncratic responses to drugs, which may be related to an unusual brain physiology. Careful empirical efforts with medications seem in order."

The agency psychiatrist at the time of this return to the rehabilitation program in 1971 also gave more credence to the neurological aspects of Sam's disorder than had been given. He wrote: "In view of the findings indicative of some form of history of seizure disorder, the possibility of existing seizure disorder, and some degree of progressive cerebral deficit, the patient deserves a complete neurological work-up, possibly including arteriogram and pneumoencephalogram. Possibility of meningioma should not be ruled out; the possibility of acute or effective brain injury because of head trauma should not be dismissed yet. If no definite evidence of any abnormality can be found, then the patient needs a systematic trial of a variety of antidepressant and anti-convulsive medications with indications to him that he may have side effects but that he will have to sit through some of them to see which is the best combination for him. With a good deal of careful analysis, work-up, and patient drug trial we will probably get the patient into a better remission. In any event the principal thing at present is to get a good neurological work-up. The fact that he has been sensitive to Dilantin in the past does not mean that he could not have a trial on other anti-convulsants in the future."

Many of Sam's symptoms are certainly congruent psychodynamically with the facts of his history. His depression could be understandable as the cumulative effect of harsh, depriving introjects, the inward deflection of rage, and the personal loss and damage to his self-esteem from giving up his intellectual interests. Castration anxiety seems inherent in his exhibitionistic and compulsive masturbation, the feelings of altering head size, the horrendous accidental death of his sibling, and his own subsequent accidental head injury. The harsh father who compelled him to give up his intellectual (head) interests might well have promoted not only the castration anxiety, but also a covertly rebellious attitude against work and authority expressed by passive-aggressive means, namely illness.

But why were nearly ten years of psychotherapy with three different therapists and much experimentation with psychotropic medication relatively ineffective? Why did they so little alter his recurrent symptomatology? One could reason properly that his ability to marry, father a child, and work effectively at a responsible job for ten years are respectable achievements for psychotherapy with a very sick person. But the causes for his changes for better or worse are all obscure, invisible, inexplicable in psychodynamic terms. Equally unexplained is his changing accessibility to psychotherapy. One may easily label these and his somatic and sensory distortion as psychotic manifestations. But to do so is to overlook the persistent fact that he has always been alienated from these distortions; they have never been real to him. Never to those who have worked with him for long periods has he seemed to be hallucinatory or delusional in the usual psychotic sense.

A first current attempt to unravel the possible neurological factors resulted in a report from a neurologist that he failed to find any EEG or neurological data of an "objective" nature. He concluded: "The history suggests that there may have been some element of seizure disorder in the past, but it is worth noting that even at the time of his evaluation forty years ago, he ended up as a psychiatric patient." Regrettably, although furnished with all of the above history, the neurologist did not offer an evaluation of its abundant suggestions, nor did he appear to weigh the fact that psychiatry had been unable to comprehend Sam's condition or to help him during the years he was considered its patient and pursued its recommendations.

Fortunately, another avenue for investigating a possible neurogenic basis for Sam's symptoms became available: a clinic department of a large hospital was found which specialized in the diagnosis and treatment of seizure disorders. There the EEG was repeated, this time with additional leads inserted through the nostrils and placed under the temporal lobes. A brain scan ruled out an expanding lesion. A diagnosis of "seizure disorder of temporal origin" was obtained from these readings. The locus was presumed to be scar tissue remaining from either a birth injury or the head injury suffered in his youth.

Mysoline was prescribed, and when he proved to be allergic and was changed to phenobarbital, he did rather well. After leaving the rehabilitation program again, two years later in 1973, when he was 59, he was unable to find employment. He became depressed, and a brief hospitalization resulted. He continued to experience strange sensations in the head, for which he now had more tolerance, and "tongue-jerking." Another doctor consulted in 1979 diagnosed this as a symptom of Parkinson's Disease and ordered him to discontinue the phenobarbital he had used for some seven years, during which no question of psychosis came to the fore, despite the depression that developed with joblessness.

Now 65, Sam belongs to a senior-citizens group, reads, draws, socializes, enjoys long and intellectual discussions with young people, and seems better able to allow himself pleasure. His life has not been long enough for the nature of his afflictions to be unravelled completely.

NEUROPSYCHODIAGNOSIS
IN PSYCHOTHERAPY

Revised Edition

I

SYMPTOMS AND SYNDROMES OF
SPECIAL CONCERN TO
THE PSYCHOTHERAPIST

While the blatant neurological disability is seldom a diagnostic concern of the psychotherapist, slight neurological disorders, difficult to evaluate, are more frequent in psychotherapeutic practice than is generally recognized.

They are easily overlooked, but their presence significantly affects learning, general adjustment, and indeed, psychotherapy itself. Failure to detect them may arise from any of a variety of reasons, among them the obscurity of what neurologists call "soft" signs (as distinct from "hard" or unquestionable signs) of disorder. Standard clinical neurological and electroencephalographic examinations do not always detect these minimal disorders. Nor do psychological tests clearly differentiate neurologic from psychogenic impairments. Moreover, the unwary psychotherapist may tend to ascribe a purely psychogenic cause to behavior that might be traceable to either psychogenic or neurological factors, or to both, such is the capacity for simulation that marks these signs and conditions.

This section is about these signs and conditions, their nature and extent, their causes, the difficulties in detecting them, and a number of syndromes in which they play a role. This role may sometimes be more suspected than established, but it is always important where it operates.

3

CHAPTER 1

Equivocal or "Soft" Signs

Equivocal or "soft" signs are those that suggest neurological pathology but result in so slight a manifestation of dysfunction or occur so inconsistently or infrequently as to create uncertainty (36). Such signs often appear without apparent relationship to other signs or symptoms. Adding to their ambiguity, they occur more frequently among the emotionally disturbed, especially children.

Ingram (34) contends that there are no "soft" neurological signs because any sign points to behavioral, emotional, or neurological etiology. The task of the neurologist is to pursue all signs vigorously, and not escape decision with a diagnosis of "minimal brain damage." Many signs miscalled soft, he maintains, can be traced to actual neurological cause, many can not. If properly pursued, the soft signs often lead to an actual neurological diagnosis. He cites examples: 1) congenital dyspraxia may appear only as difficulty in appropriately placing the tongue, lips, and hands on request or in performing tasks; 2) suprabulbar palsy may be expressed only as a mild speech deficit; 3) minimal hemiplegia may be manifested only as clumsiness and left-handedness.

Yet signs of uncertain diagnostic meaning appear in all kinds of neuropsychodiagnostic examination: neurological examination, psychological-test performance, and behavioral and mood symptomatology. They are indeed ubiquitous, and to help their victims requires our diligent effort to understand their meaning. The consequences of the many conditions signalled only by ambiguous neurological signs vary in seriousness. Perceptual deficits, for example, may cause visual neglect, scanning and distance problems, and difficulties in spatial organization. These may affect such functions of daily living as shaving,

5

dressing, eating, or time judgments. Dysphasic difficulties appearing early in life may set up limits upon communication or attempts at communication in forms that evoke harmful responses from others, and create or contribute to pathological relationships that in turn develop into what appears to be autism or schizophrenia. Persons diagnosed as having emotionally unstable character disorders or as schizophrenic with premorbid asociality were hypothesized by Quitkin, *et al.* (55) to have more evidence of central-nervous-system damage of etiological significance to their psychiatric diagnoses. They revealed more soft neurological signs than individuals with other types of character disorders and schizophrenia. Cautioning that correlations do not establish cause, the investigators cite their findings that both study groups showed a greater number of soft signs that started early in childhood and seemed "to follow a fixed course of development."

NATURE AND EXTENT OF OBSCURE IMPAIRMENTS

Studies of the incidence of neurological disorder among hospital-clinic patients, residential-treatment patients, and total child populations suggest the probability that slight but significant neurological disorders are more widespread than is now generally understood.

Neurological abnormality was found in 24 (36.9 percent) of 65 psychiatric patients by Rochford, *et al.* (58). Subjects ranged in age from 16 to 30 and were both in-patients and out-patients at three hospitals in the New Haven area. Excluded from the study were those with clear diagnoses of chronic organic brain syndrome or severe mental retardation, a history of drug abuse, or those who had received psychotropic medication during two days before their admission to the hospital. Twenty-six subjects were diagnosed as schizophrenic, 27 as having psychotic personality disorders, nine as having neurotic depressions, and three as having psychotic depressions. Diagnoses of neurological abnormality among these patients involved detection of at least one "hard" or two "soft" signs. Hard signs included: 1) lateralizing cranial-nerve findings; 2) pathological reflexes; 3) unilateral movement disorders; 4) unequivocally abnormal electroencephalographic and/or audiometric findings. Soft signs included: 1) motor impersistence; 2) astereognosis (impaired perception of objects or forms by touch); 3) agraphesthesia (impaired perception of symbols written on the skin); 4) extinction of bilateral simultaneous stimulation; 5) bilateral marked hyper-reflexia or hypo-reflexia; 6) coordination defects;

7) disturbances of balance or gait; 8) sensory abnormalities; 9) movements disorders; 10) speech defects; 11) abnormal activity; 12) score of less than 10 on an auditory-visual integration test, not identified by the author; 13) choreiform movement on an adventitious-motor overflow test, not identified; 14) cranial-nerve abnormalities, such as slight anisocoria (inequality of diameter of pupils), esotropia (convergent strabismus), eighth-nerve deficit not proved audiometrically, or mild visual-field and retinal deficits.

The finding of neurological abnormality in 36.9 percent of the psychiatric population represented a statistically significant difference when compared to the incidence of 5 percent among the controls similarly affected. Differences were even more significant for schizophrenic patients and those with personality disorders and neuroses. None of those with affective disorders were found to display neurological abnormality. No significant difference was found between psychotic and non-psychotic patients. Schizophrenic patients, however, tended to have a greater percentage of neurological impairment than the patients in other diagnostic groups. Among male psychiatric patients a greater incidence of neurological abnormality was found than among the female psychiatric patients studied.

As part of a larger study of the relationship of neurological organization to psychiatric disturbance among adolescents, Hertzig and Birch (32) studied the male adolescents admitted to the psychiatric service of Bellevue Hospital for a seven-month period. One hundred of the 115 patients admitted during this period were acceptable for the study; 12 were in the hospital too short a time to be included, two could be examined only inadequately because of language and communication difficulties, and one had a severe hearing loss. Thirty-six of the boys bore diagnoses of psychotic conditions, 64 of non-psychotic conditions. Diagnosis of neurological abnormality was again based upon the presence of any one hard sign of central-nervous-system abnormality and/or two or more soft signs. The soft signs included: 1) disturbances of speech; 2) hyperkinesis; 3) failure to maintain balance; 4) disturbances of gait; 5) inadequacies of muscle tone; 6) coordination defects; 7) extinction to criterion in response to double simultaneous tactile stimulation. Of the total population of 100, 34 were found to have neurological abnormalities. Four demonstrated hard signs; 32 presented one or more soft signs. In a normal comparison population, none were found to have hard signs and less than five percent displayed one or more soft signs. Even more significantly, Hertzig and Birch found that the hospital staff in their clinical assessment of the same group of adolescents identified only two as having signs of nervous-system abnormality, although thirty-four were found to have two or more indicators of central-nervous-system dysfunction upon intensive examination of neurologic organization. These investigators also detected no significant difference of incidence of neurologic disorder between the psychotic and non-psychotic groups of adolescents. They conclude that the risk of developing a psychiatric illness is increased by the concurrence of a central-nervous-system abnormality, but believe that the pattern of the psychiatric disorder in adolescents is largely determined by cultural and social factors.

Studies of children in a residential treatment center have identified certain children with adequate I.Q. who do not improve academically as expected. Mora *et al.* (47) tested the hypothesis that those children would display more evidence of minimal brain dysfunction in rigidity of behavior, awkwardness in motility, and hyperactivity than would children who did better academically. Fifty-seven children with an average of 9.5 years formed the study population. Six were schizophrenic, 18 showed personality-pattern disturbance, 29 showed personality-trait disturbance, and four were diagnosed as psychoneurotic. Twenty-two of the 57 manifested positive neurological signs, determined by a pediatric neurological examination comprising 85 points of inquiry. Use of the Metropolitan Achievement Test showed that there was little difference at time of admission between the organically impaired child and the child without organic impairment, but that the rate of subsequent improvement is significantly greater for the latter.

In a large-scale study of the total population (11,865) of children of compulsory school age who were not attending private school on the Isle of Wight, Graham and Rutter (27) found a very high rate of psychiatric disorder among children with epilepsy, cerebral palsy, and other neurological disorders of the brain. Their rate of psychiatric disorder, 34 percent, was five times greater than that in the general population. Previous studies had suggested many reasons for such an increased rate: "visibility of the disability, frustrations inherent in physical restrictions, negative parental reactions to the handicap, perceptual abnormalities, poor language skills which prevent the child from expressing his needs adequately, visual defects, low intelligence, effect of drugs, community prejudices, the child's reactions to his disability, and impaired emotional control resulting from a brain dysfunction." *Some of these factors are shared by children with other types of physical handicaps, while others are unique to those with brain abnormalities.*

Only the chronic physical handicap was found not to be a crucial factor. Psychiatric disorder was three times more frequent in the epileptic group than it was in children with other physical disorders. Children with asthma, diabetes, or heart disease were less psychiatrically impaired than those with cerebral palsy. The authors speculate that the severity of the physical handicap may explain this difference, but they found they could not explain the pronounced differences between the child with cerebral palsy and the blind child or one with lesions below the brain stem, both of whom tended to have less frequent psychiatric impairments. Nor could severity of physical handicap account for the high rate of psychiatric disorder among those epileptic children who were little handicapped.

Visibility of the handicap is also discredited as a major factor, since children with lesions below the brain stem resulting in physical disabilities showed no more frequent psychiatric impairment than did children with nonneurological disorders.

Community prejudice against epilepsy appears to be a probable yet equivocal factor. There was a slightly but not significantly higher rate of psychiatric disorder in epileptic children whose physical activities had been restricted. Yet psychiatric disorders were of equal frequency in children whose teachers knew the child had fits and in those whose teachers did not possess such knowledge. Although low intelligence level was related to frequent psychiatric abnormalities in children with lesions above the brain stem, low I.Q. did not account for the high rate of psychiatric disorder in epileptic children. Even when comparison was limited to children with I.Q.'s of 86 or more, the rate of psychiatric disorder in epileptic children was still more than twice that in children with other chronic physical disabilities. The authors conclude, by process of exclusion, that the most important feature relevant to the higher rate of psychiatric disorder in epileptic children compared with other physically handicapped children is the specific presence of cerebral dysfunction. Other factors are contributory, but cerebral dysfunction is the main feature.

A group of children supposedly free of brain damage, according to physical examination, were studied by Blau and Schaffer (9). They state: "Empirical evidence indicates that about 10 percent of clinical patients . . . have some critical disruption which might be described as sub-clinical intracranial pathology" despite negative results of physical examinations.

Eighty different neurological tests were administered by Peters *et al.* (53) to 82 boys (ages 8-11) with learning disabilities and/or behavioral problems and to 45 academically normal controls. The rationale for the extensive battery of tests was that no single neurological test would correlate significantly with a particular cognitive defect, but that where one or more cognitive defects were present a child was more likely to exhibit motor deviations. They found that 44 of the 80 tests significantly differentiated the populations in the direction expected. These signs tended to diminish with age in the learning-disabled children so that the older ones more closely resembled the controls. This improvement, they comment, does not rule out "subtle" brain damage as etiological.

From a wide survey of neurological dysfunction in dyslexia, Benton (7) concluded that the most frequent is some type of motor deficit. Clumsiness was most frequently observed, followed by dyspraxia, hyperkinesis, motor impersistence, and choreiform movements (irregular spasms of limbs or facial muscles). Soft signs associated with dyslexia are identified by Frank and Levinson (22) as: 1) positive Romberg (more difficulty in standing on one foot with eyes closed than with eyes open); 2) tandem walking difficulties; 3) articulatory speech disorders; 4) dysfunction in ability alternately to bring limb into opposite position (flexion, then extension or pronation, then supination); 4) hypotonia; and 5) past-point disorders in touching finger to nose, heel to toe, writing and drawing, ocular fixation, and scanning. Minimal organicity "diagnosed by psychological tests was correlated with the same diagnosis by minor" neurological signs by Klatskin *et al.* (38). They tested for: 1) general clumsiness in skipping, hopping, tandem gait, and standing on one foot; 2) poor rapid alternating movements in imitation of the examiner in opposing fingers to the thumb of each hand, and in hitting one hand alternately with the palmar and dorsal side of the other; 3) synkinesis (moving one hand unintentionally while intentionally moving the other); 4) choreiform movements; 5) agraphestia; 6) astereognosis; 7) "confused" dominance: difficulty or inability in identifying right/left body parts. (Chapter 15 discusses lateral dominance.)

I have surveyed the frequency with which soft signs appear in a mixed population of applicants to a rehabilitation agency, largely a low-income group and including those with psychiatric disorders, cardiac illnessess, and tuberculosis. One hundred applicants in sequence, without selection, were interviewed for etiological and historical factors and for present symptomatology and were given seven subtests of the Weschler Intelligence Scale for Adults. Among the applicants, 50 percent were referred from psychiatric facilities, 20 percent from community agencies, 15 percent from medical facilities, 10 percent from State rehabilitation agencies, and 5 percent from residential treatment services for adolescents.

Psychosis was the most frequent referral diagnosis, with 61 percent; 26 percent came without diagnoses of any kind; no one came with a neurological diagnosis.

Among the historical-etiological factors, significant learning problems were recalled by 57 percent; 19 percent remembered febrile episodes with temperatures around 105 degrees; 12 percent recalled comas during these episodes; 33 percent had sustained head injuries; 19 percent had been unconscious following these injuries; 19 percent had been treated with electroconvulsive shock.

Nine percent manifested gait peculiarities; 19 percent had other motor disturbances; 9 percent has some speech problem; 29 percent acknowledged visual phenomena of blurring, double vision, phosphenes, or tension experienced because of moving lights; 30 percent had been dizzy more than occasionally; 22 percent had fainted more than one time; 27 percent experienced tingling of fingers and/or toes; 19 percent had headaches unresponsive to usual medication; 39 percent experienced auditory phenomena such as ringing and high pitched sounds; 37 percent believed themselves to be clumsier than most people, falling, stumbling, dropping and bumping into things; 14 percent reported blackouts; 12 percent described episodes approximating altered states of consciousness; 39 percent manifested mixed dominance on testing.

The subtests of the Weschler Adult Intelligence Scale (WAIS) were grouped according to the three factors identified by Witkin (69, 70): Verbal, Attention-Memory, Perceptual-Analytic. Usually studies of the differences of scale scores between subtests of the WAIS produce a mean standard deviation of three scale points. In this population, on the average, 25 percent produced differences of more than three scale points between subtests within the same factor (*e.g.,* Information and Comprehension within the Verbal factor), while 35 percent produced differences of more than three scale points between subtests associated with different factors (*e.g.,* Information for the Verbal factor and Object Assembly for the Perceptual-Analytic factor). Differences of such magnitude between factors have come to suggest lateralized brain damage to the neuropsychologist.

Obviously, some symptoms found here are attributable to psychotic hallucinatory states, intense anxiety, high blood pressure, even preoccupation. But they are also associated with stabilized brain injuries or paroxysmal disorders. What is significant is their frequency in so mixed a population of patients coming largely from economically disadvantaged sectors of the community.

All the foregoing strongly suggest 1) that neurological abnormalities are more prevalent among psychiatric populations in particular than is ordinarily suspected, and 2) that among those populations showing neurological abnormalities, a higher incidence of psychiatric disturbance is likely. These observations imply that psychiatric disturbance can be intensified by brain damage and brain dysfunction or even attributable to it. One may reasonably assume, therefore, that a significant proportion of diagnosed psychiatric disturbances may have a neurological component, and that some may be primarily attributable to neurological causes rather than to psychological ones. Psychological problems, while often present in the neurologically impaired patient, are thus possibly secondary rather than primary, and unless properly diagnosed may come to be considered intractable behavior of psychogenic origin.

CAUSES OF OBSCURE NEUROLOGICAL IMPAIRMENTS

The brain is exposed to a gamut of dangers throughout life, beginning in early stages of fetal development and continuing into the declining years of adulthood. Birth itself is one of the hazards. "The most perilous journey any of us ever makes" states Apgar (2), "is the few inches from the womb to the outside world." Brain dysfunction can be caused by trauma, infectious diseases, poisons, high temperatures, and proliferating lesions, among other conditions. Often, but not always, the gross neurological disturbances caused by such factors are readily detectable in clinical examinations and electroencephalographic studies. However, as evidenced in the long ordeal of Sam, some may not be readily detectable by these standard clinical procedures. Some arise fortuitously; others are predictable. Some are readily identifiable, others are subtle and escape detection for so long that effect and cause are difficult to connect. All possible neurological contributants require our concern. A recent newsletter of a school for the learning-disabled in New York featured separate articles linking the following selected but disparate causes to learning, reading, and behavior problems: tranquilizers, antibiotics, dysfunctions of the inner ear, allergies, and food additives. There is, in short, no single cause or even group of causes for the symptoms and syndromes considered in this book.

For some decades now attention has been directed to the circumstances attending pregnancy and birth that make for subsequent cerebral dysfunction. These circumstances have come to be called "pregnancy and birth complications," abbreviated to "PBCs." Asphyxiation producing anoxia in the fetus or at birth is the major villain. As early as 1862 Little (43) saw an association between perinatal anoxia and spastic palsies. But the problem received little professional and scientific attention until eighty years later when Schreiber in 1940 (62) cited the *many* causes leading to anoxia and its neurological effects in the neonate. Shortly thereafter McPhail *et al.* (44) reviewed the known factors surrounding gestation and birth that caused anoxia and described the steps the obstetrician could take to reduce their incidence. About this time Preston (54), prompted by the neurological consequences of anoxia in two cases of the secondborn of twins, reviewed ten preceeding years of her obstetrical practice. She observed two types of later effects: *lesser* degrees of anoxia tended to result in hyperactivity, *greater* degrees in apathy. Darke (18) found retarded mental development to be significantly related to severe asphyxiation and apnea in the newborn infant without physical evidence of injury then or later.

The 1950s brought a surge of important studies. Benda (6) urged concern for the "quality as well as survival of the new born"; he reported that six of every one hundred children are exceptional in that they are not fully equipped to meet the demands and requirements of community life, and that the causes of their disability have been associated with anoxia at birth. In a series of retrospective studies from 1951 to 1955, Lilienfeld and his colleagues (40, 41, 42) found a direct association between the complications of pregnancy and labor usually accompanied by anoxia and the subsequent development of cerebral palsy, epilepsy, mental retardation, and behavioral problems. Support for their theory by other clinical researchers, however, was neither uniform nor unequivocal.

Benaron and his colleagues (5) observed that anoxia at birth affects some infants but not others. The anoxic group showed greater variability than the control group in test scores. They attributed the variability to the possibility that only a small number of individuals are affected by anoxia, not in sufficient number to produce statistical reliability when groups are compared. Nonetheless, anoxia may have serious effects in later life. A greater number of anoxic children are feebleminded, with an I.Q. below 70. Twenty percent of the anoxic group were so impaired, contrasted with an occurrence of three percent in the general population, and 2.5 percent in their control group, approximately the expected number. The anoxic group showed a persistence of infantile habits far in excess of that found among the controls, 63 percent contrasted with 26 percent. Twenty-seven percent of the anoxic children produced abnormal electroencephalograms. Among anoxic children whose siblings served as controls, 36 percent displayed EEG abnormalities, but none of their sibling controls did so. Benaron *et al.* concluded that a newborn may suffer severe anoxia without deleterious effects, that only in isolated instances will anoxia result in pathology of the brain which may result in either feeblemindedness or a condition productive of abnormal electroencephalogram.

These findings differ from more recent reports that a generalized lower proficiency is to be expected as an outcome of anoxia. Benaron *et al.* (5) reviewed and discussed the "theory of the continuum of reproductive casualty" advanced by Lilienfeld, which assumes that abnormalities of pregnancy and labor may result in brain damage varying along a gradient of injury from a point at which a lethal component results in fetal or neo-natal death to one where a sub-lethal component leads to the development of neurological disorders.

The statement that early anoxia is either lethal or that it leaves no residual effects is considered extreme by Graham *et al.* (28). They believe the question is whether any significant effects occur. Further, they question what is meant by significant. They interpret studies of defective groups to suggest a relationship between later defects and early anoxia, but consider speculation as to the extent of the relationship premature. They are, however, prepared to state that the majority of infants exposed to mild degrees of post-natal anoxia will not show gross central-nervous-system defects or mental impairment. Birth injury due to direct mechanical forces unquestionably can cause serious damage, but with modern obstetrical procedures they consider this relatively rare. Reduction of oxygen, on the other hand, occurs frequently. Five to 10 percent of newborn infants have difficulty, these authors state, in establishing respiration after birth. An unknown number have been exposed to oxygen reduction during fetal life.

It is a relatively easy exercise to associate obvious brain damage with such crippling handicaps as cerebral palsy, epilepsy, and mental retardation. But the association is more difficult with other defects, such as reading disability, particularly when it occurs along with normal intelligence. The same difficulty is present in connecting certain forms of behavior disorder with brain damage. A recognition of the range of possible effects of anoxia is required to account for such diverse phenomena. Minimal injury as well as gross, and both localized and diffuse damage, are possible. A concept that recognizes injury so slight that the adaptive capacity of the child can conceal it would both guide the obstetrician and alert the diagnostician and therapist confronting sequelae.

Some obstetricians maintain that it is difficult at birth to judge lesser asphyxia and its impact on the developmental future of the infant (14). Bowes, et al. (10), however, conclude from a wide survey of medication practices that the empirical experience of most obstetricians is that the onset of respiration is less prompt and less vigorous when analgesics, anesthesias, and sedatives are used than without them. And early post-asphyxiation neurological signs are now recognized more readily as prognostic of subsequent handicaps. These include: feeding difficulties, apnea, cyanosis, convulsions, hypothermia, persistent vomiting, a certain high-pitched "cerebral" cry. Most significant is "hypotonia or hypotonia extending to extensor hypertonus" (14).

Anoxia during gestation and at birth remains a significant problem. A majority of the 65,000 brain-damaged infants born each year in the United States (2 percent of the live births) are said to be victims of anoxia (16). Anoxia is perhaps the most important condition that can affect the brain physiologically. Many conditions can result in fetal or neonatal anoxia. Some are the results of the mother's condition, and her behavior and experiences during pregnancy. Some arise as accidents in the womb or birth canal, others may be produced by obstetrical practices. Maternal bleeding and anemia have been implicated. Recently it was discovered that a low level of placental lactogen, a hormone, results in the fetus receiving less oxygen than it needs (16). Strangulation by the umbilical chord and premature separation of the placenta from the uterine wall may occur. Prolonged labor has been cited, in difficult and delayed births or in breech presentations. As noted above, the analgesics, anesthesias, and sedatives administered by obstetricians are known to retard respiration in the newborn (10). The World Health Organization is reported (11) to be critical of two common obstetrical practices in America: the elective induction of birth by drugs or by artificially rupturing the amniotic membranes early in labor, and the practice of keeping the woman lying on her back during labor and delivery. Each uterine contraction temporarily deprives the infant of blood supply. With inducing medications the contractions tend to be stronger and to last longer, increasing the risk of oxygen deprivation.

Brain tissue is most vulnerable during periods of most rapid growth, as in uterine life, infancy, and early childhood. This vulnerability strongly suggests that the impact of known teratological agents on the fetus, neonate, and child cannot be judged by adult tolerances, as in oxygen deprivation, for example, despite the evidence that the early brain is more plastic than the later brain.

Many situations other than anoxia add stress during these periods of vulnerability. Malnutrition in the mother and/or the infant and child is a major suspect (63). In a study of 17,000 British children, low birth weight is linked to malnourished mothers and subsequently to learning disabilities (12). Birch (8) has studied the effects of fetal malnutrition extensively. Nearly all of the children born in Aberdeen, Scotland during a three-year period were studied eight to ten years later. A striking correlation between maternal height, infant weight, and subsequent mental development was obtained. In rural Guatemalan children with malnutrition plainly evident, Birch found that the shorter children were several years behind the taller in intersensory skills. This was not true in an urban middle-class population, where shortness apparently was genetic and did not represent also the effects of malnutrition.

Drugs taken by the mother during her pregnancy may alter the fetal brain. Among drugs implicated in animal studies are the major antipsychotics or tranquilizers (59). While the placental barrier appears to block most drugs from reaching the fetus, it does not block all drugs. Not enough is known to permit confidence in this matter. Bowes *et al.* (10) warn that no drug can be regarded as completely safe in the early weeks of pregnancy.

Somewhat more is known about the effects of drug abuse upon cerebral integrity and motor and cognitive functioning in adolescents and adults. Tardive kinesis is a danger in prolonged use of neuroleptic medications (17). EEG studies in salicylate (aspirin) poisoning have produced abnormal records (13). Significant numbers, 45 percent of the men, 43 percent of the women, of polydrug abusers showed EEG abnormalities and neuropsychological dysfunctions on the Halstead-Reitan Battery (29). While there is little evidence of gross neuropsychological impairment with the use of hallucinogenic drugs, there is mounting evidence of lesser degree of cerebral impairment and higher cortical dysfunction (1). Animal studies with LSD have produced defects in the offspring.

Neuropsychological studies of chronic alcoholics report a variety of dysfunctions in cognitive flexibility, spatial concept and synthesis, perceptual field orientation, planning and foresight, motor regulation, task persistence, error utilization, and learning and memory (65).

An extensive and systematic survey of the literature on neuropsychological findings in drug abuse has been made by Grant and Mohns (30). They conclude that: 1) few alcoholics suffer *severe* cerebral dysfunction; 2) many alcoholics suffer some cerebral impairment, especially of abstracting ability; 3) evidence suggests mild cerebral impairment in the long-term use of marijuana, hallucinogens, and sedatives; 4) cerebral-vascular accidents occur earlier and more frequently in amphetamine abusers; 5) intravenous use of narcotics is associated with case reports of transverse myelitis and encephalitis, but whether these are a direct effect of the drugs, of adulterants, or of infection is not known.

Trauma obviously is a source of brain damage with a wide range of degree of residual impairment. The neonate may be cerebrally injured if forceps are used in the delivery. Again, the damage and its effects may escape recognition. A recent important conference on physical trauma as a cause of mental retardation (54) heard that the incidence of undetected damage is impossible to estimate. Major surgical procedures, without directly interfering with the brain, may produce protracted anoxia severe enough to cause brain damage. Morgan (48) found that 16 of 72 cardiac-surgery survivors developed clear signs of brain damage; no accounting was made of soft signs among them.

The effect of electroconvulsive shock therapy (ECT) has been widely studied for its EEG and neuropsychological effects. Turek (66) from a survey of the EEG literature reports that generally a shift to high amplitude-slow wave activity is observed as a result of ECT. Using a neuropsychological approach, Goldman *et al.* (25) obtained significantly more error scores on the Bender and the Benton Visual Retention Test in 20 patients who had received 50 or more ECTs ten to fifteen years before the study. The known neurological effects of ECT are still being ignored, warns Friedberg (23). These include: petechial hemorrhages of the brain, gliosis, neuronal destruction, EEG change, severe retrograde amnesia, and subtle dysfunctions of memory and learning.

Some diseases make the brain especially vulnerable. Hypoglycemia is one. Brain tissue requires blood sugar to use oxygen; in conditions of inadequate blood serum, sugar levels in the brain will draw on oxygen stored in its tissue as glycogen, depriving the brain of needed oxygen. The pathological process starts with the higher cerebral levels and unless interrupted will proceed downwards to cerebellar parts (33). Serious neuropsychiatric dysfunction (mental deterioration) is reported among the sequelae of postgastrectomy hypoglycemia. Among diabetic patients Bale (3) found that non-fatal hypoglycemia may produce permanent brain damage. They appear to be subject to a higher incidence of cerebral vascular accidents, and atherosclerosis tends to develop at an earlier age and to be more severe.

A significant association between hypertension and neuropsychological deficits was obtained by Goldman et al. (26).

The expansion of knowledge about immunological disorders has established that persons, especially children, with *unidentified* immunological dysfunction are vulnerable to brain damage as a consequence of rampant infection. Glasser (24) reports that in children with such disorders unwittingly vaccinated in the usual way, toxins may enter the spinal fluid and then the ventricles of the brain, producing brain damage.

Inadvertent exposure to brain-tissue destructive agents is reported with increasing frequency. Carbon monoxide (35), food additives such as the coloring dye Red 2 (21), lead (4, 49, 50), mercury (52), hexachlorophene as talcum powder or antiseptic (19), and vinyl chloride and radiation (15) are among the culprits cited. The damage to the human organism may take place *in utero*, or at any stage of life. Awareness is increasing that occupational exposure to such hazards may damage the reproductive functions of women and to a lesser extent of men. The special vulnerability of women is not yet explained, but as more women enter the labor force the importance of the question increases (15).

Social disadvantage has been widely associated with learning and personality disorders. Vance (67) identifies three prevailing views of the cause of "social disability." The *sociological* view relates it to inequities in housing and schooling. The *cultural* sees it as a reflection of ethnic and socio-economic habits and values. The *genetic* attributes it to genotypic difference. To this should be added the *neurological* view of social disability. Montagu (46) bridges the sociological and neurological; poverty and ghetto conditions, he observes, are often marked by "physical and social malnutrition" that appear to result in serious failures in neural development and consequently in learning ability.

A widely reported study matching physical data with nutritional history estimated that more than one million children in the United States have suffered or are at risk of brain damage caused by malnutrition due to poverty (60). Malnutrition of a pregnant woman retards brain growth in the fetus; malnutrition of the infant continues the process, according to the research.

Birch (8) presents telling statistics: in the United States 13.8 percent of non-white infants weigh less than 2500 grams at birth; the percentage is 7.2 for whites. When the non-white population of Nashville was stratified socio-economically the incidence of birthweight less than 2500 grams was 23.3 at the bottom of the scale and 5.3 at the top.

A study of 17,000 British children reported that by the age of seven the children of working class parents are both shorter than and far behind middle-class peers in reading, academic achievement, and mental development. They also exhibit a higher incidence of squints, speech defects, and motor dyscoordination (68).

Conditions of poverty increase the probability that anoxia will occur at childbirth. Prenatal care is poor among the disadvantaged: delivery of newborns is notoriously more careless, less well attended. Post-natal health care is equally poor. Malnutrition is widespread. Childhood illnesses accompanied by high fevers are less well cared for. Ghetto life subjects the child to more blows and accidents physically traumatic to the brain. A newspaper story (39) reports the outcome of a nine-month study of more than 79,000 children in New York City. Black children were found to suffer from lead poisoning at a rate three times that of white children. The study concludes that lead poisoning is most common in the ghetto. Students of violence related to brain damage tend to concur that prevention through attacks upon poverty and slum living is the best answer for this problem (61).

DIAGNOSTIC DIFFICULTIES

The frequent difficulty of discriminating among schizophrenia, anxiety attacks, epilepsy, and other brain disorders is in itself a compelling argument for seeking a more effective neuropsychodiagnosis.

Studies of electrocerebral activity indicate that epileptiform patterns tend to be more frequent in patients with diagnoses of schizophrenia. Shagass (64) hypothesizes that some kinds of schizophrenia involve brain activity of a disordered nature, comparable to that found in epilepsy, and that such disorders are probably related to a biochemical lesion. Related psychological-test findings are that intra-test scatter fails to differentiate between schizophrenic patients and those with organic disease. In an inverse fashion, Nicol (51) calls attention to the frequency with which depression accompanies organic disease of the central nervous system, only to be overlooked or discounted "with frustrating and at times disastrous results for the patient." Even where damage to the brain is an accepted fact of a diagnosis, the precise influence of that damage is subject to variables which may operate independently. These variables may converge in ways of which the diagnostician is unaware, resulting in a most complicated problem. Reitan (56) in a broad overview of psychological deficits points to the real possibility "that different types of pathological brain involvement may have differential psychological effects." Another element in the complexity he observes is that any head trauma that causes brain damage may have effects far exceeding the neurological features that remain observable at some future examination, when for example, one could identify only a residual focal scar or a pattern of electrical discharge.

The practitioner may recall patients presenting states of apparent depersonalization, seeming to justify a diagnosis of schizophrenia, who fail to respond to psychotherapy or to psychotropic medication, and who begin to arouse suspicion of a seizure condition. Often EEG and neurological examination are negative for cerebral dysfunction, but psychological test findings indicate a deficit attributable either to an ego-function weakness or to a cerebral impairment. For some of these patients, trial courses of anti-convulsant medication has in my experience eliminated the states of depersonalization, which then are more accurately seen as states of altered consciousness. Thereafter, the patient is often able to benefit from psychotherapy. (Chapter 3 describes cases illustrating this clinical phenomenon.)

Hertzig *et al.* (31) concluded from studies of brain-damaged children that the effect of damage to the brain is dependent upon its location, extent, the time of life at which injury was sustained, and the developmental opportunities with which it is associated. This complex of variables results in a variety of neurological disorders accompanied by psychological aberrations, ranging from mental retardation to psychosis. Accurate neurological diagnosis in difficult-to-detect cerebral dysfunctions, they reason, will counterbalance the tendency to attribute excessive responsibility to the etiological effect of the environment or parental relationship. While these factors make their contribution to emotional disturbances, they do so "most readily in interaction with organismic patterns," the authors find.

A list of factors that may contribute to academic impairment in a child has been offered by Reitan (57): 1) familial or genetic mental retardation; 2) cultural deprivation; 3) cerebral damage; 4) adverse relationships within the family; 5) a negativistic attitude toward learning experience; 6) psychological disorders (neurotic or psychotic conditions of various types); 7) "an interaction of multiple influences" developing sequentially, with one deficit engendering consequences which promote the development of further problems in adjustment. Reitan cites the brain as the principal organ mediating adaptive behavior, whether the influences arise culturally or otherwise. Damage to this central organ, therefore, significantly influences the emergence of any one or a combination of adaptational problems.

The frequent misdiagnosis of mental retardation is assailed by Durfee (20). Acknowledging that differential diagnosis is a complicated and difficult procedure, he nonetheless finds unacceptable the all too frequent misdiagnosis by trained professionals of, *e.g.*, a language problem as mental deficiency, a neurosis as retardation, autism as mental deficiency, or a psychosis as mental retardation. Searching for causes, he identifies: 1) professional buckpassing or the tendency to accept another's diagnosis as easier than probing for new information and re-evaluating; 2) avoiding interprofessional conflicts should a current opinion based on new material contradict a former diagnosis; 3) the influence of pressure for "successful" closure exerted by many agencies; 4) the sorry fact that some trained professionals are neither careful enough nor sufficiently well-equipped to make a differential diagnosis.

The literature is full of examples of the limitation of classical clinical neurological procedures, the traditional examination of reflexes, cranial nerves, and the electroencephalogram in neurological diagnoses. A nationwide study of minimal brain dysfunction (45) comments upon the experience of a child suffering a *grand mal* seizure of epilepsy minutes after having produced a normal electroencephalographic recording. Kennedy and Ramirez (37) note how often normal pneumoencephalographic readings are obtained in many conditions of brain damage, despite the presence of pronounced psychological deficits characteristic of brain damage. They report that the great majority of children presenting evidence suggestive of brain damage produce normal or non-specific diagnostic results on physical neurological examination, and frequently on the electroencephalogram as well. Speculating about why she and her group identified seventeen times more neurologic abnormality in a psychiatric population than did the hospital staff, Hertzig (31) suggests that gross insensitivity of the standard neurological examination to neurologic abnormality, particularly in children and adolescents, is a more likely determinant of such underestimation than is the possibility that the clinical psychiatrist, intent upon a psychiatric diagnosis, is generally insensitive to neurologic abnormalities.

Reitan (56) believes that many psychological assessments of deficit have been distorted by the inadequacy of the clinical neurological examination upon which patients assigned for psychological study have been classified. He reminds us that the content of a neurological examination is quite variable from one neurologist to another; it is only crudely standardized and its data are often liable to subjective interpretation. Reitan relates that in his experience every sophisticated neurologist admits cases in which his first diagnosis based upon neurological examination and the history was found to be seriously in error when a wider variety of additional information became available from extended inquiry: electroencephalography, angiography, pneumography, surgical notes, diagnostic representations of the lesion, and findings from histological autopsy examinations.

All of this adds up to a compelling argument for the development of procedures that are both more comprehensive and more sensitive. An obvious first step is to extend the clinical examination to include a wider range of behavioral manifestations, rather than to rely upon one or two sources of information. The brain is a magnificently complicated organ. Manifestations of its disturbances are influenced by location of damage, extent of damage, nature of damage, developmental stage at time of damage, and length of time since the damage. The independent variables are so numerous that only a body of information derived from every available type of examination can be considered adequate for a proper diagnosis.

Until extensive and refined procedures are established, the psychotherapist can be guided to protect his patient by these reminders:

1) Equivocal "soft" neurological signs are found with significant frequency in so-called psychiatric populations *when they are sought.* In similar fashion, events and symptoms of neurological significance are often uncovered in a history only *when specific inquiries are made.*

2) *Normal* neurological and electroencephalographic findings have been obtained in individuals with "suggestive" symptoms in whom brain pathology, including tumors and paroxysmal disorders, was soon thereafter revealed.

3) Therapeutic cures have been obtained by the use of amphetamines, Dilantin, and other anti-convulsants in individuals with hyperactivity and seizure symptoms for whom normal neurological and electroencephalographic findings are reported.

From the actuarial viewpoint, the incidence of equivocal neurological conditions liable to be mistaken for emotional disturbances may seem of trifling importance. Statements of probability are cold comfort, however, for a long-suffering person or for a clinician who misses the boat with a single patient. Concern for individual human welfare commands our concern for the exception, the unusual. And the evidence supports the conclusion that equivocal neurological conditions in a psychotherapeutic population occur often enough to make them an ever-present minority phenomenon. They are not rare in any population. Moreover, their incidence increases in at least two specific populations: the socially and economically deprived and the psychotic. Good sense and responsibility for the patient's welfare require that equivocal neurological signs be carefully assessed along with psychogenic factors for their contribution to a patient's symptoms. These conditions are so possible, their effects individually and socially so costly, as to demand our scientific and professional attention. Techniques are at hand to improve our capacity to detect and treat them. Not to make an effort at complete diagnosis, no matter how completely one's theoretical bias accounts for the picture presented by the patient, seems in light of present knowledge to be irresponsible.

BIBLIOGRAPHY

1. *Acord, L. D.:* Hallucinogenic drugs and brain damage. Military Med., 137:1, 1972.
2. *Apgar, V.:* New promise in fight against birth defects. Reported anon in ACLD Newsbriefs, 91, 1974.
3. *Bale, R. N.:* Brain damage in diabetes mellitus. Brit. J. Psychiat., 122:568, 1973.
4. *Baloh, R., et al.:* Neuropsychological effects of chronic asymptomatic increased lead absorption. Arch. Neurol., 32:5, 1975.
5. *Benaron, H. B., et al.:* Effect of anoxia during labor and immediately after birth on the subsequent development of the child. Amer. J. Obstet, Gynecol., 80:6, 1960.
6. *Benda, C. E.:* Developmental Disorders of Mentation and Cerebral Palsies. New York: Grune and Stratton, 1952.
7. *Benton, A. L.:* Developmental dyslexia: Neurological aspects. *In* W. J. Friedlander (Ed.): Advances in Neurology, Vol. 7. New York: Raven Press, 1975.
8. *Birch, H. G.:* Fundamental effects of fetal malnutrition. *In* S. Chess and A. Thomas (Eds.): Annual Progress in Child Psychiatry and Child Development. New York: Brunner/Mazel, 1972.
9. *Blau, T. H.* and *Schaffer, R .E.:* The Spiral After-effect Test (SAET) as a predictor of normal and abnormal electroencephalographic records in children. J. Consult. Psychol., 24:1, 1960.
10. *Bowes, Jr., W. A., et al.:* The effects of obstetrical medication on fetus and infant., Monograph of the Society for Research in Child Development, 35:4, 1970.
11. *Brody, J. E.:* Some obstetrical methods criticized. New York Times, April 10, 1975.
12. *Brody, J. E.:* Low birth weight is linked to ills. New York Times, November 14, 1972.
13. *Brown, G. LaV.* and *Wilson, W. P.:* Salicylate intoxication and the CNS: With special reference to EEG findings. Dis. Nerv. Syst., 32:2, 1971.
14. *Brown, J. K., et al.:* Neurological aspects of perinatal asphyxia. Develop. Med. Child Neurol., 16, 1974.
15. *Burnham, D.:* Rise in birth defects laid to job hazards. New York Times, March 14, 1976.
16. *Chard, T.:* Reported anon in ACLD Newsbriefs, 91, 1974.
17. *Crane, G. E.:* Clinical psychopharmacology in its 20th year. Sci., 181, 1973.
18. *Darke, R. A.:* Late effects of severe asphyxia neonatorium: A preliminary report. J. Pediatrics, 24, 1944.
19. Death of 21 French babies laid to talcum powder. Reported anon. New York Times, August 29, 1972.
20. *Durfee, R. A.:* The misdiagnosis of mental retardation. J. Rehab., 35:1, 1969.
21. FDA now encourages testing of theory linking food additives to hyperkineses. Reported anon. ACLD Newsbriefs, 99, 1975.
22. *Frank, J.* and *Levinson, H.:* Dysmetric dyslexia and dyspraxia: Hypothesis and study. J. Amer. Acad. Child Psychiat., 12:4, 1973.
23. *Friedberg, J.:* Shock treatment, brain damage and memory loss: A neurological perspective. Amer. J. Psychiat., 134:9, 1977.
24. *Glasser, E.:* For Marie at 16, a birthday gift of hope. New York Times, April, 16, 1977.
25. *Goldman, H., et al.:* Long-term effects of electroconvulsive therapy upon memory and perceptual-motor performance. J. Clin. Psychol., 28:1, 1972.
26. *Goldman, H., et al.:* Correlation of diastolic blood pressure and signs of cog-

nitive dysfunction in essential hypertension. VA Hospital, St. Louis, Mo., Mimeo, undated.

27. *Graham, P.* and *Rutter, M.:* Organic brain dysfunction and child psychiatric disorder. Brit. Med. J., 3, 1968.

28. *Graham, P. K., et al.:* Anoxia as a significant perinatal experience: A critique. J. Pediat., 50, 1957.

29. *Grant, I.* and *Judd, LL.:* Neuropsychological and EEG disturbance in polydrug users. Amer. J. Psychiat., 133:9, 1976.

30. *Grant, I.* and *Mohns, L.:* Chronic cerebral effects of alcohol and drug abuse. Internat. J. Addictions, 10:5, 1975.

31. *Hertzig, M. E., et al.:* Neurological findings in children educationally designated as "brain-damaged." Amer. J. Orthopsychiat., 39:3, 1969.

32. *Hertzig, M. E.* and *Birch, H. G.:* Neurologic organization in psychiatrically disturbed adolescents. Arch. Gen. Psychiat., 19, 1968.

33. *Himwich, W. A.* and *Himwich, H. E.:* Neurochemistry. *In* A. M. Freedman and H. I. Kaplan (Eds.): Human Behavior: Biological, Psychological and Sociological. New York: Atheneum, 1972.

34. *Ingram, T. T. S.:* Soft signs. University of Edinburgh. Journal unidentified.

35. *Jefferson, J. W.:* Subtle neuropsychiatric sequelae of carbon monoxide intoxication: Two case reports. Amer. J. Psychiat., 121:4, 1976.

36. *Kennard, M.:* Value of equivocal signs in neurological diagnosis. Neurology, 10, 1960.

37. *Kennedy, C.* and *Ramirez, L. S.:* Brain damage as a cause of behavior disturbance in children. *In* H. G. Birch (Ed.): Brain Damage in Children. Baltimore: Williams and Wilkins, 1964.

38. *Klatskin, E. H., et al.:* Minimal organicity in children of normal intelligence: Correspondence between psychological test results and neurologic findings. J. Learning Disabilities, April, 1972.

39. Lead poison study finds blacks suffer at a rate 3 times whites. Reported anon. New York Times, December 7, 1971.

40. *Lilienfeld, A. M., et al.:* Relationships between pregnancy experience and the development of certain neuropsychiatric disorders in children. Amer. J. Pub. Health, 45, 1955.

41. *Lilienfeld, A. M.:* Mass Study of Reproductive Wastage in Prematurity and Birth Injury. New York: Association for the Aid of Crippled Children, 1953.

42. *Lilienfeld, A. M.* and *Parkhurst, E.:* A study of the association of factors of pregnancy and parturition with the development of cerebral palsy: A preliminary report. Amer. J. Hyg., 53, 1951.

43. *Little, W. J.:* On influence of abnormal parturition, difficult labors, premature birth, and asphyxia neonatorium on mental and physical condition of child, especially in relation to deformities. Trans. Obstet. Soc. London, 3:293, 1862.

44. *McPhail, F. L.* and *Hall, E.:* A consideration of the cause and possible late effect of anoxia in the new born infant. Amer. J. Obstet. Gynec., 42, 1942.

45. Minimal Brain Dysfunction in Children: Educational, Medical and Health Related Services. Phase Two of a Three Phase Project. U. S. Dept. of Health Service, Publication No. 2015, 1969.

46. *Montagu, A.:* Sociogenic brain damage. Amer. Anthropologist, 74:5, 1972.

47. *Mora, G., et al.:* Psychiatric syndromes and neurological findings as related to academic achievement: Implications for education and treatment. Mimeo, undated.

48. *Morgan, D. H.:* Neuro-psychiatric problems of cardiac surgery. J. Psychosom. Res., 15:1, 1971.

49. *Needleman, H. L.* and *Shapiro, I. M.:* Dentine lead levels in asymptomatic

Philadelphia school children: Subclinical exposure in high and low risk groups. Environmental Health Perspectives, May, 1974.

50. *Needleman, H. L.:* Lead poisoning in children: Neurological implications of widespread subclinical intoxication. Seminars in Psychiat., 5:1, 1973.

51. *Nicol, C. F.:* Depression as viewed through neurological spectacles. Psychosom., 9, 1968.

52. *Perlman, J. A.:* Epidemic of mercury poisoning kills 459 in Iraq, it's disclosed by medical teams. Wall Street Journal, July 19, 1973.

53. *Peters, J. E., et al.:* A special neurological examination of children with learning disabilities. Devel. Med. Child Neurol., 17:1, 1975.

54. *Preston, N. I.:* Late behavioral aspects found in cases of prenatal, natal, and postnatal anoxia. J. Pediatrics, 26, 1945.

55. *Quitkin, F., et al.:* Neurologic soft signs in schizophrenia and character disorders: Organicity in schizophrenia with premorbid asociality and emotionally unstable character disorders. Arch. Gen. Psychiat., 33:7, 1976.

56. *Reitan, R. M.:* Psychological deficit. Ann. Rev. Psychol., 13, 1962.

57. *Reitan, R. M. and Heineman, C. E.:* Interaction of neurological deficits and emotional disturbance in children with learning disabilities: Methods for differential assessment. Indiana Medical Center and Fort Wayne Child Guidance Clinic. Mimeo, undated.

58. *Rochford, J. M., et al.:* Neuropsychological impairments in functional psychiatric diseases. Arch. Gen. Psychiat., 22, 1970.

59. *Schmeck, Jr., H. M.:* Some drugs found to alter fetal brains. New York Times, March 13, 1979.

60. *Schmeck, Jr., H. M.:* Brain harm in U. S. laid to food lack. New York Times, February 2, 1977.

61. *Schmeck, Jr., H. M.:* Depths of brain probed for sources of violence. New York Times, December 27, 1972.

62. *Schreiber, F.:* Neurologic sequelae of postnatal asphyxia. J. Pediatrics, 16, 1940.

63. *Scrimshaw, N. S. and Gordon, J. E.:* Malnutrition, Learning and Behavior. Cambridge, Mass.: MIT press, 1968.

64. *Shagass, C.:* Neurophysiological studies. *In* L. Bellak and L. Loeb (Eds.): The Schizophrenic Syndrome. New York: Grune and Stratton, 1969.

65. *Tarter, R. E.:* Brain damage associated with chronic alcoholism. Dis. Nerv. Syst., 36:4, 1975.

66. *Turek, I. S.:* EEG correlates of electroconvulsive treatment. Dis. Nerv. Syst., 33, 1972.

67. *Vance, E. T.:* Social disability. Amer. Psychol., June, 1973.

68. *Weinraub, B.:* British find poor children lag. New York Times, June 6, 1972.

69. *Witkin, H. A., et al.:* Psychological Differentiation. New York: John Wiley, 1960.

70. *Witkin, H. A., et al.:* Personality Through Perception. New York: Harper and Bros., 1954.

CHAPTER 2

Minimal Brain Dysfunction (MBD)

The minimal brain dysfunction (MBD) syndrome is prototypical of equivocal neurological conditions. It presents all the problems of ambiguous criteria, and the vagaries of etiology; its very reality is surrounded by partisan controversy. Because MBD is both real and representative, and because it concerns many children, their parents, therapists, educators, physicians, and ultimately their mates and employers, the syndrome, its diagnosis, and its treatment are dealt with here at length. Much of what holds for this syndrome holds also for other conditions discussed later.

THE CONCEPT

The terms "minimal brain damage" and "minimal brain dysfunction" appear with increasing frequency in clinical discourse. They have been found necessary to describe children of "normal" or average overall intelligence in whom emerge certain characteristic signs which cannot be conclusively associated specifically or singly with any causal factor: psychogenic, cultural, familial, or organic neurological disability. Children with these signs or behaviors lag in developing specific abilities and neurological functions. These children may or may not produce abnormal electroencephalogram readings. They may or may not evidence slightly abnormal reflexes. Their impairments sometimes disappear or become less noticeable with time, but many mature with one or more apparently permanent impairments that affect reading and spelling ability, physical coordination, or depth perception, among a variety of other functions. Little wonder that a sad "in-joke" is that minimal cerebral dysfunction involves maximal diagnostic confusion.

Despite the lack of conclusive evidence of a neurological etiology, many clinical and research workers feel safe in assuming such etiology. Others are far less certain and argue that neurological etiology in particular should be ascribed only on the basis of quantifiable evidence. Some of these advocates of "more rigorous data" prefer a descriptive term for the syndrome, "learning disability," rather than an etiological one. But their argument is countered by the fact that the observed disturbances in behavior usually, perhaps always, part of the syndrome, extend beyond the learning situation. All learning and all behavior are reflections of brain function, and although the cause of this brain dysfunction usually cannot be established with present techniques, some brain dysfunction may logically be assumed as the cause of learning or behavior disability. Until the nature and cause of the brain dysfunction can be identified, however, many professionals prefer the term "minimal brain dysfunction" to the more flat-footed "minimal brain damage" to denote the situation of such children.

On the description of these children, there is something near concensus among workers. Many of these children are of near average, average, or above average intelligence (52, 78) but fail to meet the expected age-dependent, and/or intelligence dependent level in learning and behavior (53). The failures appear as disorders of motility, language, and perceptual-motor functions (78). Contributing to these disorders are signs of hyperactivity, distractibility, short attention span, emotional labileness, ease of frustration, and impulsivity. They are disadvantaged in their competition with their normal peers; they are unable to respond as rapidly or accurately in motor situations, and are less adaptable to the changing environment. To confound the diagnostic problem, the pattern is found more often among the psychologically disturbed than among those without such disturbance. This is the general description of the conditions subsumed under the rubric "minimal brain dysfunction (MBD)." In 1941, Werner and Strauss (92) differentiated the syndrome from mental retardation and suggested that it was indicative of a brain injury.

VALUE OF IDENTIFYING MBD

When sensory input is distorted or impoverished by some underlying deficiency, behavioral distortions follow because the reality sense of the young child is affected by the aberrant sensory data. Kennard (35) likens this pathological process to the observable effects of sensory deprivation. The underlying deficiency in MBD is presumed to be structural, occurring at levels of the central nervous system that integrate complex learned patterns. The earlier the diagnosis, the longer the time available for special training as an adjunct to maturation and the greater is the return usually obtained from remedial efforts. Specific training can improve functioning in reading and speech; Kennard suggests that specific training may also ameliorate both perceptual and somatic defects and increase skill in fine motor movements.

A diagnosis of MBD allows more optimism than does one of brain damage or mental retardation. When the facts are those of MBD rather than these relatively unmodifiable conditions, parents and teachers need not be discouraged by the latter terms, to the detriment of rearing and education.

Introduction of specific learning programs creates an aura of realistic optimism and has significant value as secondary prevention because it checks damage to the child's self esteem and the development of damaging reactions in the parents.

For the psychotherapist, a diagnosis of MBD gives direction to the therapy by emphasizing a treatment constellation. The treatment plan may focus upon either or both the child and the family bolstering self-esteem or structuring reality in the child, or identifying and modifying reactions of the parents, who may unwittingly burden the child. When the patient is an older adolescent or an adult in whom discerned disabilities are identifiable as persistent residues of MBD, the psychotherapist is able to pursue goals more realistic than those he might set if all behavioral problems were ascribed to psychogenic or external causes.

Finally, the syndrome occurs frequently enough to make it a major concern. In New York City a group of parents and educators attempting to design educational services to meet known needs were told recently that the incidence of MBD in the schools is between three and five percent, with a total of 36,000 to 50,000 children so impaired. Our Federal government estimate (69) conservatively places the incidence of hyperkinesis alone at about three percent nationwide.

The very fact that this and other signs associated with MBD occur in other disorders as well and in great numbers of children emphasizes the necessity for the most meticulous diagnostic procedure. That precision alone increases the probabilities that a given child's disturbance will be correctly identified so that it may be correctly treated. The importance assigned here to identifying MBD is not without opponents among therapists and educators. Some (30) argue that the individual approach suffers when diagnostic "labels" are used, and that these children need not diagnosis, but rather counseling, individual education in environments conducive to concentration, along with improvement of parental attitudes. *But this contention ignores the major goal of diagnosis postulated here: treatment designed for the comprehended needs of the individual.*

ETIOLOGY

Consideration of the etiology of the condition we here term MBD involves at least two major questions. What is the cause of the learning impairments and behavioral aberrations that constitute this syndrome? If the cause is a brain dysfunction, what is the nature of the structural defect?

Obscuring the answer to the first question is the fact that the symptoms are found with greater frequency among the emotionally disturbed, particularly children, than among individuals without psychological disturbance (35). Yet observers, following upon the experience of Werner and Strauss (92), are sufficiently impressed by the resemblance between children with known brain damage and those exhibiting symptoms of MBD to feel justified in assuming a neurological basis, and, further, that the emotional disturbances evidenced are corollaries of or secondary to the neurological deficits.

If one rejects this assumption, one need not seek a structural defect, but rather direct his efforts solely to the identification and correction of psychological contributants, environmental, familial, or individual.

But if the assumption of a neurological basis seems reasonable, a baffling obstacle to logical closure is our present inability to establish a clear-cut relationship between behavioral impairment and actual brain dysfunction.

A study of children suspected of MBD (60) could not establish a relationship among the several findings: abnormal history, neurological, electroencephalographic, intellectual, and behavioral. These investigators suggest that the clinical picture in a given child is most probably the result of the unique combination of causes, which could include innate, traumatic, psychological, and social factors. The MBD syndrome, they hold, is not homogeneous and does not reflect a single cause.

Genetic factors have been hypothesized (78). One suggestion is that

MBD derives from an autosomal mode of inheritance; another is that there is a genetically determined predisposition to the syndrome which produces vulnerability to the consequences of perinatal distress manifested in vicissitudes of later cerebral development.

Others attribute the structural defect to irregularities of biochemistry, still others to injuries to the brain resulting from direct physical trauma, high fevers poisons, or anoxia (62, 78, 83). These defects may occur, it is reasoned, during gestation, the birth process, or during the years of critical maturation of the central nervous system. As one example, 90 percent of the children who contract bacterial meningitis now survive, but 18 percent of these suffer disabling sequelae (89).

We are only now trying to assimilate the growing body of information about children who survive unfavorable fetal environment (33). A significantly greater frequency of complications of pregnancy and birth was found in the histories of behaviorally disturbed children, with the greatest frequency associated with children described as "seriously" disturbed, by McNeil et al. (46). There were, for example, more premature births and more respiratory problems at birth among the disturbed children than among the controls.

One unusual anatomical hypothesis postulates a faulty coupling of the brain stem to the cortex, thus accounting for the longer reaction time and the difficulty in making intentional motor responses observed in these children. Their distractibility and inflexibility are attributed to their decreased autonomic reactivity (83). The site of the assumed defect is located by some workers in the brain stem, particularly the reticular activating system. Such a cortical locus is considered by them to be a logical necessity to account for the high incidence of negative EEG findings in this group. One result of this anatomical reasoning is to favor use of the term "brain dysfunction" rather than "cerebral dysfunction."

Difficulties in processing and sequencing visual, auditory, kinesthetic, and haptic stimuli have been advanced by many workers as the basis of MBD (22, 67, 84, 85, 93).

Others place the etiological emphasis upon a lag in the maturation of both perceptual and motor skills that must be acquired before higher cognitive abilities can be acquired (29).

The psychological problems observed in so many MBD children are viewed by some as predating and causing their cognitive difficulties. Ney (57), for example, stresses the emotional determinants of hyperkinesis which impede learning.

THE CRITERION PROBLEM IN MBD

The MBD population is poorly defined. Rigorous criteria for whom to include are not available. Objective neurological findings, especially from EEG tracings, are scarce. Many of the symptoms pointing toward MBD are found among children with clear-cut emotional problems. The confusion about etiology is complicated by this cloudy criterion. In part, ambiguity arises from inconsistent screening and diagnostic practices. Methods for early recognition of the child with learning difficulties are still relatively primitive, and should be elaborated, tested, and standardized. Once learning difficulties are recognized in a child, characterization of his deficits is often superficial, with any diagnostic emphasis largely dependent upon the theoretical bias of the diagnostician.

Clinical neurological examination procedures were usually designed to evaluate an adult whose nervous system is established and presumably once was normal. In most instances of MBD, the presumption is reasonable that the child's nervous system was damaged at, before or soon after birth. Here the neurologic question should not be "What has been lost?" but "How much of the expected has been gained?" Techniques, criteria, and norms on a developmental scale are required.

A major difficulty in establishing criteria has been the absence of wide acceptance of that clear correspondence between the syndrome and unequivocal evidence of damage to the brain. But between the "hard" and "soft" sign advocates are workers (51, 60) who are now attempting to establish firmer, if not firm, neurological corroboration of behavioral manifestations. They have found that increasing the precision of the clinical neurological examination produces definitive evidence of neurological abnormality in almost all children diagnosed on the basis of behavioral criteria. These neurological abnormalities include tremor of the hands, dysarthria, hyperreflexia, mild choreo-athetosis, and many other signs described in Chapter 1.

DIAGNOSIS OF MBD

Diagnosis of MBD is made uncertain not only by the elusiveness of the neurological criterion but also by the heterogeneity of the elements in the syndrome. Paine *et al.* (60), among others, believe that a variety of unrelated minor dysfunctions are subsumed in the diagnostic category, some of which are neurological, some behavioral, and others cognitive. Indeed, the range of symptoms that have been associated with the diagnosis is vast. Not all occur in any single child, not all occur with the same frequency. MBD is most probably a syndrome of syndromes: hyperkinesis, dyslexia, and learning disabilities occur in many combinations of degrees and symptoms. Dyslexia, as an example, is being subdivided into "types," each identifiable with specific patterns of neuropsychological dysfunction (4, 48).

Diversity of symptoms in a range of dysfunctions of the brain is not unexpected in light of the complex brain-behavior relationship. (See Chapters 14 and 15 for a discussion of this complicated relationship.) Yet the diversity is overwhelming, as a study of the literature reveals. Schain (78) found 18 diagnostic terms in common use which are equivalent to the term "minimal brain dysfunction."

Comprehensive diagnostic procedures are essential if these often elusive disorders are to be properly identified and treated. Essential diagnostic procedures, according to one expert (58) are: a history; physical examination; neurological examination assigning appropriate importance to assessment of soft signs; psychological evaluation of intellectual and emotional functioning; assessment of small motor coordination, visual motor coordination, and auditory and tactile perception and discrimination; and establishment of base-lines for physiological functioning of kidneys, liver, and blood-forming organs for continuous comparison later if medication becomes part of the treatment.

The extensive diagnostic considerations necessary for MBD quickly overburden any clinic not geared to the complexity of the task. The task is not only time-consuming but also requires integration of data from several professional disciplines. The Sinai Hospital in Baltimore, for example, found it necessary to establish a multidisciplinary clinic for the diagnosis of learning disabilities as a special service of their Pediatrics Department (32).

Symptoms and Signs

Proper diagnosis scrutinizes each person suspected of MBD for the many symptoms that have come to be associated with the syndrome. The following description of these major symptoms, while it covers those now regarded as part of the syndrome, is not all-inclusive.

Special Learning Deficits

The child may be unable to read at grade or age level. There are dyslexic errors, spelling is poor, letters are reversed. There are omissions and substitutions. Or arithmetic presents difficulties, perhaps abstractions. Understanding of part-whole relationships may seem impaired. Any or all of these may be present. Age and grade norms are central to the diagnosis of such deficits. Estimates of the child's innate capacity and motivation, as well as of the quality or adequacy of his instruction must be considered in the diagnosis. Often a child perceives his learning difficulties before his teachers or parents do, and begins to suffer anxiety, guilt, and depression. These emotional signs may appear primary in the presenting picture when in fact they are secondary to the learning difficulty.

A child's deficits may be of so slight a degree that he will experience difficulty only when the level of complexity is increased on attaining higher grade levels. Or the deficits may decrease slowly and progressively as maturation proceeds.

The deficits often persist into adulthood, along with the secondary emotional problems of anxiety, guilt, and depression. Any adult presenting himself for psychotherapy and offering a history of persistent learning difficulties should be scrutinized diagnostically for evidences of MBD.

Motor Impairments

Motor impairments give a variety of clues. Writing, printing, and drawing may be poor. The fingers when extended may tremble. There may be tremors when intentional movements are requested—touching a finger to the nose, touching a finger of one hand to a finger of the other hand, touching a finger to the heel and then the knee. Or the movements may be inaccurate when executed rapidly. Clumsiness, tremor, and ataxia may be tested in children as early as three years of age by having the child place marbles in a cylinder whose diameter is only slightly larger than the marbles. Smoothness of movement and fair rapidity are usual by three years (53).

Balance may be poor when visual cues are absent, as when the person is asked to stand with eyes shut without moving.

Minimal abnormalities of gait, with asymmetry of associated movements, may be noted. Tics or grimacing may be present (35). Apraxia of the face or tongue may be observed. In rest, muscle tone may be abnormal, or peculiarities of the resting position or posture may indicate persistence of a dominant avoiding reaction. Evaluation of the rate of alternate motion in the fingers and toes is of great value in identifying the neurologically impaired child (55).

The presence of choreiform movements—slightly jerky movements occurring suddenly and of short duration—among MBD children has been noted (78), but their diagnostic import is questioned (73). Differentiation from a psychogenic tic is necessary.

Hyperkinesis—high activity level—is most frequently cited as a motor sign. High activity level and impaired coordination are viewed by Wender (91) as the principal motor abnormalities of the syndrome. Underactivity and listlessness also have been observed in MBD children (1, 91) but with far less frequency than hyperactivity. As compared with controls, brain-damaged children spend more time in locomotion and engage in more motor activity when required to do a difficult task, according to Pope (64).

Motor abnormalities are likely to disappear with maturation, and thus signs of them are rarely evident in the adult suspected of MBD. Ozer (59) has found focus upon the pattern of complex patterned responses and associated movement to be the most discriminating approach in detecting "neurological immaturity," but cautions that such measures are less useful after the age of nine, by which time the child may have matured through his lag.

Sensory Impairments

Disorders of visual perception (depth perception, spatial orientation of self, others, and objects) have received attention because of their association with dyslexia. Reversals and difficulty distinguishing between figure and ground are among the disorders noted. In addition, a variety of end-organ defects have been associated with MBD (53, 78): nystagmus, pupillary inequality, extraocular movement. Some visual-perceptual defects become apparent through motor-expressive tasks, as in copying figures (in the Bender Gestalt test), or in constructional tasks requiring the assembly of parts with and without guides, in the Wechsler Intelligence Scales. (See Chapter 11 for a discussion of these intelligence measures.)

Equally important in the genesis of learning disabilities are disorders of hearing. Kennard (35) reported auditory deficits with associated "soft" neurological signs in 25 percent of emotionally disturbed children. The importance of hearing in language and speech development is obvious, but the complexity of the process if often neglected, as emphasized by Sabatino (74). The auditory-perceptual function involves 1) recognition of sound as meaningful, 2) retention of the sounds as informative, 3) integration of the symbols into syntactical units, and 4) comprehension of the units. Effective audition therefore consists of recognition, retention, integration, and comprehension. Sabatino incorporated these measures into the Test of Auditory Perception, so that each area may be assessed differentially. His study emphasizes the necessity to test audition as well as vision to avoid overlooking many bright under-achievers.

Reading ability also requires integration of both visual and auditory perception. Investigating the ability to integrate two stimulus modalities simultaneously is more diagnostically productive than is the testing of single sensory modes. Birch and Belmont (5), through an ingeniously simple test (Auditory-Visual Pattern Integration) demonstrate that learning to read "requires the ability to transform temporally distributed auditory patterns into spatially distributed visual ones." Disturbance of ability to integrate these two sensory modalities was at the root of reading problems among their population of children, all of whom were without a significant hearing impairment or uncorrected visual defect.

A related process involves the haptic (touch) ability to recognize the presence of two stimuli presented simultaneously. With the child's eyes shut he is touched simultaneously upon: 1) both hands, 2) right hand and left cheek, 3) left hand and right cheek, 4) both cheeks. An additional measure of sensory integration requires ability to rule out an irrelevant stimulus (sound) while identifying the simultaneously relevant stimulus (touch).

Impairments of Attention

Shortness of attention span, limited concentration, easy distractibility, and poor memory are characteristics of many MBD victims. Parents will report, and in the playroom it will be observed, that the child does not stay with one task or play for very long, and cannot sustain concentration in the face of an intruding stimulus. These symptoms tend to diminish with age, although they may be discerned in the formal psychological testing of adults. Some observers (21) believe that deficits in learning are caused by impairment of ability to attend and concentrate rather than a deficit specific to the material or process to be learned.

Other Maturational Lags

A history of generally slow development may be reported by parents, or a history of differential rates: "He spoke at an early age but didn't walk until he was two." Bowel and bladder control may lag.

Defects in right-left discrimination may persist beyond the usual age of seven or eight. This may be associated with the presence of mixed dominance, or with the delayed acquisition of laterality.

Impairments of Language, Speech, and Conceptualization

Kennard (35) observed a high frequency of speech defects among children with soft neurological signs. These ranged from lisping to stammering and stuttering. Lags in language and skill development are early and sensitive indicators of a disability (53).

Language skills may not only be slow in developing but also remain restricted throughout life, as evidenced in poor reading and use of spoken vocabulary.

Impairment of capacity for abstract conceptualizations expected for age and I.Q. has been noted.

Behavioral and Emotional Problems

The consequences of brain damage, as we have seen, can be most diverse. No single sign or cluster of signs appears in all brain-damaged persons in the same way or in similar degree. The consequences vary from almost unobservable behavioral disturbance to severe disorganization of social, interpersonal, and intellectual organization almost indistinguishable from psychotic conditions. Damage to the brain may initiate a series of changes in behavior that beget each other, so that in short order the original etiological factor is obscured by consequent emotional and behavioral problems. Distortions of sensory data may produce disturbances of body image, and misperception of body boundaries and of external reality, and in turn lead to alienation and maladaptation of a degree resembling the functional psychoses.

The child with MBD is impaired in some measure in his basic developmental task of establishing a sense of competency. He is exposed to repeated frustrations and failures. He experiences considerable anxiety while having lowered ability to tolerate anxiety. Increased pathology of defenses is only to be expected.

Impulsivity and emotional lability are frequently observed in the MBD child. His ability to inhibit appears decreased. He cannot restrain himself from touching and handling objects; gratification cannot be delayed. New environments therefore are frequently overstimulating. Aggressive outbursts, sexual displays, and antisocial behavior are frequent: lying, stealing, fire-setting, destructiveness, verbal outbursts.

Difficulty in inhibiting leads to poor judgment and inadequate foresight; the press of impulse obscures consequences of behavior for the child. He is reckless.

Rapid changes of mood and affect occur. The child easily cries or becomes irritable, sweet, or angry. He may appear high-strung and overly-sensitive. Anxiety is likely to escalate to panic with slight provocation.

The *hypoactive* child by contrast is more likely to be even-tempered, cooperative, and less likely to react to failure and frustration in an obviously disturbed way. Some such children nevertheless have been recognized as belonging within the MBD diagnosis (9, 91).

Some children resort to denial of impairment and become grandiose in their efforts to avoid detection of their disability. They may seek to control with bossiness and demandingness while at the same time they are stubborn and unyielding; they tend to resist control by adults and so are hard to socialize, acculturate. Wender (91) describes them as "obstinate, stubborn, negativistic, bossy, disobedient, sassy, and imperious."

The child asserts his independence in efforts to mask his disability, yet his anxiety increases his dependency. This is the characteristic and painful dilemma for the MBD child and his parents. Its negotiation is the central task of the child's upbringing.

The MBD child may make friends easily in an outgoing mood, but lose them quickly as he becomes irascible, or as his deficits impress themselves upon his peers so that they reject him, or he withdraws to hide his depression or protect his self-esteem.

Wender (91) associates four qualities of dysphoria with the MBD child: anhedonia (diminished pleasure in things, activities, relationships), depression, low self-esteem, and anxiety. Long after maturation has overcome some of the lags, socialization has improved, and skills have developed around assets that serve to mask deficits, these dysphoric qualities may persist.

The MBD child grown into young adulthood may have trouble with those age-specific tasks that now confront him: vocational choice and development, and peer and sexual relationships. These difficulties are likely to evoke the major emotional symptoms of anxiety, depression, lowered self-esteem, and anhedonia, although in the absence of symptoms of motor, sensory, and attentional impairments that characterized his childhood. It is these states for which the MBD adult may seek psychotherapy. Then if his situation is not perceived, the pursuit of essential psychodynamic causality in masochism, or inward deflection of rage, for example, may well lead to failure of the therapeutic effort.

Perhaps more than any other syndrome of equivocal neurological basis, the possibility of MBD demands of the diagnostician an attitude of skepticism and a thorough scrutiny. All persons in whom MBD can be suspected who present themselves for psychotherapy deserve no less.

Diagnostic Methods

The many permutations of symptoms suggest the various professions involved in the complete diagnosis of MBD. On the full team would be teachers, pediatricians, neurologists, psychologists, psychiatrists, electroencephalographers, social workers, audiologists, and ophthalmologists. Assessments should be made of the patient's processing of sensory data—visual, auditory and haptic, the integration of sensory data, memory, symbolic operations, auditory language, reading, writing, and qualitative concepts, personality, motivation, emotional state, and peer and family relationships.

Systems Analysis as a Model

Mark (53) concludes that a systems-analysis procedure is the only rational approach to the complexity of diagnosis in patients suspected of MBD. The diagnostic examination must be specifically sensitive to the major systems of communication, learning, memory, localization, and perception, and it must be sensitive to disorders in these systems. Mark lists the variety of "organic learning disabilities": acalculias, dyslexias, aphasias, concept-formation disorders, conditioning disorders (agnosias and apraxias), disorders of resolution, disorders of discrimination, disorders of arousal, and disorders of habituation.

Diagnosis of a disorder within an area of potential disability must have "adequate resolution." By this, Mark apparently means that the diagnosis must be able to discriminate between levels of skill in the hierarchy of a particular channel of learning. Thus, a language test administered with instructions largely in pantomine will fail to identify either young children or adult stroke victims who have central language disorders of a major nature, such as the agnosias or aphasias.

Difficulties with standard test batteries are cited by Mark. Rote memory may *imitate* success in processing of new information of which the patient is fundamentally incapable; limitations upon time and testing conditions may result in the assignment of a failing score to skills which are less than optimal in a patient, but which nonetheless are useful and could be employed in teaching him to solve new problems as they arise in his life. Diagnostic examination, therefore, should always include limit-testing to determine how far up in a ranked list of systems in all channels a person *can be taught* to achieve success.

Hearing and vision are the major channels of learning. To view the complexity as simply as possible, one would have to remember that an auditory stimulus may require either a gross or fine motor response or a verbal motor response, that is, through speech. The auditory stimulus may be spoken language or it may be spoken language involving mathematics. This very primitive complication extends the line of required inquiries. Mark estimates that there are 132 potential learning disabilities, and that each of them may or may not be amenable to improvement through teaching interventions. Differential diagnosis, he maintains, must be pursued at least to the point which permits the differentiation of disorders which will respond to teaching interventions from those which are incapable of doing so.

Mark's systems-analysis approach identifies a total of 42,432 data points derived from a set of hierarchical systems. To operate most efficiently, his approach starts with the "most complex system" in a test channel. If success is encountered there, minimal-level success is presumed in all the underlying subskill data points. If failure is encountered, the system just below in level of complexity is tested. At the Johns Hopkins Center, Mark has developed a formal systems-analysis approach to both diagnosis and treatment, and has trained technicians in the use of a digital paper-and-pencil computer system. The technicians begin with the administration of standard tests in the standard fashion, and move to "channel-specific, system-specific, limit-testing techniques" when a "significantly deviant score" is obtained in the standard testing.

Such a complete systems-analysis approach is not now taught elsewhere by any professional discipline. But it is through professionals presently at work that the MBD victim seeks relief. The good diagnostician probably uses an informal and crude systems-analysis approach. His investigation covers as many processing systems as are feasible, and he interprets a child's response in terms of age-specificity. In addition he tries to integrate all of the varieties of data—sensory, motor, learning, attentional, maturational, behavioral, emotional, and social—into a statement of probable cause and a prediction of subsequent response to appropriate treatment.

An informal systems-analysis approach is essentially that of neuropsychodiagnosis (as set forth in the third section of this book). The major components of that approach as it applies to the MBD syndrome are presented here.

The History

The history searches the life experience of the individual for evidence of symptoms of MBD—in the maturational lags, behavioral abnormalities, educational impairments, and for any event of potential etiological significance during the mother's pregnancy, the birth, and the child's early development. With children, the parents and teachers may be recruited as informants. Teachers can furnish accurate data: they are less involved emotionally, their observations are current, and they have comparative norms in a classroom of children. The reports of parents suffer from memory attenuation, shame, denial, and overprotectiveness. They may recall only symptoms that were important to them, but which throw no light upon the probability of MBD. Physicians may have protected the parents from a candid discussion of a critical illness or of ominous sequelae. Nonetheless, the history should be pursued as carefully as possible with all informants.

Wender has a special enthusiasm for the history that is not shared by many neuropsychodiagnosticians. He states (91) "The history is the most important diagnostic tool . . ." This comes after an equally enthusiastic derogation of psychological testing and neurological evaluation, ". . . most extra-historical information is of limited value." His put-down is based in large part upon the inability of non-historical methods either to confirm or rule out the presence of the neurological. But Wender does not apply the same rigorous demands to the historical method.

Menkes *et al.* (51), who have demonstrated the diagnostic efficacy of extended neurological examination, found that for only one-third of 83 children, all of whom showed some neurological abnormality, could the history produce evidence suggestive of MBD.

A view of the value of the history more realistic than Wender's is provided by DiLeo (17). The history, he emphasizes, suggests and directs the attention of a good clinician in developing a diagnostic impression. The history in itself does not make the diagnosis, but is an essential part of the diagnostic process. In many cases, the cause of the dysfunction cannot be located, even though there may be a clearcut neurological deficit, for example in cerebral palsy. DiLeo is impressed by the frequency with which the history in impaired children reveals complicated pregnancy, bleeding from the womb, long or interrupted labor, difficult birth, instruments employed in birth, premature birth, underweight at birth, the use of resuscitation to start breathing in the child, visible damage to the head, convulsions, twitching, and restlessness. To these may be added signs of cyanosis and jaundice in the first ten days of life, or surgery for corrective or life saving reasons. Yet as DiLeo points out, many children with histories including potentially positive influences for pathology are normal in every way. The clinician must understand that the history may or may not support a diagnosis. Such is the lot of every diagnostic method. Any one if used alone can produce indefinite findings when equivocal neurological conditions are being diagnosed.

Diagnostic merit of the history is further attenuated when the patient is adult. Parents and teachers are usually not available, the patient's memory is usually unreliable for facts of his childhood, and he can offer only hearsay about events of his gestation and birth. Yet a thorough history of the adult patient should be pursued. With the adolescent and adult patient, the *entire* life history requires exploration, not only the events surrounding birth and development. Traumas, febrile episodes, poisonings, and prolonged anesthesias occur at all ages; the subtle harms called MBD may be incurred at any age.

The Neurological Examination

The value of the classical neurological approach in the diagnosis of MBD is extensively questioned (53). This skepticism is discussed in Chapter 12. However, there is evidence (35, 54) that the neurological procedure becomes more productive when extended beyond its classical assessments to include equivocal signs, finer signs, and age-specific assessment of sensory, motor, integrational, and cognitive functions.

In similar fashion, the value of the EEG here is questioned (78). Many children suspected of MBD produce normal EEG tracings yet function abnormally on psychological examination. These discrepancies are not necessarily contradictory. They may reflect differences in the type of brain function measured by each method and the relative sensitivity of each of the assessment methods.

Yet the neurological examination procedures cannot be overlooked in the presence of suspicion of brain dysfunction. Through its evaluation of sub-cortical levels of behavior, the neurological examination tests for the presence of brain conditions or progressive disease that may require immediate therapy. It may detect non-progressive diseases such as seizure disorders requiring regular continuous treatment. Further, the neurological examination may contribute to confidence that the behavioral, perceptual, and motor dysfunctions observed are not due to such conditions as parietal-lobe tumors, which tend to cause very similar behaviors.

Increasingly the emphasis in the neurological examination of children suspected of having MBD is upon "soft" signs. These are discussed at length in Chapter 1. Benton (4) observes that little "hard" data appears in the EEG patterns of dyslexic children. Here, too, innovative departure from traditional procedures show promise of improved diagnosis. An interesting innovation in the use of the EEG (87) suggests that continuous EEG recording made while a child is performing a task may show that disruption of learning is correlated with transient EEG abnormalities.

Psychological Testing

Psychological tests may make important contributions to the diagnosis and treatment of the MBD patient. They can identify and assess specific disabilities to which remedial efforts should be directed. They can identify and assess strengths and assets in the disabled person to be used in circumventing dysfunctions. And they provide a baseline reference for evaluating change through treatment and maturation.

The diagnostic power of the complete Wechsler Intelligence Scale for Children (WISC) in the assessment of MBD is stressed by Clements and Peters (10a). (The contribution of psychological tests to the diagnostic process is discussed in Chapter 11.) The value of this instrument rests in the pattern of subtest scores which a child-patient achieves, rather than in the total Verbal or Performance scores or the Full Scale I.Q. A minimal test battery generally includes the WISC, Bender Visual Motor Gestalt Test, Human Figure Drawings, and reading tests. Projective techniques, especially the Children's Apperception Tests, the Thematic Apperception Test with adults, and clinical interviewing all contribute to the psychological assessment of the emotional status of the patient. However, confidence should not be placed in the power of the classical battery to do more than arouse suspicion of MBD. The many symptom clusters possible in this syndrome require that the wider-ranging neuropsychological test battery be the next step in the psychological test investigation. These batteries differ in many respects from worker to worker (48, 68, 72). They all seek to assess a variety of brain-behavior relationships. Psychological testing is one of the three essential methods properly employed in the diagnosis of MBD, no one of which may be excluded without impairing confidence.

TREATMENT

The effective treatment of MBD proceeds from identification of specific deficits to efforts to correct them by means focused as specifically as possible on each deficit. Several principles guide the treatment program of the MBD child:

1) Multiple efforts are needed, encompassing all available types of intervention: remedial learning, perceptual training, environmental manipulation, counseling of parents, counseling and/or psychotherapy of the child, and medication.

2) Specific needs of the individual child must direct an individual plan based upon a detailed assessment of the child's specific impairments; MBD children cannot be treated as a homogeneous group.

3) Strengths can almost always be identified and developed as compensation for deficits.

4) Treatment approaches and plans should be reviewed periodically to exploit developmental progress in the child.

5) The complexity of the treatment plan and its multimodal nature require that one professional among the treatment team act as overseer and coordinator.

The treatment programs of 100 disadvantaged children with learning disabilities in The Learning Disability Clinic at Sinai Hospital in Baltimore reflect the range and variation that grow from careful, multidisciplinary diagnosis. The educational recommendations include: placement in a learning disability class, a special education class, or a special education school; a change of class within the regular school; continuing at present grade level beyond the usual progression time; tutoring by the staff of the clinic, the class teacher, or a teacher's aide; consultation with the regular class teacher by the diagnostic and remedial teacher. Medication was recommended for 36 children. Social recommendations for 67 children included family counseling; in six cases medical or psychiatric care was advised for other members of the family whose problems were affecting the child. Protective changes in living arrangements were made in seven cases, and 12 referrals to other social agencies were advised. Individual counseling was arranged for 32 children; five received group counseling. Speech therapy was recommended for 13 children, eye examinations for 19, while one child received a hearing aid.

Experience with such complicated treatment programs of MBD children increasingly stresses the importance of the coordinator. This central person should be in regular touch with the child in order to assess changes, alter plans, intervene in crises, and serve as communication center between child, parents, and other treatment personnel.

As the reports of various treatment methods—remedial and special training, environmental modification, medication, psychotherapy—are surveyed, the impression is strong that no central guiding core of theory has yet emerged about how interventions work to improve the functioning of the MBD child. But the impression is even stronger that the MBD child does respond to input of remedial efforts, that growth in any child is a function of "input x time x development," and that the MBD child needs more inputs, very carefully selected. While remedial workers differ in orientation and emphasis, they are alike in innovative and dedicated response to the special needs of special children.

Remedial Instruction and Special Training

The most effective treatment for MBD and for the emotional impact of that disability is the earliest possible correction of the patient's dysfunctions. When specific learning disabilities—impairment of reading, writing, and speech—are recognized, remedial learning programs often provide valuable adjuncts to any gains that will accrue through maturation. The remediation efforts, or deficit training, may be coupled with programs for developing alternate cerebral pathways. This is the functional reorganization described by Luria as reported in Chapter 17. Careful diagnosis is worthwhile if it leads to rehabilitative programs based upon assessment of each child's assets and liabilities. For the child to benefit from remedial instruction, the point at which such instruction is begun is of great importance. Developmental studies and theories suggest that normal progression is toward greater differentiation, accompanied by integration. This underscores the value of age norms in diagnosis, and indicates that work based upon learning should first establish the child's basic level of capability, and then advance upward from that stage. Too often, remedial efforts, because of a child's obvious brightness, begin at a level too advanced for some aspects of his functioning.

Remedial instruction should take into account the process by which the child learns a task and be based upon an analysis of the components of the task. An effort should also be made to determine how well a child learns through each of his sensory modalities and how well he integrates the data received from two or more sensory modalities (e.g., the integration of visual and auditory stimuli necessary to learn to read). The focus of instruction then will be less upon content of subject matter and more upon the processes involved.

Johnson (52) has suggested that a learning task be analyzed to determine:

1) whether the task is primarily intra- or inter-sensory;

2) the sensory modalities involved—vision and audition are most frequently employed in learning but the haptic modality must also be considered;

3) whether the task is primarily verbal or non-verbal;

4) the *level* of the task—does it involve primarily perception, memory, symbolization, or conceptualization?

5) the expected mode of response—is it to be pantomimed (pointing, gesturing, manipulating objects), or expressed in speech, or writing?

The purpose of the analysis is to enable the worker to facilitate the child's ability to comprehend and to respond; success contributes positive reinforcement to the learning experience.

Length or size of units of instruction is adjusted to the attention span of the individual child. Repetitive drill usually is avoided so as not to foster the emergence of perseverative behavior, although patient repetition of information is helpful with hyperkinetic children (80). Remedial instruction may focus upon a specific brain function: perception, categorization, peripheral motor manipulations, for example. Encouraging manual manipulation of parts may abet a child's ability to focus on the task at hand, as in learning numbers by using a number wheel.

Treatment of a perceptual and concept-formation disorder is described by Levi (40). Through persistent peripheral prodding, primarily auditory, an 11-year-old boy was taught over a year of special training to understand the notion of category, to acquire a set of categories, and to scan categories in order to select from them. Improvement after a year was significant and was accompanied by improvement in school grades. Initial introduction of concrete rather than abstract material within a structured program in which changes are introduced slowly and carefully is recommended with hyperkinetic children by Schrager et al. (80).

Operant conditioning is being used increasingly in remedial instruction (59). The child is started with a step already within his repertoire. Graded steps are introduced successively, producing gradual alteration of the child's set. Reinforcement at each step makes the next step possible.

A latency concept in responsiveness has been developed by Belmont (3) into a perceptual-motor training principle. The portion of the brain that is impaired responds more slowly to excitation than does the rest of the brain. Where a dysfunction is unilateral, stimulation may be applied to the impaired side before it is introduced to the intact side, or the stimulation to the impaired side may be intensified, while that to the intact side is kept at a lower degree.

Some remedial instructors prefer to work on the development and improvement of skill in attention as such, prior to the introduction of any particular content, since such skill or ability is prerequisite to learning anything.

The effectiveness of remedial instruction in general is questioned by Luria (44, 45). His studies suggest that intact systems should be encouraged to take over the tasks of impaired systems, and he demonstrates ingenious use of visual for auditory abilities and vice versa in developing competence when one has been impaired. Electronic and mechanical developments are being used in remediation programs to circumvent dysfunctions instead of seeking to correct them. The severely dyslexic person may learn by listening to tapes rather than by reading. Similarly, the dysgraphic deficit may be overcome by use of the typewriter rather than pen and paper. Dyscalculia may be minimized by use of the hand calculator. It is important that educators overcome any rigid adherence they may possess to traditional teaching methods or modes of expressions of learning.

Environmental Manipulation and Structuring

Alteration of the environment may facilitate the ability of the MBD child to learn. Distractibility and hyperkinesis may be decreased somewhat by removing distractions as much as is feasible and protecting the child from intrusions while under instruction. Some workers reason that the MBD child is more likely to experience sensory deprivation through too much stimulation than through too little. The quality of the sensory experience is improved when the MBD child's concentration can be sustained in time upon a single stimulus or task. Hence, reducing the number of objects in the room, removing clocks which audibly tick or visually move, disconnecting bells that may ring, removing the telephone, locking doors, facing the child to a screen, blank wall, or corner of a room are devices to facilitate ability to attend and reduce impulsive behavior.

These maneuvers are based upon a "stimulus overload" concept of hyperkinesis, a concept contested by Zentall (93). He argues that hyperkinesis is an effort to increase stimulation in all sensory modalities and so represents a state of stimulus deprivation. He attributes the paradoxically quieting effect of stimulant drugs to their provision of the needed stimulation, and the paradoxically hyperkinetic effect of barbiturates to their causing stimulus-deprivation.

Medication

Accumulated evidence now supports the judicious use of drugs to reduce hyperactivity and irritability, increase attention span and improve performance in tests of motor coordination (9, 10, 10a, 12, 13, 16, 65, 66, 91). The drugs used include the amphetamines, magnesium pemoline, and methylphenidate. Improvement is measured variously by teacher "before and after" ratings of classroom behavior, parents' ratings of home behavior, and performance on tests of attention, motor behavior, and cognitive functioning.

Wender (91) reports that about 25 percent of MBD children have a "specific therapeutic response" to amphetamines that is more than merely quieting. He found that these drugs promote psychological growth through decreasing activity and impulsivity and improving social behavior and cognition. A conference of the federal department of Health, Education and Welfare (69) estimated that among children for whom use of the drug is warranted—those who have not responded to educational and environmental-manipulative interventions—beneficial results are obtained in one-half to two-thirds of the cases. Wender's clinical experience was also that often a child who has not responded satisfactorily to amphetamines does so when the dosage is increased, and that many children need and are able to tolerate relatively large doses without evidence of side effects. He is convinced that the "hard" data makes medications the treatment of choice in hyperkinesis, while there is no comparable support for individual or family therapy (90). He likens the possibly lifelong need of some hyperkinetic persons for the stimulant drugs to that of those afflicted with epilepsy or diabetes who also require medications all their lives.

Satterfield (77), while finding support for the use of medications, also observes that hyperkinetic children differ in their response to them, so that they should not be used indiscriminantly with this group.

Indiscriminate use of stimulant medication has led to concerned scrutiny by professionals and government agencies. In part, the concern is caused by the wide use of "uppers" by adolescents as well as adults. A "speed" culture has developed around the abuse of these medications, with an increase in frequency of addiction and health impairments. In part also, the concern is provoked as a reaction to the strong advertising campaigns by drug companies, the casual, injudicious manner in which some physicians have prescribed the drugs, and the increasing number of school children who are given these drugs (36) as a quick and easy solution to the problems caused by their hyperactivity, without concomitant interventions (76). Walker (88), a physician, contends that society is cavalier about drugging the hyperactive child. He cites treatable causes of hyperkinesis seldom explored by physicians: improper oxygenation, glucose intolerance, inadequate levels of calcium. He notes that methylphenidate is an hallucinogen more potent than LSD, and that its long-term effects have not been established.

Considerable criticism of the research design reporting favorable outcomes from use of drugs has emerged. Especially the use of teachers ratings (56, 71) can be seriously subjective in that they may reflect a teacher's preference for quiet rather than overly-active children, overshadowing a concern for improved learning. Studies are criticized for being short-term (19), and for being unduly casual about possible side effects. DiMascio (18), a severe critic of medication research with children, notes that few studies have been made on large numbers of subjects, dosages have not been systematically explored, adverse reactions have not been well documented, and little is known about the effects of the drugs on the maturing organism. Further he charges that important patient-factors are often ignored, including severity and chronicity of the behavior, the age, maturational level, and sex of the child, and diagnostic homogenity in study populations.

In a middle-ground stance, some workers seek to maximize benefits from drugs, while minimizing the hazards. They emphasize extensive diagnosis to assure the applicability of the drug to the specific child, careful monitoring and management once treatment is begun, and objective data rather than anecdotal reports (38). Others stress a more realistic view of the potential benefits of the medications, as providing some stabilization, but not a cure (41), or that in their use the goal be limited to improving a child's behavior enough to elicit a more favorable response from his teacher (71).

The controversy continues. Psychotherapists, teachers, counselors, remedial personnel, parents, all need some basic facts about the drugs. The principal side effects possible are irritability, appetite loss, weight loss, growth stunting, blunting of affect, insomnia, headaches, elevated blood pressure and heartrate, and a potential for abuse of the drug. The *Physician's Desk Reference* (63) provides details on the effects to be expected with a drug prescribed, effects to which all concerned should be alerted.

Certainly the physician, usually a pediatrician or child psychiatrist, who prescribes a stimulant medication for a child should have experience in using the medication.

A careful diagnostic process should precede drug treatment and should consider the full range of possible physical, psychological, environmental, familial and social causalities of the child's symptoms, including especially those in which stimulant medication is not indicated or might be contraindicated.

Stimulant medication should not be presented as the sole or primary treatment intervention, but as a potentially useful adjunct to other important measures. The physician should be aware of the availability of special education, environmental manipulation, and psychotherapy and counseling for both parents and child. The physician should also prepare both parents and child in a realistic way for the drug regimen, setting realizable goals. Any inflated expectations should be curbed with realistic information about what has been achieved by others in behavioral changes and improved attention, learning, and social behavior. They should be told that the child's response to the medication is impossible to predict, that only a trial can establish this. The parents should know that the hyperactivity must be mitigated before other treatments can begin to take hold, although if the child is already depressed, withdrawn, or learning-disabled the drugs alone are not sufficient therapy.

The possibility of side effects should be discussed with the parents, with care taken that the physician's bias does not influence the parents' elections. It is their right and responsibility to decide which is most undesirable, the child's present behavior or the possible side effects. They need information to guide their choice. This should include the fact that the possible side effects are not necessarily probable in each case, and that any side effects dissipate quickly when the medication is discontinued. The risk of evoking ideas and fears stimulated by suggestibility in some parents is outweighed by their right and responsibility to make a determination for their dependent child while knowing the essential facts about the medicine proposed. They should be informed that, counter to the general belief that hyperactivity improves at puberty, there is a group of children who retain the symptoms into young adulthood and may require continued medication.

Parents should be made responsible for administering the medication, regardless of the age of the child. The child should be told the compelling reason: that evaluation of the effectiveness of the medicine depends upon certainty that it is being taken exactly as prescribed. As the child becomes adolescent this requirement is likely to collide with the youth's need for autonomy and individuation. The physician's ability to establish a working alliance with his teenage patient reduces the possibility of careless or rebellious mistakes.

Exactly established dosage is critical to success of this drug regimen, and here the physician's experience should govern. Effective dosage does not necessarily correlate with the age, height, and weight of the child. Individual manipulation of timing of administration as well as dosage is a major factor in maximum response. Some children do best with alternating periods on and off the medication. Others do well with week-ends as medication-free periods. Still others may do well when the drug is suspended over the summer (although arrangements for resumption if necessary should be made in advance, at camp, for example.) Generally, a "titrating" approach to each child's dosage level is advisable, beginning with a low level, and slowly increasing the dose to the point where either benefits or side effects appear. Each MBD child is best considered to have an idiosyncratic responses to any drug, so that he is carefully tested for the drug and dosage most suited for him. Withdrawal from medication should also be titrated, to avoid any rebound or "crashing" response. Feighner and Feighner (20) find that it usually takes four to six weeks to establish the maintenance dose for a child, with doses adjusted at one to two week intervals. Ideally, according to Laufer (39), the effects of a single morning dose should last through the homework period without a rebound at pre-bedtime. Some children may need an afternoon dose as well. In some cases doses required to calm the child are so high that learning is inhibited (82). In such cases it may be advisable to schedule instruction three to four hours after the drug is administered, when the blood-serum level is decreasing. The desired level is one where the child is in control of his activity and attention, neither incapable of control nor excessively controlled.

Obviously, this desired response is not always attained, but it should be the physician's goal. The effort to attain it requires a dedication of time and interest. The hyperactive child and his parents should not undertake a stimulant-medication regimen without continuous monitoring accepted by the physician. Monitoring includes seeing the child regularly and frequently until maintenance dosage is reached, and at longer intervals thereafter to check response and side effects. The program should incorporate periods of suspension of the drug during the school year, to test the continued need for it. Regular serological and other laboratory tests are essential as safeguards. Periodic objective testing of cognitive functions, attention, and motor skills should be scheduled, along with regular and frequent occasions for feedback from parents and teachers. Here again, objective rather than anecdotal data are essential if sound decisions are to be made. Monitoring is an indispensable feature of a medication regimen in order to adjust dosage to both short-term and long-term changes in responses. Where medications may be administered over a period of years, the need for continuous check is obvious.

A conference on the use of the stimulant drugs with behaviorally disturbed children, convened under the auspices of the Department of Health, Education and Welfare (HEW) in January, 1971, cited the value of drugs in those children who did not respond to remedial instruction, operant conditioning, family counseling, or environmental control (69). Stimulant drugs, methylphenidate and amphetamines, known for several decades now to have a paradoxically quieting effect upon many hyperactive children, may be utilized in the well-planned treatment of the MBD child.

My experience is that, cautiously used after careful diagnosis and with the continuous medical safeguards essential to any long-term drug use, these medications are a reasonable part of the therapy with MBD, and sometimes indispensable.

Behavior Modification

Procedures developed to modify behavior are used increasingly in the non-medical treatment of hyperkinesis. The critical basis for these applications varies according to one's view of hyperkinesis. Krop (37), for example, specifies three general classes of behavior as most antagonistic to being able to focus attention: locomotive behavior, communicative or quasi-communicative activity interfering with a task assignment, and distraction.

Operant conditioning is perhaps the most frequently used behavioral method to combat hyperkinesis. Prout (65) reviewed the literature describing these methods and cites studies of operant conditioning to shape new behaviors and extinguish undesirable ones, using token systems and systematic programming of adult social reinforcement. Almost all behavioral intervention involves the parents as surrogate therapists. They become co-therapists with the primary therapist, extending the training time and continuing it in the home.

Recently biofeedback procedures of many kinds have come into prominence. Braud and his colleagues (7, 8) used electromyographic (EMG) biofeedback successfully to reduce hyperactivity in a six-and-one-half-year-old boy in 11 sessions. Some deterioration (erratic behavior) observed seven months after the last training session was attributed to a lack of reinforcement by parents and teachers. This observation was coordinated by Lupin et al. (43) with the notion that the hyperkinetic child is also emotionally tense, and that tension can produce the very symptoms identified as hyperkinesis. Since EMG is a laboratory procedure, they used a relaxation technique that permits treatment at home under the direction of the parents.

Behavioral methods *a priori* appear promising in the treatment of hyperkinesis. Their application may reduce or eliminate the need for stimulant medication; they flag success for the child with tasks (arranged by levels of difficulty as to not overwhelm him), and they often permit parents and child to become involved in a mutual effort that can counteract the divisive impact of hyperkinesis upon a family. While as Prout (65) concludes from his survey, the literature is "dominated by case studies," hence small populations, the techniques appear capable of providing access to some hyperactive children otherwise reachable only when medicated or the many who react to medication with side effects that vitiate seeming accessibility.

Parents in the Treatment Process

Parenting, muses Frostig (23), is the most difficult of the professions. For the parents of a victim of MBD, the difficulty is increased enormously. The demands on them multiply: providing direct aid to their child in both educational and emotional ways; participating in social, political, and communication activities that foster the welfare of all MBD children including their own; and examining their own reactions and those of their other children to their MBD child in order to try to change these reactions when they are pathological. Parents who make these efforts can help their child directly and indirectly. To do this they in return require much help.

Parents may struggle against recognizing and accepting their child's condition or the family pathology that aggravates that condition. They may denigrate any school achievement, actively or by implication, and by identification the child is discouraged from making efforts to overcome disabilities. Severe intra-family psychopathology may block or minimize the motivation of the vulnerable child and keep him from the very experiences he needs.

The quality of parental management influences the self-esteem of the MBD child. Good parent management supplies both support and controls. Poor managers are rejecting, neglectful, overprotective, or overindulgent (42).

The symptomatic behaviors of their MBD child may distress parents to the point where their reactions are harmful to the child. Intel-lectually oriented parents or those who stress goals may not be able to tolerate their child's low academic achievement and react in a way that seriously attacks the child's self-esteem. Parents may become upset by the ceaseless repetition of a question by a child, or, in a youth, the expression of a wish for an activity such as automobile driving that seems dangerous, or a developing sexuality, or the child's or adolescent's negativism, anger or inaccessible depression. Rejecting sentiments and actions of the child's siblings may further burden the parents.

Differences between father and mother in understanding of the child's limitations and reactions may lead to differences in expecta-tions, and anxiety, guilt, and anger in relationship to the child. Con-ceivably a child could benefit from these differences if one parent's understanding and patience offset the other's anger and disappoint-ment. But the child may well be made more bewildered and more conflicted, more uncertain that he himself is acceptable, where such differences are marked.

Parents need help in understanding realistically and in tolerating what they reasonably may and may not expect from the child now and later. They benefit from knowing that while intensive positive invest-ment in their child may not produce immediate significant gains, their efforts are likely to forestall the development of negative acting-out and delinquent behaviors, leave the child accessible to future rap-prochement, and increase his response to normal developmental changes.

When the parents are accessible, either family therapy or individual psychotherapy for them may be indicated. Videotape feedback is used by Feighner and Feighner (20) to record the parent-child interaction. The tape is edited to shorten and focus the family interaction, and played back. Parents are then counseled around desirable changes.

Some hyperkinetic children, Ney (57) reports, are "conditioned" into their behavior by the depression of their parents, usually a single mother. The child seeks the attention of the depressed parent that he gets only when he is hyperactive. Ney utilizes a behavioral approach to treat the mother, not the child. She is taught to recognize and respond to the child's efforts to please her, and to reinforce him when he is quiet. Presumably, other factors may contribute to her depres-sion, factors that might require, for example, financial aid, psycho-therapy, or a different personal situation.

Most constructive, of course, is mobilization of the parents as treatment resources for their child. They may serve as co-therapists in behavior modification programs for hyperkinesis under the direction of the professional therapist, or as adjunct remediation teachers under the direction of the education specialists, helping with homework according to the plan prescribed for their child. They can apply the principles of special education to many life tasks within the home and to the child's social life, outside the provinces of the several specialists, the teachers, pediatricians, optometrists, speech pathologists, or other professionals. Effective discipline is kept short, firm, non-negotiable.

Structuring the child's activities is urged by Gordon (31) to give the child a sense of the future, combat feelings of disorganization, and encourage a sense of stable environment. He advises that parents not fear robbing their child of his independence as some may fear. Children with MBD have trouble making and keeping friends, and benefit from having their social experiences outside the classroom organized for them. Indicated as sources are associations with other MBD children, special camps, clubs, and play groups, or selected activities with normal children in which the MBD child's dysfunctions are not differentiating and isolating to too great an extent. Also advised is carefully teaching the child social skills and leisure activities with gradual step-level methods: shopping, eating at restaurants, using public transportation to move about, sports, theatre, museums, cooking, and sewing.

Attention is now directed more to modifying the parent-child relationship and somewhat less to specific behaviors of the child, observes Cantwell (8a). He cites the work of G. Patterson of the University of Oregon where parents are offered courses over ten to twelve weeks that require mastery of certain successive levels of parenting, one after another. This customary behaviorist method is modified by the use of two group leaders: one concentrates on psychodynamic, interpersonal issues, the other on parent training.

Obviously such programs can be demanding. They can overburden parents facing other heavy demands and responsibilities such as other children, elderly parents, illnesses, job problems or personal emotional problems. Such programs are a strain upon any parent, even without these additional problems. Parents of the MBD child need the support of information and advice about diagnostic and treatment resources in their community. Ideally, pediatricians, day-care and nursery-school personnel, and first-grade teachers would be trained for the early detection of the vulnerable child and equipped to move parents and child toward these resources. But such informed sensitivity and knowledge of helping resources are not always locally available. The federal government has in recent years undertaken a nationwide effort to help parents find services needed for a handicapped child. The Office of Education of the U.S. Department of Health, Education and Welfare initiated television and radio advertising for its newsletter, *Closer Look* (available from Box 1492, Washington, D. C. 20013) that keeps parents informed about resources, laws, and developments.

Many national or state membership organizations are available to parents. Among these are: Association for Children and Adults with Learning Disabilities (ACLD), 5225 Grace Street, Pittsburgh, Penn. 15236; Orton Society, 80 Fifth Avenue, New York, N. Y. 10011; California Association for Neurologically Handicapped Children (CANHC), P.O. Box 4088, Los Angeles, California, 90051; New York Association for Brain Injured Children, and the Association for Children with Learning Disabilities, P.O. Box 710, Grand Central Station, New York, N. Y. 10017.

The groups publish newsletters, list resources for special education, list and review new books, print special articles, advise on sources of financial aid through state governments, inform of new laws and interpret them, issue directories of special services, sell informative pamphlets and books, hold meetings, conferences, and workshops. The parents of the MBD child are well advised to join one or more of these organizations.

Exploration may turn up local groups of parents working together to develop and improve services to their MBD children, to obtain and modify state and federal laws, to provide advocacy for the whole MBD population and for individual children, and to provide support and understanding for each other. And where these groups do not exist, parents can make no better contribution to the treatment of their child than to find other parents with MBD children and form such a group. An example of the kind of help available in a group is that needed by parents of hyperkinetic children who must make decisions about whether to initiate medication or continue it should side-effects appear. In a parents' group they are likely to find members whose experience can be helpful in rounding out the information available to the parent who must make the decision.

Such groups provide peer associations for MBD children. They can extend horizons that otherwise might be drastically limited, increase the child's sense of mobility, and do much to restore self-esteem lowered by social isolation, ostracism, and feelings of being unique and bizarre.

Parents, we see, must be intimately involved in the treatment of their MBD child. Their contributions may come from their role as teacher, co-therapist, social and political activist, or as patient in individual or group psychotherapy in an effort to modify their own pathological interaction with their child.

Psychotherapy

The pragmatic therapist emphasizing the use of drugs—Wender (91) is a most outspoken advocate of this approach—asserts that psychotherapy is without real value in the treatment of MBD. The often quick and dramatic effects of the stimulant medications in reducing hyperactivity appear to have lured many professionals to believe that psychotherapy is not needed in these disorders. Some moderate this position by limiting their interdiction to the use of psychotherapy with younger children while accepting it for adolescents and adults in whom maladaptive behavior is long-established (74) or hyperactivity has lessened and the patient is more accessible to psychotherapy (65). Even where hyperkinesis is viewed as a disorder of heterogeneous etiology, as by Ney (57), psychotherapy is regarded applicable only to those with parents whose depression is believed to promote hyperactivity in the child trying to get their attention, or to those children who must be removed from chaotic homes while the parents also undergo psychotherapy. Gardner, who has written extensively and positively on psychotherapy in MBD (24, 25, 26, 27, 28), nonetheless ranks psychotherapy at the bottom of his list of therapeutic modalities, giving first position to medication. Overall, the view of moderate workers is that psychotherapy in the younger child is at best adjunctive, but that it moves to a position of primary importance for MBD adolescents and adults.

The positions of both the moderates and the more rigidly pragmatic seem to me to neglect the psychodynamics of MBD whatever its manifestations, the inevitable interaction of organic deficits with the psychological and emotional aspects of personality development. Focus is confined to the most prominent symptoms: motor dysfunction, learning disability, hyperactivity. If recognition is given to psychological concomitants it is usually with the secure belief that these will disappear if the "primary symptom" is treated. Probably their neglect of the psychological is partially justified by the relative ineffectiveness in MBD of traditional psychoanalytic work that emphasizes uncovering of unconscious material, resolution of conflicts, and the unfolding of a transference neurosis. But their neglect goes beyond a down-grading of the ability of classic psychoanalysis to help the MBD child. Their position ignores the specific psychodynamics of MBD in the developing child, dynamics that produce symptoms similar to those in the child whose disturbance is on emotional basis solely, but have a much different evolution and require a different kind of psycho-therapeutic intervention. Delaying psychotherapy until adolescence often allows psychopathology to encroach upon extensive aspects of the personality and to ossify defenses, denial particularly, so that the MBD adolescent and young adult become more difficult to treat as well as likely to reject treatment altogether. Psychotherapy is important in the treatment of children, adolescents, and adults with MBD. With children, its importance cannot be overstressed; their relative flexibility makes them amenable to its help, and receiving help in their youth strengthens them for their years ahead.

A condition of "object inconsistency" in the MBD child has been related by Schechter (79) to the physical disruption of perception. The perceptual dysfunction, he postulates, prevents formation and mainte-nance of a "constant immutable internal image" of stimuli. These children do not relate to parents and other people in a usual way be-cause their mental image of these others is variable and inconsistent. A significant result of this process is the increasing development of superego lacunae that underwrite impulsivity, cruelty, disobedience, anti-social behaviors. These behaviors then cause people to treat the MBD victim inconsistently, adding to the disruption of the child's control of affects, thoughts, and impulses. The MBD child's inner language doesn't make sense, doesn't "add-up," Schecter believes, with damage to all his interactions with others and to his self-image.

Many professionals regard a negative self-image to be the major psychological damage in MBD. Palombo (61) observes that in children with perceptual deficits from birth the impaired area is never experi-enced, resulting in an incomplete, distorted body image. Seldom di-rectly understood by the child, the deficit distorts his perception of reality and of social relations particularly. Anxiety levels are high. This may arise from feelings of physical vulnerability and appear in psychosomatic complaints. Separation anxiety is also prominent, often expressing a fear of abandonment by the parents, who are perceived as disappointed in the child's attainment. The anxiety may find ex-pression in frank phobias (school, dark, insects, among others), or in more disguised forms of stubborn school refusal or sleep and appetite disturbances. Tics are also frequent motor evidences of the child's tension and anxiety.

Protracted eneuresis is also reported (79). Gardner (28) views this as a sign of either failure to progress in maturation (fixation) or regression. Other signs of these developmental abnormalities are clowning, clinging, avoiding age-appropriate responsibilities about dressing and home chores, preferring to associate with younger children, or a boy's choice of play with less aggressive, less competitive girls.

Anxiety evokes anger as the MBD child feels ceaselessly pressured to confront anxiety-arousing and frustrating situations. With poor inner controls, the child is likely to react impulsively and inappropriately, further impairing his relations with others and intensifying his feelings of humiliation. Already burdened with inhibitions to growth because his conflict-free energy for learning is inadequate, the child's impulsiveness creates additional blocks to learning (63).

Negativism is another possible impediment to growth and learning in the MBD child. The negativistic child avoids opportunities out of fear of failure or relationships out of distrust of others, expecting rejection and denigration. Negativism sometimes expresses rejection of the values, judgments, requests, demands, and expectations of elders, a rejection arising from the MBD sufferer's belief that he has been deceived in a significant way by his parents.

Little wonder that depression is so often observed in the MBD victim. Battered by low self-esteem, an extremely negative self-image, by a persistent sense of loss of respect and love, by the inward deflection of anger, he often reveals increased depression as he moves into adolescence and adulthood. Depression and anxiety without impulsivity and hyperactivity are remarked as major symptoms in adults with MBD.

At all ages, the MBD person is likely to encounter crises: severe depression, intensified withdrawal, acting out of aggression and antisocial behavior, episodes of increased hyperactivity, refusals to cooperate or to try. These may reflect internal or external pressures: a continued series of failures, a transitional lifestage confrontation, a reaction from a parent, teacher, or employer that is sadistic or chaos-producing.

Adolescence, a well-recognized crisis in normal development, is painfully intensified in the MBD child. The major tasks of adolescence carry double burdens of anxiety and conflict for him. Many dysfunctions do not become manifest in the MBD child until the age-appropriate demands in a certain new level of development are reached. So the MBD child's social aversiveness may have been only a minor problem before, but in adolescence the internal and external pressures for dating and sexual exploration are so enormous, persistent and ubiquitous that they can not be glossed over.

Denial is a major defense in MBD: there are no deficits, there is no problem, so there is no need for worry. Where concern is grudgingly admitted, the need for long, hard work to overcome the problem may be denied. Faith, in these cases, is placed in the magic cure: new glasses, eye exercises, macro-molecular diets, in tomorrow. Denial is often fostered by the parents who themselves need to believe all is well. It may be fostered also by teachers or pediatricians who assure that the problem is transient, that the child will "grow out of it." The child reacts to the parental denial or secretiveness with distrust and negativism, with feelings of being deceived, or the fear that his disability is too terrible to talk about. Rationalization often emerges when the child, forced into recognition of a problem, denies its cause and cure: "I could do it if I wanted to, but I don't want to." Wanting to and trying not only mean long, hard work with gratification delayed but also threaten failure and disappointment.

The MBD child may resort to displacement. Anger over failures or rejection at school may be brought home, to be wreaked against parents or siblings with whom he feels more secure. Or it may be acted out in anti-social behavior such as destructiveness or stealing. Or the child who maintains a seemingly involved or cheerful facade at school may sink into a slough of depression as soon as he is home.

Escape into daydreaming is frequently observed. With severely damaged self-esteem the child regresses into the overcompensation of grandiosity. But not all daydreams are grandiose. The MBD child lost in thought may be searching for an understanding of his difficulties.

Obsessional qualities develop in some MBD children, particularly those who recognize their problems and seek to control them rather than correct them through remediation or reduce their impact through psychotherapy. To protect against the anxiety of cognitive failure these children may become so concerned with every possible alternative that they are unable to progress to a solution. Or the premium placed on control of affects and impulses can become so great in the child whose superego lapses are ego-alien that classical compulsive and obsessional behaviors emerge.

Another major defense associated with MBD is aversive withdrawal.

Seeking to avoid a repetition of failure and shame, the child withdraws from confrontation with tasks or associations with peers. Allowed to progress, this defense is likely to result in a typically schizoid pattern in adolescence and adulthood.

The immediate and principal task in the psychotherapy of the MBD patient is the establishment of a positive transference. Always there is therapeutic benefit for the child who feels understood by at least one adult while most other important adults in his world find him irascible and incomprehensible. Such a kernel of understanding may prevent an abysmal pessimism and keep alive a thread of hope for change or realistic improvement.

Equally important, the positive transference enables the therapist to evolve a "working" or "therapeutic alliance" (81) with the child that is simply not strong enough to tolerate it. Accordingly, negative trans-confront himself and undertake the arduous task of remediation. To establish such an alliance, the therapist presents himself as an understanding person who wants to help and has ways of helping not usually available through parents, teachers, or physicians. Accessibility of the therapist at times of special need or crisis is especially important for a patient with MBD.

A transference neurosis in the classical psychoanalytic sense should not be allowed to develop; the ego of the MBD patient of any age is simply not strong enough to tolerate it. Accordingly, negative transference features are brought immediately to the surface and discussed. With some MBD patients the positive transference is difficult to achieve and to maintain. "Object inconsistency" (79) may be so great that the child is unable to attach to anyone, parent, teacher, or therapist, in the usual way, to see the therapist consistently as a helping person. Perseverance is needed in such cases. The therapist must make himself available after being rejected by the patient should he want to return to therapy. Careful attention to negative countertransference is also required of the therapist.

The therapist must also avoid viewing the dynamics of the MBD patient in traditional ways applicable with non-organic patients. Traditional psychoanalysis often sees failure in a patient as a fear of success or a wish to fail. Obviously, these may exist in an MBD patient, but more likely to operate is a profound pessimism that any success is possible even when reasonable goals are set. Or the therapist's wish, like that of the parent, to see the child succeed may lead him to expect more than the child can do at the time.

The interpretation is a major technique in the psychotherapy of MBD, moderated by two important conditions: 1) Many MBD patients suffer a complicated set of dynamics that involves anger, anxiety, masochism, negativism, acting-out, and avoidance. When these are developed in the context of impulsivity and emotional lability, the direct interpretation is likely to weaken impulse control further; 2) Some MBD patients are dysphasic, with difficulties in comprehending or expressing symbolic or abstract concepts, and may find interpretations bewildering. The therapist may adopt a step-by-step approach to interpretations, so finely focused as to be almost titrated. He can put out a partial interpretation and test the patient's reactions before proceeding further, or wait for the patient to make the leap himself. At a point where some insight into self appears, the emphasis may be shifted to a didactic one helping the patient to become aware of the many clues that guide social exchange so that he can respond to them. The insight need not be pursued to its ultimate end, and indeed should not be pursued. Insight, at whatever depth, must be linked with practical, achievable steps for correction or control. Otherwise it is likely to overwhelm the patient, or seem only to repeat what he has been told often by parents, peers, and teachers, and further convince him of his unworthiness.

Some MBD patients are dysphasic, a situation usually determinable early in the diagnostic interviewing and testing. (See Chapters 10 and 11.) For them, simple concrete terms should be used and repeated as necessary. Verbal illustrations that evoke visual images or very simple auditory ones are helpful, the crowing cock, for example, or the player who hits a home run and basks in the roar of the crowd. Visual thematic material may be used as well, such as a comic-strip character who tells a story or makes a point without using words. Sessions may be tape recorded and important ones replayed by the patient alone or with the therapist.

A primary goal with many MBD patients is to break through denial in order to improve reality perception and testing. Care is necessary to test the patient's ego strength, and his willingness and ability to tolerate this process without undue intensification of anxiety and threat of regression, both of which induce resistance. Where the parents foster the denial, work with them is a necessary prelude or accompaniment to the patient's therapy. This may require some sessions with the parents alone, and then together with the child, or the parents may require individual treatment by other therapists.

Improved reality perception and testing here center on the patient's dysfunctions, their possible causes, and, above all, the many steps the patient can take to circumvent or remedy his dysfunction, and the assets he has available to help him in the effort. Chess (9) recommends giving the child a clear concept of his handicap in age-specific terms. The child is helped to recognize situations in which he competes on an equal basis with peers and those in which he can participate only partially. For some children there may be activities that are best avoided all together.

Improved reality perception and testing help the patient become more accessible and responsive to the help that is available. It removes the dysfunction itself as a rationalization for not trying, and opens the door to therapeutic work with other pathological symptoms. The aversive, withdrawn patient can be helped to see his retreat as an effort to escape repeated humiliation in failure which need not be generalized to avoid also those many situations in which he could be successful and enhance his self-esteem.

Increasing tolerance for anxiety can be obtained, again through step-by-step procedures. Especially helpful is developing an understanding of the "vestibule" anxiety experienced by most people on the threshold of a new situation which relents on entry into the situation.

Most important is the fact that improved reality perception and testing allow the patient to use such didactic interventions in his psychotherapy as he becomes willing to seek improvement through effort. The therapist can promote more impulse control by teaching a "stop-think-wait" guideline. This is most effective when a similar program is being taught simultaneously in remedial work. There the benefits of the "pause on the threshold" can be made immediately and concretely evident to the child, who can be helped in this way to differentiate between "feelings" and "actions" and ultimately to control the actions. In similar fashion the parent can be trained in stimulus avoidance and tolerance.

As the patient's ego strengths improve through the combination of remediation and improved reality testing, more attention to the role of affect-experience becomes possible within the framework of the therapeutic alliance. Ventilation and catharsis can be encouraged with less danger of acting-out. Self-assertiveness can be fostered as self-esteem improves. Fantasies can be explored at greater depth, to expose feelings of bizarre uniqueness or of insurmountable inadequacy and inferiority.

Naturally, psychotherapy seldom proceeds in the smooth linear fashion that may seem implied here. Crises, as noted earlier, are to be expected as the patient is asked to give up his essentially phobic defenses. Often before reality testing can be improved, the MBD patient may have to use the support of the therapeutic alliance in order to allow himself to give way to a depression he has been warding-off for years, to grieve for himself, to live out affectively the despair he feels, to expose the wounds to his self-esteem, to ventilate the anger he has flagellated himself with, or to allow to erupt the paroxysms of anxiety he has struggled to contain.

Working through in MBD is a long process. A termination of psychotherapy is less likely than a discontinuance (61), or a series of discontinuances, brought about perhaps by summer vacations and camp stays, or by the preferability of a real-life experience such as a job over psychotherapy at the time. Or psychotherapy may become episodic as the youth completes high school and goes away to college, to return for brief therapeutic contacts on holidays.

Gardner has specialized in the psychotherapy of children; his somewhat redundant publications (24, 25, 26, 27) emphasize the techniques he developed or adapted to evoke and combat fantasy in these children in order to develop controls. He seeks to strengthen the superego rather than develop insight by providing the child with a model he anticipates the child will emulate, and with directive guidance he expects the child will follow. His sessions with children are structured rather than open-ended. He reasons that the MBD child needs organization, that open-endedness evokes anxiety and counteracts the development of controls. As much as possible he has a parent (usually the mother, presumably) sit in on sessions, maintaining that confidentiality is irrelevant to the pre-adolescent, a presumption that many therapists would challenge. His rationale is that the arrangement avoids the we-they schism, and guides the parent in handling the child. He tape records and videotapes sessions for reinforcement through feedback, and to utilize intersensory stimulation through which some MBD children best learn. He also uses intersensory stimulation in the pictures, toys, and games he has developed and adapted.

In his "Mutual Storytelling Technique," Gardner (26) seeks to communicate with the child at the child's level. A story is evoked from the child; its dynamic content is assessed for pathology. The therapist, using the characters in the child's story, tells his own story but with a "healthier" resolution. He has no reticence about letting the child know how he reacts to his behavior or to mirroring the child's behavior in games and play. On hearing that a child patient has pulled the leg off a frog, Gardner rolled upon the floor screaming with pain, emphasizing that such acts hurt and kill. Many therapists will feel that this technique might leave the child with feelings of shame, fears of being bizarre, and more deeply humiliated than before. They would mitigate such demonstrations with an ego-sharing technique, telling the child that they too, have had these kinds of feelings and pointing out better ways to deal with situations that arouse the feelings. Pointing out a different way of coping is precisely how Gardner attempts to derive therapeutic progress from the emotional confrontations he arouses, showing that there is a better way, while believing that his technique helps the child learn about himself and how to make himself better. He emphasizes a "work ethic," and also seeks to help the child express feelings more appropriately, and to be able to do so before mounting tension touches off acting-out behaviors.

Schechter (79) tends to work more closely within the insight-interpretation model of psychotherapy. In one-to-one psychotherapy with an MBD child or adolescent he explains the unconscious processes that lead to anxiety and interprets impulsivity as a search for punishment, hence for control from the outside. He teaches better internal control by encouraging a stop-look-listen technique before acting. Deficits are logically and clearly explained. Families are drawn in when their conflicts contribute to or aggravate pathology in the child.

Both approaches demonstrate the incorporation of didactic methods and the principles of special education with those of traditional insight therapy.

For the adult patient with MBD for whom psychotherapy is considered, the clinical picture is different. Hyperactivity is less frequent, but frequently impulsivity is equally pronounced, and depression is more likely to be frank. Need for concrete evidence of acceptance and affection often leads to sexual adventures in which the patient is likely to be exploited and rejected. The dependence-independence conflict has not been resolved, parents are weary and perplexed, the patient is demanding, yet easily infuriated and hurt if parents "pry" or "overprotect." Jealousy of siblings who have been successful in education, work, and marriage is prominent.

The successful psychotherapeutic approaches to adults known to have MBD are similar to those practiced with children. They benefit from a stable relationship and understanding; they require careful instruction in the consequences of behavior and control of impulse. Often with young girls, it is advisable to insist upon contraceptive instruction and practice at once, even before initiating impulse-control therapy. The sagging self-esteem of adults with MBD requires repair and bolstering; most often they benefit from achieving success in paid employment, with emphasis upon physical activity and social exchange, if they prossess the specific verbal or spatial skill required, as determined by diagnosis. Vocational counseling, placement services, and vocational training programs developed by rehabilitation specialists may be precisely appropriate for them. Many benefit from being supported in establishing their own living quarters away from parents and siblings. Care, however, must be exercised to establish that the patient is sufficiently mature to tolerate the separation. One cannot indiscriminantly pursue the usual psychotherapeutic goal of contributing to individuation through separate living, since the adult patient with MBD may appear more mature than is the fact.

Group therapy with adolescent and young-adult MBD patients is often fruitful, especially if the probability of the minimal brain dysfunction is made explicit and is accepted by the patient as a likely determinant of some of his other difficulties. In such groups goal-directed discussion fruitfully centers around an exploration of the following subjects: differences from other people because of the minimal brain dysfunction itself; that these differences may arise because their emotional experiences have been and are different from most people; the possibility that some aspects of their characteristically intense emotional responses may be of specific value to the person with an organic impairment; and that they are not helpless to modify or restrain their emotional expressions and acts, whatever may be the cause of their feelings and behavior. Gordon (31) favors a group-therapy focus on solving practical problems of living rather than on feelings. One might add, however, that feelings are problems of living and that in many instances practical ways to deal with them can be found.

As we have seen, the involvement of parents and/or family in the psychotherapy of the MBD patient is frequently necessary to promote the growth of the patient, whether child, adolescent or adult. Family therapy may be feasible if patient and parents can tolerate the stress. A colleague of the patient's therapist should be enlisted either for family therapy or for work with the parents, since the adolescent or adult MBD victim with emotional problems severe enough to need psychotherapy requires the exclusive and undiluted support and the unbreachable confidentiality of his own therapist.

For the adolescent resistant to psychotherapy, placement in a special school where all the students are coping with emotional and/or learning problems is often helpful. The presence of fellows helps to "reach" the unwilling person and turn him toward the helping potential in psychotherapy and remediation. This outcome is especially likely if the school offers remediation facilities without pressure to use them, but many of the students do so, and are in individual or group psychotherapy, and talk about their experiences in discussion sessions both formal and informal.

Finally, bibliotherapy can be useful with the resistant adolescent or adult. There are biographical accounts of children burdened with MBD handicaps in learning who became successful adults (10), newspaper accounts of famous people who are said to have had MBD (47), or simple direct exposition of what MBD is and what can be done about it (2).

PROGNOSIS

Conflicting conclusions are drawn from the available research on the prognosis of MBD.

Wender in 1972 (91) concluded from an extensive survey of the literature that the disorder could be an early precursor of serious psychiatric disturbances in adolescence and adulthood, including infantile and impulsive character disorders, sociopathy, and schizophrenia. Later (90) he modified this to the slightly more reassuring conclusion that a "fraction" of MBD children do not outgrow their disorder with age.

His conclusions find some support. Katz, et al. (34) caution that a group of MBD children remain significantly symptomatic beyond puberty and that their parents should be made aware of this possibility. Safer and Allen (75) in a study of the age at which medications were introduced (before 8 or 13 and over) found that while aggressivity decreased, hyperactivity and inattentiveness remained problems.

More optimistic prospects are offered by many pediatricians who assure parents that their child will probably outgrow his disturbing symptoms or by reminders, usually in newspaper accounts (47), that many accomplished and famous persons were identified as manifesting learning disabilities. Louise Clarke (10) has published a moving, more realistic account of the painful, often discouraging progress of her dyslexic son from being diagnosed as mentally retarded by an outstanding private school to a Ph.D. in mathematics.

What is the truth about prognosis in MBD? Does a single prognosis exist? Can it be gleaned from among conflicting research outcomes and professional attitudes? A review of some of the major research picks out a torturous path through a maze of research design that never seems adequate to the complexity of the problem.

Favorable modification over time of some MBD symptoms in the syndrome—presumably as the result of maturation and learning—has been demonstrated by Menkes, *et al.* (51). Fourteen individuals were located who had been patients a mean of 24 years earlier at a children's psychiatric clinic. All 14 originally had I.Q.'s of over 70 and had shown hyperactivity, short attention span, and neurological abnormalities such as visual motor dysfunctions, poor coordination, and impaired speech. Eleven of the 14 were available for complete re-examination, and information was obtained about the others. Two of the subjects were neurologically normal, definite abnormalities were found in eight, and abnormalities were suspected in one. Hyperactivity was present in three subjects aged 22-23, but had disappeared in the others between the ages of 8 and 21. Eight subjects were self-supporting; two were mentally retarded and were supported by their families; four were institutionalized as psychotic. The I.Q. emerged as a major prognostic factor: all but one of the eight self-supporting subjects had scored an I.Q. above 90 during their initial contact with the child clinic. Low I.Q. and established brain damage were found to be prognostically unfavorable. An I.Q. above 90 when first seen appeared significantly associated with the status of self-supporting adult.

The findings in this now classic study of 1967 are what is most generally reported, rather than sweepingly optimistic or pessimistic conclusions: some symptoms in some children improve.

A two-year prospective follow-up (70) of 72 hyperkinetic boys (mean age = 10.2 years) and a matched control group found 65 percent still on medication. Classroom and home behaviors had improved, but no improvement was noted in academic achievement, peer status, or depressive symptoms.

A longer follow-up (two to five years) is reported by Mendelson *et al.* (50). Fifty-five percent of 83 patients formerly treated for hyperkinesis were judged to be improved, while 35 percent were the same or worse. The basis of findings was interviews with their mothers that inquired into behavioral symptoms, school records, family history, police record, and the mother's opinion of the effectiveness of the treatment. This study highlights the design defects inherent in research in this complex problem. No uniform criteria for selection are reported; 92 percent of the children had been on drug treatment but neither the length of such therapy nor its congruence with psychotherapy is reported, except for the notation that most of the children still attending psychiatric clinics were those who had improved on drugs. The authors make a point that merits emphasis: low self-esteem and defeatism remain serious aspects of the MBD child's problems and have a crucial effect on prognosis.

A 12-year follow-up of drug-treated hyperactive subjects by Laufer (39) sought to answer many more questions than are usually incorporated in these efforts. One hundred former patients who had been treated for hyperkinesis with amphetamines or methylphenidate were asked to complete a wide-ranging questionnaire; 66 responded. At the time of treatment their age ranged from 3 to 18 (M = 8 years); at follow-up the range was 15 to 26 (M = 19.8).

Twenty-four took medication for less than six months, 31 for six months to five years. Of 57 reporting, 10 were continuing on medications (anti-convulsants, minor and major tranquilizers). None were taking stimulants or anti-depressants. Two had had an overdose experience; 96.5 percent had not. Five acknowledged using pot or LSD, 91.2 percent had not. No addictions were reported. Three of 56 had used "speed," Benzedrine, or Dexedrine; 94.6 percent had not. Four of 50 were excessive drinkers; 92 percent were not.

Hyperactivity had stopped in 27 respondents. Most of these (61 percent) reported cessation of this symptom between the twelfth and sixteenth year. Seventeen percent acknowledged that they were reckless drivers; 82 percent said no. Sixteen (30 percent) had had trouble with the police, but none were jailed.

Five of 56 responding to the question indicated that they had had a psychiatric hospitalization; only one person had been hospitalized more than once. None of the 56 respondents had made a suicide attempt. Twenty (35 percent) had psychiatric treatment after the period of medication, most of these during adolescence. Five (9 percent) were in psychiatric treatment at the time of follow-up.

Of the 37 respondents 19 years of age or older, 18 were employed, 14 were in universities, one in graduate school. Of ten who had been or were in military service, one had a bad conduct record.

Most of the respondents (no figures given) were described as pleasant, meticulous, having friends. The minority were moody, loners, subject to outbursts of violence and feelings of persecution.

In an extensive survey of the literature on prognosis in dyslexia Benton (4) describes these major typical patterns: 1) the majority improve slowly over time; the dyslexic child grown into early adulthood is a slow reader and a poor speller, with great difficulty learning foreign languages. 2) Some make a "remarkable spurt" over a year or two, usually about 13 or 14, with modest improvement thereafter. 3) A small number make only a slight improvement over time and in adulthood are seriously disabled readers.

No single general prognostic statement about children with MBD, hyperkinesis or dyslexia can be made. A number of major factors make for this ambiguity and should be understood by all concerned with these children.

The symptoms and behavioral sequelae of MBD, as in frank brain damage, are most diverse. They range from little or almost none through neurotic disorders of various degrees of severity to serious disruptions of social, intellectual, and personal functioning (86).

Not all symptoms disappear, either with time and/or with treatment. Spontaneous remission is not to be expected in most cases. Indeed no data tell which symptoms are most likely to remit with time or with which treatment. Degrees of remission cannot be predicted.

Patterns of change are as diverse as those of symptomatology. Some general trends are observed, as in Benton's study of dyslexia (4) which identified patterns of improvement described as slow-steady, sudden spurts and very little change. Another general trend appears in most studies of hyperkinesis, where medications suppress hyperactivity and improve attention in some children without assured concomitant improvement in academic achievement, peer relations, and self-esteem in these same children. Individual reports (10, 47) verify the possibility of development of outstanding capabilities in the adulthood of MBD children. In some children, dysfunction may become obvious only as increasing age brings types of tasks or levels of difficulty or abstraction not required of them earlier or that they had been able to escape. For them it is as if "chronological age" catches up with the limit of their "mental age" in a specific function, revealing the deficit fully for the first time. Gender appears to influence prognosis to some extent, an effect that may result in some measure from a difference in social reaction to the appearance of the same behavioral characteristics in boys and girls. The forces of social interaction and their potential influence on outcome are not sufficiently understood.

The effects of various treatment interventions either singly or in combination are obscure. Most studies of the treatment of hyperkinesis, for example, focus on the use of medication. We know little about the comparative outcomes of medication alone, medication in various combinations with psychotherapy, behavioral modification, environmental manipulation, special education, vocational training, teacher counseling, and parent counseling or psychotherapy. We are equally uninformed about the effects of length and timing of treatment, although consensus favors the earliest possible diagnosis and intervention.

There is little doubt that prognosis is improved by inputs of concern, time, and determination. Benton makes this point in his survey of dyslexia (4). And Clarke attributes the successful outcome for her son to his family's *refusal* to accept the verdict of the educational system, his opportunity to get the kind of schooling that proved effective, and to his indominable personality (10).

The basic personality and temperament of the child are major factors in prognosis if these can be distinguished and separated from pathological behavioral characteristics. Parental input and interaction are as enormously significant in the personality formation of the MBD child as in all children. Consistency, acceptance, and support will allow favorable temperament to emerge; denial, rejection and excessive demands will erode the constructive aspects of temperament.

Findings from work with children with more clearly established brain damage contribute to reasonable hypotheses concerning prognosis with MBD children. Temperamental organization was found by Birch *et al.* (6) to be the single behavioral feature with the greatest prognostic value. A favorable organization is manifest in ease of adaptability, ready modifiability, predominantly positive mood, and predictable rhythmicity. The arhythmic child, negative in mood, markedly unadaptive, with a low response threshold and short attention span has a less favorable prognosis.

Chess (9) followed three brain-damaged patients from early infancy into school years. Each child's developmental course was differently influenced by brain damage in early life. In each case, Chess concluded that temperamental organization of the child was prognostic of the developmental course and that the interaction between the child's temperament and the environment was the crucial factor in the outcome. These conclusions were reaffirmed in another follow-up ten years later (86).

These hypotheses stress implicitly that the MBD child born and reared in social, cultural, and economic disadvantage must carry an enormously negative burden. There seems no escape from this conclusion or from society's responsibility. If many MBD children of the middle and upper social classes slip unnoticed and neglected between the chairs to emerge later with major personality, emotional, and behavioral pathologies, one can only imagine with horror the numbers of such children in socially deprived groups.

Discernible changes are slow in the MBD child. But developmental and maturational changes when they bring improvement are greatly enhanced by all the fostering conditions cited. Everyone concerned with and for the MBD child must be aware that the prognosis can improve only with multiple services to meet the multiple needs of the MBD child over a long period of time. "Wait and see" without action is tantamount to denial and neglect.

CASE ILLUSTRATIONS

The four young people whose cases follow were all seen by the author when they were between the ages of 15 and 19. Because my clinical experience with this syndrome has been with adolescents and young adults, I do not describe younger children here. However, the problems that children and their families encounter are all here: learning difficulties, behavioral problems, damage to self-esteem, depression, and aversive behavior. Many of the symptoms described are common to both children and adolescents, as are the etiological possibilities considered.

CASE 1. *An under-achieving girl of 15, of intact family with supportive parents, is seen for psychological assessment for admission to a therapeutic school, where her parents hope she will be able to catch up academically.*

In making arrangements, her father communicated that T. is considered an under-achiever, that she is very anxious to succeed, but seems unable to, that she does not read well, her written material is poor, and her concentration span is short. She has had tutoring but it doesn't seem to meet her needs. He described home life as very happy, and said T. had not manifested any need for psychotherapy.

T. is a charming girl, rather tall, athletic looking, slim. Her love for clothes is immediately apparent; her choices seem appropriate to her age. There is a slightly soporific quality to her eyes; their surface placidity is in contrast to the signs of tension manifested as her legs move in fairly constant jerking activity.

T.'s highest intellectual level appeared to be in the ability to conceptualize (with a prorated I.Q. of 106 in Similarities) and in the awareness of logical thematic relationships (prorated I.Q. of 107 in Picture Arrangement). In light of this High-Average level, she manifested considerable deficits in a number of areas. Information was relatively poor at a prorated I.Q. of 81; the sun, she said, sets in the East, and oil floats on water because it is greasy, and there are 100 pounds in a ton. She tended to offer a response when it seemed quite clear that she did not know the answer. She seldom said "I don't know," but almost always offered an answer as if to discharge her responsibility to the questioner. Asked where turpentine comes from, she said, "You want me to tell you the mixture? It is alcohol and benzine." Comprehension is somewhat better at a prorated I.Q. of 94. Her performance here was inconsistent and extended over the entire range of the subtest, so that she obtained partial answers on difficult items while failing others of lesser difficulty.

In Arithmetic she reached her level at a prorated I.Q. of 81, and thereafter offered incorrect responses in a voice of authority. When unaware of the correct response, she often answered by association or position, so that the similarity for mountain and lake is "sometimes a mountain is next to a lake." Liberty and justice "are the pursuit of happiness." This tendency emerged vividly on the Vocabulary subtest in which she achieved a prorated I.Q. of 87. She had difficulty achieving and maintaining cognitive focus, so that her answers often tended to be peripheral; one felt that she was close to the content but not able to bring it sharply into consciousness. She defined "affliction" as "bad between." Asked for an explanation she said, "I don't know, I just felt like saying that." No personal association to the idea could be obtained from her.

Difficulty in maintaining concentration is demonstrated in the Digit Span subtest, in which she achieved a prorated I.Q. of 81. She was able to recall seven digits forward, but when the difficulty was increased with the requirement for reciting them backwards, her capacity was two digits. She cut off contact quickly when her capacity level was reached and she was over her depth; she then appeared to resort to mechanisms of denial to mask feelings of inadequacy or failure. This capacity was highlighted on the Object Assembly subtest. On the Auto, she omitted parts four and five which she pushed to one side, and said, "I am finished." Given an opportunity to change her mind, she did not do so.

The nature and extent of the intellectual deficits here are manifested in a comparison of average scale scores for various areas of functioning: the Verbal area produces an average scale score of 8, attention-memory 8, and perceptual-analytic 6. These, viewed in contrast to the 11 she obtained on ability to conceptualize, indicate clearly that T.'s tools for cognitive focus, concentration, and perception were not commensurate with her basic ability to conceptualize. These deficits most probably were the cause for her academic difficulties.

Her susceptibility to failure when the level of difficulty passed a particular point was clearly manifested in the Bender Visual Motor Gestalt Test. Under conditions of reproduction from memory she made a triangle out of a diamond, and it penetrated the circle, instead of abutting it. When she drew the figures from direct copy this error was not repeated; however she tended to collide the figures, and lost the Gestalt when directional forces of the lines took her eyes in different directions, as if she could not order a perception in the face of conflict. This impression was further reinforced by evidences of figure and ground reversal on the Block Design. There was a basis for conflict of lateral dominance: she was right-handed and footed, but left-eyed.

The Rorschach suggested an undercurrent of anger checked by massive denial. There also was some evidence for a tendency toward passive-aggressivity, with a display of mild negativism. Affect appeared to be held strongly in check; she limited her responsiveness, but even so a mildly critical attitude emerged.

The Thematic Apperception Test highlighted the denial. This extended particularly to sexuality; she called the frankly sexual card (13MF) a "dirty picture." There was evidence of a strong wish for achievement and success, and a feeling that this could be accomplished only by magic. This suggested that she was giving-up on the possibility of achieving success by the usual methods. Important to note was the suggestion of a depressive tendency, also buried under denial. Thus, she portrayed a man on the depressive card (3BM) who killed himself because of problems; this was said in a rather sweet, light voice. Immediately following this story, for the card portraying an idyllic country scene, she portrayed the end of the world. It was a sad picture to her because there were no people in it. A theme emerged here that appeared clearly in her responses to projective queries: she was fearful of being deserted and deceived, and clung to the family which is portrayed as happy, close, and loving, for protection against her anxieties about the external world.

Much of her fantasy life was at a relatively simple level, not regressive in the sense of psychotic, but childish: things, objects, clothes, money, having one's wishes.

Feelings of incompleteness, inadequacy, and depression were indicated by her figure drawings. She drew a female first; the figure lacked hands and feet; she wore a long gown; her features were not complete; her eyes were small, almost closed, and there were no ears, as if to shut out awareness and perception of certain realities. Her handwriting was clear and well formed; she made spelling errors in some rather simple words ("here" was spelled "hear").

Her responses to projective queries in content were at the childish level of acquisition and gratification. She remembered dresses she wore when she was a little girl; she dreamed of achieving wishes: going to Disneyland, getting a Jaguar car, having a party.

T. appeared to be of High-Average basic intellectual capacity, she had suffered impairments in the verbal, attention-memory, and visuomotor areas. There was no evidence of psychosis or of undue anxiety to explain these impairments. The suggestion left open as an alternative was that these impairments were caused by a cerebral dysfunction. On interview there was no indication of any events in her life of neurological import. The possibility of a birth genesis remained open for consideration. On the emotional side, she was somewhat regressive. She was interested in sports, and apparently was competent; she liked clothes and with her great figure this had reward for her. She had studied many musical instruments, but was unable to achieve mastery in any of them. Depression and moderate passive-aggressivity were noted. One suspected that her close and loving family had sought to deny their perception of impairments in T.'s development, and strove to bulwark her by demonstrations of love and acceptance. T. appeared to fearful of having to leave the protection of this family, and so was caught in a developmental bind. An expert mixture of support, protection, and gentle push to autonomy was needed by her. Individual and/or family therapy appeared indicated.

CASE 2. *Learning difficulties and a suicidal attempt in an 19-year-old man with a history strongly suggestive of a neurological etiology.*

P. was born in Puerto Rico. While pregnant with him (during the fifth month) his mother fell from a horse and because of uterine bleeding was confined to bed for one month. P. weighed 12 pounds at birth, and forceps were used to deliver him. His mother left him in Puerto Rico under the care of another woman when he was one and one-half years old; he rejoined her in the United States when he was eight and she had remarried. He is described as a slow developer, walking and talking at a slower rate than most children. When he was four or five he fell down some stairs, hit his head against stone, and was hospitalized in an unconscious state. No other information is obtainable from the mother or the patient about this event, except that he now has a bump on the back of his head as a result. He has had a great deal of trouble learning. Public and private schools and a tutoring experience have all resulted in failure. Depressed about his future, under pressure from his mother to take a job, he took a quantity of tranquilizers that had been prescribed for his mother and was admitted to a psychiatric hospital. P. cannot read Spanish or English. The hospital referred P. to a vocational rehabilitation agency for vocational training under protected circumstances. His diagnosis was Minimal Cerebral Dysfunction.

The psychiatrist associated with the agency reported:

"P. is a pleasant young man who appears considerably limited in his capacity to communicate with me. There were few things that he was able to remember, not even the month that he was at St. J.'s Hospital, though it happened as recently as two months ago. There was confusion about current items of information but he was able easily to recall his own home address and things that happened in the past. When asked the Mayor of the city, he said Mayor Nixon. He became quite confused when attempting to recall even four digits, but improved on this after the first attempt. There was a good deal of forgetting and denial. There was no gross thinking or affective disorder apparent. He is a friendly young man who describes everybody in his building as being his friend, and I would believe this. He has drifted from one menial job to another and he seems interested in a program that would help him to improve his working skills.

"Diagnostically, my impression is mild mental retardation. I would also seriously consider minimal brain damage, but I feel that has to be more carefully evaluated through psychological testing. A neurological would be indicated to evaluate this "accident" that he described at the age of four or five; at present the trauma to his head is covered up by a hairpiece. I do not feel that this young man is presently suicidal and I would recommend that he be brought into the program. It is necessary to include his mother in casework that may follow."

My report as the agency's psychologist follows:

"Psychodiagnostic testing at the hospital in October of this year, attributes to P. a Full Scale I.Q. of 86, Verbal I.Q. of 77 and a Performance I.Q. of 101.

"P. is a nice looking, gentle-appearing lad, who has barely managed to grow a moustache. He has a baby-like quality about his skin and manner, heightened by large limpid brown eyes. There is a speech difficulty, a slur, a problem in forming words that may be peripheral, rather than central to the nervous system.

"The overall intelligence figures today (Verbal I.Q. 73, Performance I.Q. 101, Full Scale I.Q. 84) correspond closely to those obtained in the past. However, there is a remarkable spread in prorated I.Q.'s from a high of 140 on the assembly of familiar objects to a low of 49 on Digit Span. This is a remarkable difference of 15 scale points (16 and one) and 91 I.Q. points. His next highest function after the assembly of familiar objects is Comprehension at a prorated I.Q. of 103. Here there is a clear indication of ability to understand and exercise judgment at a higher level, so that he is able to understand and state why it is that a deaf person cannot speak and what is the purpose of licenses for marriages. In abstract conceptualization, he operates at a mental defective level with a prorated I.Q. of 67 in Similarities. He gives evidence of an anomic difficulty, when for a dog and a lion he says that they both eat meat. I asked if he knows the word for meat-eating animals, and he says, "I can recognize the word, when I see it, but I can't say it." There is an even more significant problem with attention and memory in modalities of auditory stimulus and oral expression, so that he can retain only three digits forward and two in reverse, for a prorated I.Q. of 49, his lowest function in the entire test.

"Finger dexterities indicate that attention-memory in the peripheral motor-control area is moderate with a prorated I.Q. of 81. He is able to increase speed slightly on retesting. He achieves the same prorated I.Q. of 81 in the recognition of essential details. His perceptual-analytic ability in the assembly of familiar objects is absolutely superb. He achieves the highest score possible for both accuracy and speed on two of the items and the next highest on the other two items.

"The Bender Visual Motor Gestalt Test administered under conditions of reproduction of memory and direct copy confirms his good perceptual-analytic abilities, and indicates that his psychomotor problems have to do with peripheral motor control, and that this is a relatively moderate impairment contrasted with this attention-memory one and the one for abstract thinking. This holds true on the Heimburger-Reitan Test as well. We must add here that he has a great spelling difficulty; he can not spell square or triangle or cross, though he can name these figures. He can repeat and explain the meaning of the expression, "He shouted the warning," but he cannot write it. It is clear that his self-esteem is tremendously damaged in relationship to these impairments.

"The central emotional feature is his anxiety about his ability to achieve and succeed, to comprehend and master. This makes him phobic of a large number of situations and contributes to the development of a schizoid personality. He withdraws out of shame and is unwilling to express a wish for personal relationship, focusing first on the wish for achievement, seeing this as the key to improved social relationships. There is depression rising out of tremendous damage to his self-esteem as a result of his impairments.

"I agree with the referring diagnosis of minimal cerebral dysfunction evidenced in major impairment of abstract thinking, concentration, and memory, particularly in the auditory area which affects his ability to read, to write, to retain information.

"It is possible that his impairments will prevent him from using his superb psychomotor and perceptual-analytic ability in the machine shop trade because of the mathematics involved. If this is the case, then it is possible that some kind of assembly work of a fairly complicated nature, that does not require computations, could be his goal. It would be worth exploring whether anti-convulsive medication would improve his attention span."

CASE 3. *Learning difficulties are encountered by a girl on entering high school. A history of high fevers accompanied by disorganized behavior is paralleled by a constructional apraxia.*

M., 16, is referred for psychodiagnostic assessment by the special school to which she is applying for admission. She has been in psychotherapy for several months. M.'s mother said that M. had been cutting school with resulting failures. M. states that she had done very well through the ninth grade, making mid-80 grades, and that she ran into trouble very soon after starting high school. She felt that she was the dumbest student in the class, and became increasingly ashamed of going to school and exposing what she took to be her limited ability. So she would leave school and sit in a luncheonette across the street. She acknowledges feelings of depression and much damage to her self-esteem which she hides under the pretense of carefreeness.

M. says, and her mother confirms, that she has been subject to very high fevers, and that a year-and-a-half ago, close to the end of her first semester of high school, she contracted a strep throat, nephritis developed, and M. was sick for about two weeks. In the course of this, she ran a fever as high as 104, of unspecified duration. The mother says that M.'s behavior very rapidly becomes disorganized and erratic as a fever starts and that this has long been a warning sign to the mother.

M. is a medium-sized girl of mature body but with youthful facial characteristics that are heightened by slack lips and jaw and small teeth. Her nails and cuticles are bitten. She experiences what best might be described as eruptions of anxiety, and bursts of intense feeling of other kinds. There is a slight speech slur and an apparent slight convergent strabismus. She is open, responsive, cooperative, humorous, and hard working.

M.'s basic capacity for abstract thinking and conceptualization appears to be in the Above-Average range, with a prorated I.Q. of 111 in Similarities. Information, Arithmetic, and Vocabulary are all fairly close to that level. Comprehension is a bit down at a prorated I.Q. of 99. Several features of M.'s verbal performance are noteworthy. She tends to fail easier items after having passed more difficult ones, suggesting an inherent capacity for higher-level functioning than she is currently manifesting. She often has enormous difficulty zeroing in the concept she requires. This might be identified as a problem of cognitive focusing. Thus, she knows that the Vatican is a religious center, ponders whether it is Catholic or Protestant and chooses the wrong answer. She knows that the similarity between the eye and the ear is that are both sense organs but she is unable to make that specific. She says, "They are both important to help you and are needed to see and to hear." She is very conscious of this difficulty with cognitive focusing. At times it seemed to be aphasic but this could not be clearly delineated. In attempting to define the word "terminate," which she was unable to do, she pounded her thighs and exclaimed, "I hate it when I know it and I can't think." It was characteristic of her performance that she seldom named specifically the core item in a task: when asked to identify missing parts in pictures she would always call the missing part "the thing" instead of identifying it as a nose, for example.

Her best function appears to be in attention and memory tasks when the memory function is limited to recent material; for example, her highest performance is finger dexterities at a prorated I.Q. of 128. This specialization is seen in a comparison of averaged scale scores. In the verbal areas these averaged to 10, in attention-memory functions they are 12, in perceptual-analytic functions they dropped to an 8. In the latter area she achieves a prorated I.Q. of 82 in both Block Design and Object Assembly. There is indication here of a moderate perceptual-analytic impairment relative to her verbal and attention-memory capabilities.

Dual administration of the Bender Visual Motor Gestalt Test shows that a slight constructional apraxia is heightened when memory is introduced to make the task more difficult. On the Heimburger-Reitan Test there is a slight difficulty in naming objects, but with perseverance she was able to arrive at the correct answer.

Her difficulties with cognitive focusing lengthen the time necessary for all tasks, so that she took well over the usual length of time for completion of almost everything. On several tasks she failed to arrive at a correct answer within the time allowed, but when allowed to go beyond the standard time permitted she succeeded, although she could not be credited. The impression is very strong, therefore, that her performance level improves in quality as she is allowed more time for cognitive focusing.

The Rorschach protocol heightens the impression of more capability than the overall intelligence test scores would indicate. Her mode of perceiving is qualitatively well above the average level.

There is indication on the Rorschach that she is pent-up emotionally, that the exercise of denial has resulted in accumulation of feelings, that she experiences intense affect as eruptive, possibly explosive, and goes to great length to curtail and contain it.

A support for this latter statement is obtained by the evidence of highly developed altruism in M. She prides herself in sacrificing for other people, and says that it reaches such a degree that it is a fault, involving self-sacrifice on her part. She cannot stand anger or hatred either in herself directed toward other people or in other people directed toward her; she must move to change these feelings in herself or in some way placate the other person.

There is a clear undercurrent of depression in M. Her T.A.T. depicts themes of neglect as a child, of parents seemingly not interested in spending time with or in teaching her. She communicates a sense of sadness and loneliness, of absence of support. The idea of suicide appears to occur at a deeply unconscious level. Consciously, M. denies that it ever occurs to her. However, she admits that she masquerades in order to hide depression, and there is, as indicated, evidence of denial of feelings of sexuality and aggressivity. She expresses unconsciously a great need for help, and portrays herself as calling for help in a covert fashion by upset and disturbed behavior. There is indication of phobic qualities which were more intense years ago but traces of which still can be observed. Also, there is a regressive tendency which highlights the appeal for help, her need for support, her dependency.

There are indications that M. felt anxious, even deserted as a child. Her mother returned to work by the time M. was five when she was entered in public school, perhaps even before that. M. recalls in the early years of school that there was always a baby-sitter to whom she went after school. It is also possible that the mother and father had difficulties between themselves for some years, which may have contributed to anxiety in M. and the development of phobic responses. This is not verifiable from the data at hand; it is suggested. She gives indication of strong rivalry with her mother of an oedipal nature, and at the termination of testing today she manifested some anxiety about her father. She greeted her mother in the waiting room by asking, in an apprehensive manner, "Where is daddy," to which the mother replied, "What do you mean, 'where is daddy?' " There is indication that the relationship between M. and her mother was quite stormy when she was very young, of an argumentative, possibly sadomasochistic nature.

No data suggestive of a neurological impairment are obtained on interviewing.

The data obtained are difficult to interpret in the causal sense. Actual data relating to her school history would help in the diagnostic process. If indeed her performance was much higher before high school than it is now, it is possible that she simply may have reached the limit of her intellectual capability, and as a result encountered situations damaging to her self-esteem. Or, it is possible that the high fever associated with her strep throat and nephritis resulted in minimal brain dysfunction responsible for her difficulty in cognitive focusing particularly, and for the perceptual-analytic impairment noted. On the other hand, if her school work always demonstrated difficulties similar to those she is now having, the case for or against a febrile causation is neither proved nor disproved because of the history of high fevers in the past.

In any case, M. shows evidences of a higher-level capability than she is presently functioning at; her present functioning level is in the High-Average area verbally. Central to her learning difficulties appears to be impairment of cognitive focusing. It might be helpful to obtain achievement levels in reading rate and comprehension in both timed and untimed trials.

Regressive, dependent features appear to be related to disruptive influences in her upbringing. These combine with her present difficulties to produce depression and damage to her self-esteem.

CASE 4. *A difficult diagnostic problem: pronounced deficits in a bright, highly verbal lad with a history of psychiatric hospitalizations because of assaultive behavior.*

A. is referred for vocational training by a community psychotherapy agency. Now 17, he has had three psychiatric hospitalizations since his twelfth year for assaultive behavior to younger boys. An adopted child, he often fought with his younger "foster" sister, also an adopted child. He was adopted when he was four months, and told this by his adoptive parents when he was four years. His development is said to have been rapid, he talked at an early age, was articulate by three. He read by four, but was extremely sensitive.

Rapidly escalating anger has always been a characteristic. He started school when five, and it is reported that he either was reading or fighting while there. Because of his temper he was taken to a therapist when he was eight; at twelve he was hospitalized because he threatened to kill a boy; on another occasion he thrust his hand through a pane of glass during an argument. He has had four hospitalizations in all. His relationship with his adoptive parents has improved during the last year, and he has been able to live with them, but not to attend school. The treatment plan is that he now work, live at home, and continue psychotherapy. His hospital records bear the diagnosis Anxiety Neurosis.

At this point of referral, I saw A. as the psychologist of the vocational agency; my report follows:

"A. immediately makes his high-level verbal ability apparent. He is testwise; he says he has had the test a million times. He achieves a perfect score on the Information subtest for a prorated I.Q. of 157+. However, ability to conceptualize is considerably below this level at a prorated I.Q. of 117; the suggestion is either that he has over-compensated to anxiety by the acquisition of knowledge beyond his general conceptual ability, or that there is actually some impairment of abstract functioning, with a tendency toward the concrete. I believe the latter is more likely to be the case. Comprehension is rather good at a prorated I.Q. of 129, but considering his high-level Information functioning, this too seems somewhat impaired. Traces of an impulse disorder are evident. If he discovered a fire in the movies, his response is 'Don't yell, just walk out; if you yell, you will cause a panic.' His superb verbal ability is evident in responses such as "Do you want me to give you the whole sociology of the child-labor laws?" He prefaces his perfect explanation of the meaning of 'Shallow brooks are noisy with 'If you were to anthropomorphize. . . .'

"He has marked impairment of ability to attend to and retain recent materials. This is true when the material is both auditory and visual, but especially so when the material is visual. Thus he achieves a prorated I.Q. of only 105 in ability to retain digits forward and backwards, but drops to a low of 69 on finger dexterities; he can improve his speed slightly to achieve a prorated I.Q. of 75 on this test. Recognition of essential details is superb at a prorated I.Q. of 128. Assembly of familiar objects at a prorated I.Q. of 95 suggests that there is a perceptual-analytic deficit as well.

"The 30-point superiority of the Verbal I.Q. (128) over Performance I.Q. (98) is strongly suggestive of a cerebral dysfunction. This impression is reinforced by the marked deficit of attention-memory, where he achieves an average scale score of 8 in contrast to the average scale score of 17 in the Verbal area. A perceptual-analytic difficulty is observed, but it is not as great as the attention-memory one, with an average scale score of 12.

"Dual administration of the Bender Visual Motor Gestalt Test suggests that whatever perceptual-analytic deficit is present is of moderate degree. He reveals a great deal of impatience, as he does in fact throughout all of the tests. His tension mounts rapidly when concentration is requested from him. This may be a major problem in vocational training, so that giving him freedom to move about may be important.

"There is some indication of poor graphomotor control, but it is difficult to tell whether this is inherent or a reflection of his impatience. He has a rather good gross motor control; in going through the motions of kicking at a ball he showed remarkable coordination and ability.

"The Rorschach data call attention to a perceptual-analytic deficit in a more dramatic way than either the Bender or the WAIS does. Despite his verbal ability and above-average conceptual ability he finds it very hard to organize visual material into larger Gestalts, so that most of his responses are relatively fragmented. In addition, there appears to be considerable withdrawal from object relations, and with a great deal of denial of pressing drives of sexuality and aggressivity.

"Denial is indeed a major defense; it appears rather dramatically in all of his responses to projective queries. He finds it difficult to name good and bad features about himself, and tries to transcend personal, ego-oriented drives, so that given three wishes, he becomes quite altruistic.

"On interviewing for evidences of possible neurological implication, he reports severe headaches in, as he says, 'the frontal lobes.' He reports ringing in his ears on occasion.

"My favored diagnosis would be cerebral dysfunctions of minimal nature, possibly as a result of the birth process in the absence of other etiological events, which created difficulties with concentration and in the perceptual-analytic area. This set up conditions for his feeling different from other children and promoted aversive behavior and intensification of anxiety as he moved into competitive areas. His tension under conditions of concentration needs to be emphasized. He encountered great difficulty assembling the Elephant on the Object Assembly subtest, and expostulated about the inability of the pieces presented to make something; he said, 'I know it is an elephant, I have seen a lot of elephants. If I were paranoid, I would say that these pieces were not designed to fit together, but I am not paranoid.' "

BIBLIOGRAPHY

1. *Aaronson, L. J.:* Mea culpa: A confession about minimal brain dysfunction. The Clin. Psychol., Spring, 1968.
2. *Anderson, C.:* Society Pays: The High Cost of Minimal Brain Dysfunction in America. New York: Walker & Co., 1972.

3. *Belmont, I.:* The relation of afferent change to motor performance in the rehabilitation of cerebrally damaged patients. Bull. N.Y. Acad. Med., 42, 1966.

4. *Benton, A. L.:* Developmental dyslexia: Neurological aspects. *In* W. J. Friedlander (Ed.): Advances in Neurology, Vol. 7. New York: Raven Press, 1975.

5. *Birch, H. G.,* and *Belmont, L.:* Auditory-visual integration in normal and retarded readers. Amer. J. Orthopsychiat., 34, 1964.

6. *Birch, H. G., et al.:* Behavioral development in brain-damaged children. Arch. Gen. Psychiat., 11, 1964.

7. *Braud, L. W., et al.:* The use of electromyographic biofeedback in the control of hyperactivity. J. Learning Disabilities, 8:7, 1975.

8. *Braud, L. W.:* The effects of EMG biofeedback and progressive relaxation upon hyperactivity and its behavioral concomitants, Mimeo, undated.

8a. *Cantwell, D. P.:* Early intervention with hyperactive children. J. Operational Psychiat., 6:1, 1974.

9. *Chess, S.:* An Introduction to Child Psychiatry. New York: Grune and Stratton, 2nd Ed., 1969.

10. *Clarke, L.:* Can't Read, Can't Write, Can't Takl Too Good Either. New York: Walker & Co., 1973.

10a. *Clements, S. D.* and *Peters, J. E.:* Minimal brain dysfunction in the school age child: Diagnosis and treatment. Arch. Gen. Psychiat., 6, 1962.

11. *Comly, H. H.:* Cerebral stimulants for children with learning disorders. J. Learning Disabilities, 4:9, 1971.

12. *Conners, C. K., et al.:* Magnesium pemoline and dextroamphetamine: A controlled study in children with minimal brain dysfunction. Psychopharmacologia, 26, 1972.

13. *Conners, C. K.:* The effect of stimulant drugs on human figure drawings in children with minimal brain dysfunction. Psychopharmacologia, 19, 1971.

14. *Court, J. H.:* Psychological monitoring of interventions into educational problems with psychoactive drugs. J. Learning Disabilities, 4:7, 1971.

15. *David, O. J., et al.:* Lead and hyperactivity. Behavioral response to chelation: A pilot study. Amer. J. Psychiat., 133:10, 1976.

16. *Denhoff, E., et al.:* Effects of dextroamphetamine on hyperkinetic children: A controlled double blind study. J. Learning Disabilities, 4:9, 1971.

17. *DiLeo, J. H.:* Early identification of minimal cerebral dysfunction. Acad. Ther., 5:3, 1970.

18. *DiMascio, A.:* Psychopharmacology in children: Problem areas, methodological considerations, and assessment techniques. Mimeo, 1969.

19. *Douglas, V .I.:* Are drugs enough to treat or to train the hyperactive child? Int. J. Ment. Health, 4:1-2, 1975.

20. *Feighner, A. C.* and *Feighner, J. P.:* Multi-modality treatment of the hyperkinetic child. Amer. J. Psychiat., 13:4, 1974.

21. *Fisher, L.:* Attention deficit in brain-damaged children. Amer. J. Ment. Def., 74:4, 1970.

22. *Frank, J.* and *Levinson, H.:* Seasickness mechanisms and medication in dysmetric dyslexia and dyspraxia. Acad. Ther. Pub., 12:2, 1976-77.

23. *Frostig, M.* and *Pascale, M. A.:* Children with Learning Difficulties. Los Angeles: Marianne Frostig Center of Educational Therapy Newsletter, Fall 1974.

24. *Gardner, R. A.:* Psychotherapy in minimal brain dysfunction. *In* J. H. Masserman (Ed.): Current Psychiatric Therapies. New York: Grune and Stratton, 1975.

25. *Gardner, R. A.:* Techniques for involving the child with MBD in meaningful psychotherapy. J. Learning Disabilities, 8:5, 1975.

26. *Gardner, R. A.:* The mutual story telling technique in the treatment of psy-

chogenic problems secondary to minimal brain dysfunction. J. Learning Disabilities, March 1975.

27. *Gardner, R. A.:* Psychotherapy of minimal brain dysfunction. *In* J. H. Masserman (Ed.) Current Psychiatric Therapies. New York: Grune and Stratton, 1974.

28. *Gardner, R. A.:* Psychotherapy of the psychogenic problems secondary to minimal brain dysfunction. Int. J. Child Psychoth., 2:2, 1973.

29. *Gearhart, B. R.:* Learning Disabilities: Educational Strategies. St. Louis: C. V. Mosby, 1973.

30. *Goldberg, H. H.:* New procedures "yes" but a "no" vote on "minimal cerebral dysfunction." J. Clin. Issues in Psychol., 2:2, 1971.

31. *Gordon, S.:* The "brain-injured" adolescent. New York Association for Brain Injured Children, March 1966.

32. *Kappelman, M. M., et al.:* Profile of the disadvantaged child with learning problems. Ment. Health Digest, 1971.

33. *Katz, M. M., et al.* (Eds.): The role and methodology of classification in psychiatry and psychopathology. Public Health Service Publications No. 1584. Washington, D.C.: U.S. Government Printing Office, 1965.

34. *Katz, S., et al.:* Clinical pharmacological management of hyperkinetic children. Int. J. Ment. Health, 4:1-2, 1975.

35. *Kennard, M.:* Value of equivocal signs in neurological diagnosis. Neurol., 10, 1960.

36. *Krager, J. M.* and *Safer, D. J.:* Type and prevalence of medication used in the treatment of hyperactive children. N.E. J. Med., 291, 1974.

37. *Krop, H.:* Modification of hyperactive behavior of a brain-damaged, emotionally disturbed child. Training School Bull., 68:1, 1971.

38. *Lambert, N., et al.:* Hyperactive children and the efficacy of psychoactive drugs as a treatment intervention. Amer. J. Orthopsychiat., 46:2, 1976.

39. *Laufer, M. W.:* Long-term management and some follow-up findings on the use of drugs with minimal cerebral syndromes. J. Learning Disabilities, 4:9, 1971.

40. *Levi, A.:* Treatment of a disorder of perception and concept formation in a case of school failure. J. Consult. Psychol., 29:4, 1965.

41. *Levine, E. M., et al.:* Hyperactivity among white middle-class children. Child Psychiat. Human Devel. Xerox, undated.

42. *Loney, J., et al.:* Parental management, self-concept, and drug response in minimal brain dysfunction. J. Learning Disabilities, 8:31, 1975.

43. *Lupin, M., et al.:* Children, parents, and relaxation tapes. Acad. Ther., 12:1, 1976.

44. *Luria, A. R.:* Psychological studies of mental deficiency in the Soviet Union. *In* N. R. Ellis (Ed.): Handbook of Mental Deficiency. New York: McGraw-Hill, 1963.

45. *Luria, A. R.:* Restoration of Function After Brain Injury. New York: Macmillan, 1963.

46. *McNeil, T. F., et al.:* Pregnancy and birth complication in the births of seriously, moderately, and mildly behaviorally disturbed children. J. Nerv. Ment. Dis., 151:1, 1970.

47. *Mangel, C.:* The puzzle of learning disabilities. N. Y. Times, April 25, 1976.

48. *Mattis, S., et al.:* Dyslexia in children and young adults: Three independent neurological syndromes. Develop. Med. Child Neurol., 17:2, 1975.

49. *Mauser, A. J.:* Learning disabilities and delinquent youth. Acad. Ther., 9:6, 1974.

50. *Mendelson, et al.:* Hyperactive children as teenagers: A follow-up study. J. Nerv. Ment. Dis., 153:4, 1971.
51. *Menkes, M. M., et al.:* A twenty-five year follow-up study on the hyperkinetic child with minimal brain dysfunction. Pediatrics, 39, 3, 1967.
52. Minimal brain dysfunction: A new problem area for social work. National Easter Seal Society for Crippled Children and Adults. Chicago: 1968.
53. Minimal Brain Dysfunction in Children: Educational, Medical and Health Related Services. Phase Two of a Three-Phase Project. U.S. Dept. of Health, Education, and Welfare. Public Health Service Publication No. 2015, 1969.
54. *Mora, G., et al.:* Psychiatric syndromes and neurological findings as related to academic underachievement: Implications for education and treatment. Mimeo, undated.
55. *Mordock, J. B.* and *DeHaven, G. E.:* Interrelations among indexes of neurological "soft signs" in children with minimal cerebral dysfunction. Proceedings 76th Annual Convention Amer. Psych. Assoc., 1968.
56. *Neisworth, J. T., et al.:* Naturalistic assessment of neurological diagnoses and pharmacological intervention. J. Learning Disabilities, 9:3, 1976.
57. *Ney, P. G.:* Four types of hyperkinesis. Can. Psychiat. Assoc. J., 19, 1974.
58. *Oetinger, J.:* Learning disabilities, hyperkinesis, and the use of drugs in children. Rehab. Lit., 32:6, 1971.
59. *Ozer, M. N.:* The use of operant conditioning in the evaluation of children with learning problems. Clin. Proc. Childrens Hospital, 22:8, 1966.
60. *Paine, R. S., et al.:* A study of "minimal cerebral dysfunction." Dev. Med. Child Neurolog., 10:4, 1968.
61. *Palombo, J.:* Perceptual deficits and self-esteen in adolescence. Clin. Soc. Work J., 7:1, 1979.
62. *Parsons, O. A.* and *Klein, H. P.:* Concept identification and practice in brain-damaged and process-reactive schizophrenic groups. J. Consult. Clin. Psychol., 35:3, 1970.
63. Physician's Desk Reference. Oradell, N. J.: Medical Economics Co. Published annually.
64. *Pope, L.:* Motor activity in brain-injured children. Amer. J. Orthopsychiat., 40:5, 1970.
65. *Prout, H. T.:* Behavioral intervention with hyperactive children. J. Learning Disabilities, 10:3, 1977.
66. *Quay, H. C.* and *Werry, J. S.:* Psychopathological Disorders of Childhood. New York: Wiley, 1972.
67. *Quiros, J.* and *Schrager, O.:* Neuropsychological Fundamentals in Learning Disabilities. San Rafael, California: Academic Therapy Press, 1978.
68. *Reitan, R. M.* and *Boll, T. J.:* Neuropsychological correlates of minimal brain dysfunction. Ann. N. Y. Acad. Sci., 205, 1978.
69. Report of the Conference on the Use of Stimulant Drugs in the Treatment of Behaviorally Disturbed Young School Children. Washington: Dept. of Health, Education and Welfare, 1971.
70. *Riddle, K. D.* and *Rapoport, S. L.:* A two year follow-up of 72 hyperactive boys. J. Nerv. Ment. Dis., 162:2, 1976.
71. *Rie, H. E., et al.:* Effects of ritalin on underachieving children: A replication. Amer. J. Orthopsychiat., 46:2, 1976.
72. *Rourke, B. P.:* Issues in the neuropsychological assessment of children with learning disabilities. Can. Psychological Rev., 17:2, 1976.
73. *Rutter, M., et al.:* Interrelationship between the choreiform syndrome, reading disability and psychiatric disorder in children of 8-11 years. Develop. Med. Child Neurol., 8, 1966.

74. *Sabatino, D. A.:* Auditory and visual perceptual behavioral function of neurologically impaired children. Percept. Motor Skills, 29:10, 1969.
75. *Safer, D. J.* and *Allen, R. P.:* Stimulant drug treatment of hyperactive adolescents. Dis. Ner. Syst., 36:8, 1975.
76. *Sandoval, J., et al.:* Current medical practice and hyperactive children. Amer. J. Orthopsychiat., 46:2, 1976.
77. *Satterfield, J. H., et al.:* Physiological studies of the hyperkinetic child. Amer. J. Psychiat., 128:11, 1972.
78. *Schain, R. J.:* Minimal brain dysfunction in children: A neurological viewpoint. Bull. Los Angeles Neurological Societies, 33:3, 1968.
79. *Schechter, M. D.:* Psychiatric aspects of learning disabilities. Child Psychiat. Human Devel., 5:2, 1974.
80. *Schrager, J., et al.:* The hyperkinetic child: An overview of the issues. J. Amer. Acad. Child Psychiat., 1966.
81. *Small, L.:* The Briefer Psychotherapies. Revised Edition. New York: Brunner/Mazel, 1979.
82. *Sprague, R. L.* and *Sleator, E. K.:* Dose-related effects of methylphenidate in hyperkinetic children. Sci., 198, 1977.
83. *Stevens, D. A., et al.:* Reaction time, impulsivity, and autonomic lability in children with minimal brain dysfunction. Proc. 76th Annual Convention Amer. Psychol. Assoc., 1968.
84. *Strauss, A.* and *Kephart, N.:* Psychopathology and Education of the Brain-Injured Child. Vol. II. New York: Grune and Stratton, 1955.
85. *Straus, A.* and *Lehtinen, L.:* Psychopathology and Education of the Brain-Injured Child. Vol. I. New York: Grune and Stratton, 1947.
86. *Thomas, A.* and *Chess, S.:* A longitudinal study of three brain damaged children: Infancy to adolescence. Arch. Gen. Psychiat., 32:4, 1975.
87. *Tymchuk, A. J., et al.:* The behavioral significance of differing EEG abnormalities in children with learning and/or behavior problems. J. Learning Disabilities, Nov., 1970.
88. *Walker, S.:* Drugging the American child: We're too cavalier about hyperactivity. Psychol. Today, 8:7, 1974.
89. *Webb, W. W., et al.:* The sequelae of acute bacterial meningitis: A possible clue to early school problems. J. Spec. Ed., 2:4, 1968.
90. *Wender, P. H.:* The minimal brain dysfunction syndrome. Ann. Rev. Med., 26, 1975.
91. *Wender, P. H.:* Minimal brain dysfunction in children. New York: Wiley-Interscience, 1971.
92. *Werner, H.* and *Strauss, A. A.:* Pathology of figure-background relation in the child. J. Abnorm. Soc. Psychol., 36, 1941.
93. *Zentall, S.:* Optimal stimulation as theoretical basis of hyperactivity. Amer. J. Orthopsychiat., 45:4, 1975.

CHAPTER 3

Epilepsy: The Less Obvious Forms

Confusion between psychiatric and neurological diagnoses seems more prevalent for epilepsy than for any other disorder, according to Sherwin (62). Possibility for confusion certainly exists, a confusion all the more important because of the frequency of occurrence of epilepsy, in contrast to no less ambiguous but far rarer disorders, such as Gilles de la Tourette Syndrome.

Epilepsy is now regarded as a disturbance of the central nervous system that involves episodic failure to maintain the metabolic equilibrium of some nerve cells. The state of disequilibrium produce excitation of the cells involved, which, depending upon their location in the brain and hence upon their function and the speed with which the excitation spreads, results in symptoms ranging widely in severity, from convulsions with loss of consciousness to momentary lapses of attention. Many cases of epilepsy do not involve frank seizures, but instead are manifested as disturbances of behavior and mood, often misdiagnosed as purely psychogenic, to the detriment of any psychotherapy undertaken. Detection of this less readily identified type of epilepsy is not an easy matter.

All phenomena associated with seizure disorders do not fit neatly into categories. Not all epileptics have sudden fits. "Odd" behavior, for example, which is in fact epileptic, may endure for years without proper diagnosis. Epileptic phenomena shade imperceptibly from frank convulsions toward normal behavior, and as the normal end of the continum is approached, the certainty of diagnosis diminishes markedly. (This may be the case also with psychological-test data. One study (61) found it necessary to create a diagnostic category, "Questionable Convulsive Disorder," to accommodate the variations in neuropsycho-

90

logical deficit observed: minimal in children without convulsive disorder, somewhat more obvious in questionable cases, and prominent in children with established epilepsy.) Yet it is exactly in this area that weighing of probable causes is most important to the welfare of the patient.

TYPES OF EPILEPSY

Epilepsy is sometimes categorized according to whether its cause has been established. *Symptomatic epilepsy* is the term which refers to seizures of known origin. *Idiopathic epilepsy* is the title used when no definition of abnormality of the brain or body system can be found and the locus of origin of the seizures cannot be determined.

Symptomatic epilepsy is further separated into two kinds. In one, a definite brain disease irritates specific brain cells, which in turn gives rise to electrical discharges; when these discharges "spread," a "fit" or convulsion results. The point of origin of electrical discharge is called a focus. In the second category of symptomatic epilepsy, the disease process is located elsewhere in the body, not in the brain. For example, a deficiency of oxygen because of heart or lung disease may interfere with the flow of oxygen to the brain, and a fit may occur.

Four major types of epileptic attacks have been described. A victim usually experiences only one kind, though some few sufferers on occasion experience one or several of the types of seizures.

The *grand mal* attack is the commonest type of fit, and accounts for about 50 percent of all epileptic seizures. It is usually preceded by a warning period, either a long-lasting prodrome or a brief aura. The prodrome is described as a sensation (a feeling of depression and tension, less frequently of excitement or elation) which may last for several hours before an attack. The brief aura occurs more frequently than the prodrome. Electroencephalographic studies of the brain have shown it to be the very beginning of the attack itself. In the aura, the patient may experience a strange smell, or tingling in the hands. This soon passes into the tonic phase of the fit, in which the muscles of the body are rigidly contracted, often accompanied by an automatic cry. In the clonic phase which then follows, there are jerkings and muscular contractions. A period of unconsciousness ensues, and the attack ends usually with a deep sleep which may last from a few minutes to several hours.

The *petit mal* is the simplest and briefest kind of attack; it usually occurs without aura or prodrome, and there is no recognizable period of recovery; it is essentially a brief lapse from full consciousness. The person may stop in the middle of a conversation, seem momentarily inattentive, and there may be fluttering of the eyelids. There may be slight jerking of the arms and legs; in some cases this behavior may be quite pronounced. The patient's confusion and disorientation often lead to a psychiatric diagnosis (50).

In the *Jacksonian* attack, the patient does not lose consciousness or awareness of his surroundings as he does in the *petit mal* or *grand mal,* but he experiences lack of control of an extremity. He may be able to give an account of his experience since he is alert throughout it. The Jacksonian attack may begin with a tingling in the hand or the involuntary movement of a finger and spread throughout the extremity. The limb affected may remain weak for a few hours or as long as a few days.

The *psychomotor* attack is second in frequently to the *grand mal* fit, representing 35 to 40 percent of all epileptic seizures. It begins in a small part of the brain, often found in the temporal lobe. The electrical discharge may spread slowly in the brain without causing a convulsion. The psychological and emotional manifestations are now more extensively recognized than they were twenty years ago, when the person in a psychomotor seizure state was described as ". . . conscious but amnesic. Usually engages in bizarre, often aggressive behavior, completely alien to his ordinary character" (72). The phenomena now recognized as associated with this type of seizure are more varied and seem to depend upon the part of the temporal lobe affected (24). The patient may have the sensation of smell or of hearing; he may notice an unpleasant odor, hear familiar voices, a ringing or high pitched sound: he may report complex events, often *déjà vu* (sensations involving vivid scenes from childhood which are relived) or *jamais vu* (the sensation of unfamiliarity even though the person is at home). The observer may be uncertain as to what is going on with the victim of the attack; the victim may stop what he is doing, stare vacantly, and then begin some repetitive, automatic movement. During these attacks the victim is in a kind of a dream that may develop into a fugue state. He may travel a considerable distance or perform complicated acts without being aware of what he is doing, and is unable to recall what he had done once he returns from the dreamlike state. It is this form of epilepsy in which psychological factors contribute most clearly to the pattern of an attack. It is also the form of epilepsy which should be of most concern to the psychotherapist, since so many of the neurological symptoms of this disorder may be incorrectly diagnosed as having purely psychological origins.

Closely related are the *subictal* states—epilepsies without seizures—which have occupied the attention of Jonas (34, 35) among others. These states may be equivalents of psychomotor seizures, manifested in rages, tantrums, acting out, and character disorders. As *petit mal* equivalents, they appear as forgetfulness and absent-mindedness. *Grand mal* equivalents may be observed as tic-like gestures, restless convulsive movements during sleep, and isolated muscle contractions. The personality manifestations of subictal states are frequently bizarre and may arouse tremendous anxiety in the patient. Singly or together these manifestations may lead to misdiagnosis as "malingering, hysteria, hypochondriasis, psychopathy, pseudo-neurotic schizophrenia, and schizo-affective psychosis" (35).

Physicians are frequently confused by the symptoms of epilepsy and led into misdiagnosis. So-called *abdominal epilepsy,* usually occurring in children, is a case in point. Visceral pain and other abdominal sensations have long been associated with the epileptic aura preceding seizures, and for some time abdominal epilepsy (established by EEG patterns) without seizures has also been recognized. This type of epilepsy is marked by a sudden onset of pain in the mid or upper abdomen, lasting usually for only a few minutes. The pain disappears until the next episode, which may be days or weeks later. During the attack the child does not lose consciousness, but suffers nausea, vomiting, confusion, and disorientations, as well as loss of appetite. After the episode the child usually falls asleep to wake feeling well (4, 51). Frequent visceral sensations have been observed both in individuals with psychomotor epilepsy and those with episodic behavioral disorders (48). Inappropriate surgery must be guarded against (1).

Gelastic or "laughing" epilepsy is another of the so-called "types" of seizure disorder. Rare, it occurred in 0.32 percent of 5,000 cases of epilepsy (10).

Hysterical seizures are reported fairly often in the literature (33, 56, 66) and are not infrequently diagnosed by neurologists. Their etiology (see the section on *Etiology* below in this chapter), even their existence is vigorously debated. Psychotherapists may attempt to pursue the origins of so-called hysterical epilepsy in deeply unconscious motivations, sexual expressions, avoidances, and the like, with little effect. Extreme diagnostic skepticism is recommended (56). Some observers believe that hysterical seizures occur mostly among individuals of low intelligence or in more primitive cultures, but also find a double etiology—emotional and organic—to be likely or even essential (66).

The misuse of the psychoanalytic concept of determinism, of cause and effect in symptomatology, when applied to the emotional sphere while ignoring the physiological, has contributed to the danger of misdiagnosis of epileptic equivalents by psychotherapists. The danger is decreased considerably when the therapist approaches causality in terms of probabilities applied to soma as well as psyche, and considers the full range of physical and emotional causes and their possible combinations.

The persuasiveness of this argument is reinforced by a review of the symptoms observed in non-convulsive epilepsy by Gibbs and Gibbs (23): headaches, dizziness, nausea, vomiting, syncope, parathesias, behavior disorders, mental retardation, unconsciousness, severe abdominal pain, unprovoked rage, amnesia, distorted vision, speech heard as a roaring sound, numbness of hands and lips, severe nightmares, shivering on a hot day, loss of consciousness after a bowel movement, spells of food-gorging, insomnia, temporary incontinence of bladder and bowel, sweats and hot flashes, momentary failure to recognize people, inability to talk, rapid panting.

Significant studies of the relationship between ictal activity and behavioral manifestations have been conducted by Monroe (48), a psychoanalyst and electroencephalographer, employing an activating drug (alphachlorolose) to amplify electrical activity from subcortical structures usually not accessible to the electroencephalograph. He finds two basic behavioral patterns associated with ictal phenomena: 1) Episodic inhibition accompanied by torpor, apathy, loss of initiative, dulling of affect, confusion, disorientation. These are most likely to be associated with ictal or postictal EEG recordings characteristic of centrencephalic epilepsy. 2) Episodic disinhibition characterized by intense affect, impulsive actions dictated by these affects, psychotic symptoms such as hallucinations, delusions, depersonalization, altered states of consciousness, or loss of awareness. These patterns are likely to be associated with rhinencephalic epilepsy. Monroe finds some creditability in associating the inhibitive and disinhibitive episodic types of behavior with Delay's findings on the Rorschach of the coarctative and the extratensive personalities.

ETIOLOGY AND PRECIPITANTS

The pursuit of etiology is essential in every case of epilepsy, since the possible causes include a life-endangering brain tumor or other serious disease that may result in grave permanent functional impairment.

The underlying disease conditions that cause seizure symptoms have been succintly described by Goldensohn (26). In addition to brain tumors, they include: injury to the brain during gestation, at birth or at any subsequent time in life; congenital defects; common infectious diseases of childhood; meningitis; encephalitis; abscesses of the brain; parasitic invasions; degenerative diseases; cerebral vascular accidents; endocrine disorder; and metabolic abnormalities.

Heredity is often citied as an etiological factor in epilepsy: Alvarez (1) emphasizes this causal source while failing to list traumas, fevers, and toxemias. He cites studies by Lennox and the Gibbs which reported 65 to 70 percent of epileptics as having relatives with epilepsy, and 67 to 94 percent incidence for both twins among monozygotic twins with only 3 to 24 percent for both twins among fraternal twins. Equally compelling are the data for perinatal factors (maternal complications during pregnancy, toxemias, bleeding, anoxia, instrument injuries, etc.) reported by Lilienfeld and Pasamanick (40, 41). Beaussart (6) argues that the determination between an hereditary and an organic cause is obscured by the variety and complexity of epileptic disorders. Both possible origins should be considered.

The underlying disease condition may not be the factor that precipitates a specific seizure. Psychological stress, for example, may precipitate a seizure, as it frequently does, but the epilepsy is the cause.

In an interesting and seemingly valid speculation, Jonas (34) suggests that the advent of tranquilizers has been responsible for an increase of manifest epileptic symptomatology. In pre-tranquilizer days, barbiturates—which happen also to be one of the earliest effective anti-convulsant agents—were used primarily as sedatives and soporifics. With their discontinuation for people regarded as "nervous," some of these patients have lost their protection against seizure equivalents, and now reveal the symptoms. Within the present cultural phenomenon of widespread drug use and abuse, it is useful to ask patients in whom epilepsy may be suspected what their favorite medication is or has been. When barbiturates are cited, it may be reasonable to investigate for a form of seizure disorder. The same considerations apply when a patient reports having relied upon amphetamines, which also have an anti-convulsant effect.

The precipitants of seizures are many and varied. Moving lights or hyperventilation touch off episodes in some people. Alcohol, aspirin, and marijuana have been implicated in several patients within my recent clinical experience. A possibility exists that in some cases the "bad trip" phenomenon, and its repeated recurrence without further drug ingestion, may be due to the irritation of susceptible brain tissue by marijuana or LSD. Among other precipitating factors reported are: emotional and physical stress (20), sexual orgasm (48), unconscious sexual strivings (48), sleep deprivation (29), loss (48), demands (48), specific visual, auditory, or cutaneous sensations (48), severe burns causing cerebral edema (30), fear (1), tricyclic antidepressant drugs (14), phenothiazines (48), lithium carbonate (18), eye movements as in reading or watching television (25, 59, 79), immersion in hot water (67), and hyperventilation.

EMOTIONAL AND BEHAVIORAL CORRELATES
OF EPILEPSY

The damaging effects of epileptic seizures upon the emotional adjustment of children was vividly demonstrated by a large-scale epidemological study on the Isle of Wight by Graham and Rutter (27). Children with epileptic conditions manifested five times as many psychiatric disorders as did children in the general population, and three times as many as children with chronic physical handicaps not involving the brain. While the epileptic children showed a normal I.Q. distribution, psychiatric disorders were twice as common among those epileptic children whose I.Q. was less than 85 as among those whose. I.Q. was higher. The authors attribute the high rate of psychiatric disorder in the neuroepileptic children to specific dysfunctions of the brain. Contributing to the psychological effects of the brain dysfunction are: visibility of the disorder, frustrations inherent in physical restrictions, adverse parental reactions, perceptual abnormalities, frustrations arising from the child's inability to express his wants adequately because of poor speech and language skill, visual defects, low intelligence, the effects of drugs, community prejudices, the child's individual reaction to his disability, and impaired emotional control produced by the brain dysfunction.

Chess (11) observes that the first experience of convulsive epilepsy frequently occurs during adolescence, and that this timing has serious psychological consequences which affect the adolescent's relationships with his peers.

There appears to be some relationship between epilepsy and the subsequent development of schizophrenia. Slater and Beard (64) observe that patients suffering from epilepsy will develop schizophrenia-like psychoses with greater frequency than chance expectations would suggest, and that epileptics are more likely to become schizophrenic than are schizophrenics to become epileptic. The symptoms demonstrated by epileptic individuals who become schizophrenic differ slightly from the usual schizophrenia patterns. Catatonic phenomena of gross degree are rare. Decrease of the affective response does not occur as early nor become as marked as it does in the typical schizophrenic patient. By and large, this type of epileptic schizophrenic is described as friendlier, more cooperative, and less suspicious.

The length of time an individual has suffered from epilepsy is regarded by some (55) as the main factor leading to the development of schizophrenia in the epileptic person. Years of attacks may produce clouded consciousness, which leads to confusion of reality and autistic thinking.

Hallucinations, laughter, involuntary obscenity, assaultiveness, perceptual illusions, disturbances of mood and affect, forced, obsessional thinking, *déjà vu, jamais vu,* hypo- and hypersexuality, depersonalization, derealization, withdrawal may all arise from epileptic disturbances of cerebral function. These are all too readily confused with psychogenicially derived symptoms. A psychologically-oriented therapist may be led to consider a diagnosis of schizophrenia, severe neurosis, or a borderline condition, rather than to further explore a history to check for possible seizure phenomena.

Whitten (78) has reviewed these phenomena extensively, and finds that they are most specifically associated with temporal-lobe disease: 45 percent of non-institutionalized patients with temporal-lobe lesions reported hallucinatory experiences. He remind us that Hughlings Jackson called attention to "dreamy" states that involved symptoms such as chewing movements, and experiences of alteration in apparent size and distance of external objects. These may be important diagnostic indices of epilepsy rather than trifling matters. They may appear as part of an emotional disorder, or they may constitute the sum total of a seizure phenomenon. Full investigation is necessary in order to differentiate between emotional expressions and symptoms of epileptic or paroxysmal disturbance.

Hallucinatory seizure equivalents are symptomatic of a discharging focus in the temporal lobe. The content of such hallucinations usually refers to past personal experiences. The patient most often is aware of the hallucination and of his real surroundings, and may report it as a waking dream state. The hallucination may involve any of the sensory modalities: smell, taste, hearing, vision. He may hear voices, see people, feel pleasure or fear upon recall of past events.

Perceptual illusions resemble the hallucinatory phenomena in that they are brief, paroxysmal, stereotyped, and involve transient, partial impairment of cerebral functions. They are false interpretations of real sensory stimuli; they take many forms and involve any sensory modality; the *déjà vu* phenomenon is a common occurrence. Often patients report a brief feeling of loneliness, strangeness, or a dreamy state. A patient may describe feelings of depersonalization, of being "out of this world," in a silly situation, a spectator at an event, or not part of it. Objects may appear to be either very small or very large. There may be distortions of hearing. Such events, particularly, are likely to be diagnosed as schizophrenic phenomena unless the clinician explores carefully for evidence—or a history—of cerebral pathology.

Mood and emotional changes occurring alone are less frequently reported than hallucinations and illusions. These may include feelings of fear or of well being. Depression also has been associated with temporal-lobe seizures.

Obsessional thinking may be evidence of a seizure disorder, to be checked especially in the absence of the psychodynamic basis of a neurosis. The thought process often has a quality of being forced and of excluding control by the patient of his own thoughts. The affect is usually unpleasant; sometimes it may not be remembered by the patient.

It has amused some writers to refer to the temporal lobe as "libidinous." Excessive activity of the limbic system is believed to cause decreased release of gonadotropic hormone, resulting in hyposexuality which may involve diminished arousal, failure of arousal, inability to maintain intercourse, or decreased fantasy and erotic discourse. Inhibited activity of the limbic system stimulates hypersexuality (7, 75).

Even seemingly prolonged psychiatric states may be ictal phenomena. Patients without motor seizures but having abnormal electroencephalograms have demonstrated protracted emotional behavior that is confused, hostile, negative, withdrawn, foggy, or dreamy, as well as intellectual changes (78). Both onset and termination in these patients were rapid.

The studies of children on the Isle of Wight (27) indicated that states of partial consciousness seem to be more threatening psychologically to a child than is the total loss of consciousness that accompanies a *grand mal* seizure.

An upsurge of concern about the roots of violence in the United States (44, 60) has called attention to the tendency to associate assaultiveness with epilepsy, especially temporal-lobe seizures. There is reason to believe that modulating influences are exerted within the brain by the limbic system which includes the temporal lobes, so that a seizure disorder in these areas may prevent them from modulating the attack reflexes which originate in the brain stem. In short, *some*, but far from most, persons with temporal-lobe epilepsy exhibit assaultive and violent impulses. The manifestations of epilepsy arising in these areas are multitudinous, and their association with violence is the exception, not the rule. Nonetheless, violence may be a symptom of epilepsy and its outbreak in an individual should be investigated for a neurogenic cause, as well as for other causes, including the patient's culture and personality (39).

The psychodynamically oriented psychotherapist must by careful not to attribute seizure phenomena solely to an insufficient repression of ego-alien aggressive drives, with the aggressive affect being discharged in the seizure behavior (63). The task is made more difficult by the occurrence of disturbed behavior between episodes of identifiable seizures—so-called interictal behavior. Patients with such behavior have sometimes been diagnosed as functionally psychotic, only to later have EEG establish temporal lobe foci (76).

The relationship between seizure phenomena and behavioral manifestations has been and is being rewardingly investigated by Monroe (48). He distinguishes between non-episodic and episodic disorders or maladaptive behavior. The former includes the usual psychiatric diagnosis of psychoses and neuroses. Some episodic behavioral disturbances are characterized by inhibition and result periodically in narcolepsy, catelepsy, mutism, catatonia, or *petit mal*. Others are marked by loss of inhibition or control, a group for which Monroe has developed a rather elaborate classification. Two major subgroups constitute this episodic dysinhibition category. One is characterized by episodic *reactions* that are intermittent, periodic, and remitting. These include:

psychotic episodes attributable to schizophrenia, brain syndrome, or depression; and sociopathic, neurotic, or psychophysiologic reactions. The second subgroup—episodic dyscontrol—within the episodic dysinhibition category in turn breaks down into two other subgroups: primary dyscontrol and secondary dyscontrol. Within the primary dyscontrol subgroup, two further divisions are recognized: *seizure dyscontrol* and *instinct dyscontrol.*

Seizure dyscontrol: the pattern of expression in this group is marked by explosive affect, and diffuse, chaotic motor behavior so uncoordinated that the act seems to have no object, or the object appears to be an accidental utilization of the nearest thing at hand. There is little or no delay between stimulus and act. Often the act is so maladaptive as to be incapacitating. There is some possibility that the act may be utilized to divert the urge from an object-directed impulsive act. The act discharge tensions and is typical of ictal behavior.

Instinct dyscontrol: Again there is little delay between stimulus and act. But the affects expressed are differentiated, and gratification of specific needs is apparent in actions upon specific objects. The acts are primitive and relatively undisguised: fight or flight, reaching out for contact, closeness, sexuality. Nonetheless they are coordinated, efficient and their associational linkage, their intention, can be discerned. Need gratification rather than tension relief characterizes the act.

The *secondary dyscontrol* category is also further subdivided into the *impulse dyscontrol* and *acting out* subgroups. *Impulse dyscontrol:* In their primitiveness, intention and object directedness the acts here are similar to those of the *Instinct Dyscontrol* group, except that they are preceded by mounting tensions about maintaining control or letting go. The act occurs when the tension becomes unbearable. There is little affect manifest during the act, but great relief afterwards, with manifest gratification. *Acting out:* These are circumscribed, complex, dynamically significant acts that involve unconscious premeditation and planning. The intent of the act is usually disguised and the need gratification indirect. The act is out of character for the personality of the actor. This last factor distinguishes this behavior from neurotic actions in general, from acting on psychotic fantasy, acting out as a way of life, and from acting out as a form of communication among those with limited capacity for introspection.

To return to the first distinction made within the episodic dysinhibition group, Monroe describes differences between the episodic dyscontrol act and the episodic reaction, especially the episodic psychotic reaction. In both there is usually an altered state of consciousness and awareness, and the psychotic reaction is linked significantly with convulsive disorders, or at a minimum with an epileptoid phenomenon, marked by precipitous onset and abrupt remissions. The episodic psychotic reaction usually has a more persistent morbidity, while episodic dyscontrol behavior usually involves a single act or a short series of acts. Monroe found many such patients who produced normal baseline EEG recordings but after activation with alpha-chlorolose exhibited epileptoid abnormalities. Transient ictal psychosis is also described by Wells (77) as correlated with cerebral epileptiform discharges that do not produce other clinically recognizable seizure activity.

Monroe identifies an ictal depression characterized by abrupt onset and remission, little motor retardation but intense anxiety, only mild feelings of guilt and inferiority, but more frequent hypochondriasis, depersonalization, and simple compulsive behavior (laughing and crying). The episodes are of short duration, lasting several hours or days.

This review may convey something of the complexity that characterizes the relationships between epilepsy, anatomical localization of pathology and behavior. Temporal-lobe epilepsy has been challenged by Taylor (71) as being merely a location, not a clinical concept, as is psychomotor epilepsy, for example. He contends that temporal-lobe epilepsy is an overly simplified nosological category, rendered imprecise by the inclusion of a variety of EEG and neurological findings, psychological disturbances, and symptoms. He suggests that metaphorically epilepsy is like a fire, a process that is not discrete and cannot be made concrete, that is a varying complex relationship among phenomena.

NEUROPSYCHOLOGICAL CORRELATES OF EPILEPSY

Where epilepsy is definitively associated with established lesions of the brain, the usual neuropsychological correlates are readily obtained. As the case illustrations demonstrate, sub-clinical epilepsy of unknown or difficult to establish etiology is frequently associated with neuropsychological test patterns suggestive of minimal brain dysfunction.

A high frequency, about 70 percent, of learning disabilities associated with minimal brain dysfunction that includes dyslexia and dysgraphia is reported in epilepsy (32). Impairment of attention is also frequently associated with ictal disorders. These episodes may be of short duration as in *petit mal*, or more prolonged as in confused states following seizure attacks, or in the subtle manifestations of subclinical seizure discharges (22, 70).

The presence of epileptiform activity in EEG recordings has been significantly related to lower intelligence levels as measured by the Wechsler Adult Intelligence Scale by Dodrill and Wilkus (16, 17). Frequency of seizure activity has also been connected with lower intelligence and other neuropsychological levels in a study of identical twins (18).

Perhaps the most ambitious efforts to identify neuropsychological correlates of epilepsy is reported by Klove and Matthews (36), who sought to ". . . investigate cognitive impairment in a series of increasingly refined classifications of patients with epilepsy." Using the WAIS and the Halstead Neuropsychological Test Battery, their effort was to determine whether seizures themselves or their underlying causes (brain damage or disease) are most important in producing cognitive defects. They were able to establish a gradient of impairment that strongly suggests that seizures arising from established causes (brain damage and disease) are more impairing than are seizures of unknown etiology, and that major motor seizures are more impairing than psychomotor seizures. The authors find that the literature shows that the surgical removal of epileptic foci fails to establish specific patterns of cognitive impairment due to epilepsy. The major determinants of measurable neuropsychological impairment are: 1) the lesion, its nature, location, and extent; 2) the type and frequency of seizure caused by the lesion; 3) the patient's age at onset; 4) the patient's personality, and 5) the social forces operating upon the patient.

DIAGNOSIS AND MISDIAGNOSIS

The likelihood of misdiagnosis by mistakenly attributing psychological causation to temporal-lobe phenomena is underscored by a number of investigators. For example, Slater and Beard (64) state that a striking feature of a series of epileptic patients with schizophrenia-like psychoses was the preponderance of temporal-lobe abnormalities. Misdiagnosis is common because psychological factors tend to mask organic symptoms and mislead the unwary clinician. This is particularly likely when convulsions are not prominent in the clinical picture.

Then the clinician may be most impressed and misled by evidences of neurosis, anxiety, depression, hysteria, confusion, disorientation, paranoia, schizophrenia, even exhibitionism and fetishism (5, 9, 19, 35, 47, 50, 56). Alvarez (1) believes that medical experts largely ignore the nonconvulsive aspects of epilepsy which are more common than the convulsive forms.

Misdiagnosis may simply delay the application of proper treatment until the psychotherapist finally realizes that psychotherapy is unproductive, or that factors other than emotional ones appear to be operating. Gradually he may be struck by his inability to discern precipitants for the patient's schizophrenic-like experiences. He may become convinced that the patient's usual behavior, mood, and manner are so clearly devoid of the stigmata of schizophrenia that he comes at least and at last to question his original diagnosis and seek other causes.

Hysteria, though relatively rare in contemporary clinical experience, may complicate the diagnostic picture here. It is sometimes difficult to differentiate from epilepsy. Many of the emotional, sensory, and motor phenomena of ictal equivalents arouse panic and exaggerated reactions in some individuals (35). One reported attempt at differentiation is based upon the presumption that one is able from the "outside" to interrupt the hysteric fit, but not to interrupt the epileptic fit (56). Hysterical patients are supposedly responsive to external intervention during a seizure, to talk, obey commands, and make and maintain eye contact. They rarely hurt themselves during a seizure, and certain neurological signs associated with true seizures (the absence of pupillary and extensor plantar responses) are not found. Onset in the hysterical seizure is found to be gradual, in contrast to the abrupt beginning and ending of the epileptic seizure (33). But where there is no loss of consciousness, differentiation is extremely difficult. To compound the difficulty, hysterics, reports Jonas (35), may show "theta rhythms, slow waves on overbreathing, and a low convulsive threshold" on the EEG. The difficulties of diagnosis are complicated further by the frequent failure of the EEG to identify a clinically established seizure disorder, or the absence of clinical phenomena in the presence of abnormal tracings. There is a slow but steady accumulation of cases in which evidence of seizure was obtained *only* under special conditions, such as sleep readings, or with use of nasopharyngeal leads, which are not always used in electroencephalographic examination. (See Chapters 16 and 17 for discussion of the EEG as a criterion of cerebral disease.) Brain damage has been definitively associated with the development of seemingly hysterical seizures by Standage (66), who warns, however, that *both* organic and psychosocial pathology may be necessary to produce such seizures.

The worst consequences of misdiagnosis in these cases of presumed hysteria, schizophrenia, or another psychopathology are disastrous for both the patient and the therapist. Failing to benefit from psychotherapy, the patient becomes pessimistic, self-esteem is damaged, despair may set in. The therapist also may become pessimistic and consider or prescribe heavy doses of psychotropic drugs or electroconvulsive treatments, or he may abandon the patient as being so resistant as to be untreatable.

The effort to differentiate between ictal and non-ictal or seizure and motivated behavior has concerned Monroe (48). The extremes—*grand mal* and the complex acting out of a psychoanalytic patient—present little difficulty, but in between there is a gray area where often a definitive diagnosis is extremely difficult, if not impossible. Monroe found that the clinical criteria for a seizure disorder proposed by Lennox—abrupt onset without apparent cause or explanation; abrupt cessation of the disturbed behavior; fragmentary awareness of what took place during the attack; a family or personal history of more typical epileptic seizures; an abnormal EEG; and a favorable response to anti-convulsive medication—were *not* reliable in established clinical practice.

Monroe proposes these criteria for diagnosing an episode as epileptic:

1) Stereotyped, repetitive patterns of behavior during an episodic disorder whatever the environmental situation may be. The usefulness of this criterion increases with the richness and variety, flexibility, spontaneity, and intelligence of the patient's behavioral patterns between episodic disturbances.

2) The more emotionally and symbolically neutral the environmental situation in which the attack occurs, the more likely is the episode to be caused by excessive neuronal discharge. If the precipitating circumstances are emotionally overwhelming and the patient responds with reduced consciousness, the likelihood of psychodynamically motivated behavioral discharge is increased.

3) The seizure behavior is more likely to be lower in the hierarchical level of response. The validity of this criterion increases with the

disparity between the level of motor integration during the attack and that characteristic of the intervals between attacks.

4) The absence of secondary gains. Caution is required here as the epileptic is not immune from the temptation to manipulate people with his illness.

5) The epileptic is more likely to assume responsibility for his actions, to report feeling driven beyond his control. He is more likely to ask for help and restraint, more willing to accept hospitalization, to feel less guilt and shame, to manifest less denial. The non-epileptic tends to renounce responsibility, and resorts to denial and amnesia and portrays himself as a helpless victim, since he unconsciously perceives the intention of his acts as alien to his superego. Monroe cautions that where the response—however emotionally or symbolically overwhelming the precipitating circumstances—involves a dissociated state, altered state of consciousness, or primary-process thinking, both a motivated and an epileptic etiology must be considered.

Obviously the psychotherapist, unless trained in neurology, is not equipped to diagnose an epilepsy. But this does not release him from the responsibility to investigate carefully the patient's behavior and history (See Section II: Application for the Psychotherapist) for neurologically significant data and to refer those with suggestive behavior for specialized consultation.

TREATMENT

The psychotherapist is most likely to become responsible for the treatment of individuals who present both behavioral-emotional problems and *subclinical* epilepsy. Such individuals are more likely to benefit from a combination of therapeutic approaches selected from among the drug, the psychotherapeutic, and the behavioral interventions. Where the troubling behavior is closer to the epileptic end of the continuum from the organic to the emotional, medication alone may be preferred. Conversely, psychotherapy alone may be preferred for the patient who appears closer to the psychodynamic end of the continuum. But even when a single course is elected, the therapist should prepare the patient for the probability that other types of therapeutic intervention may have to be introduced. When different approaches are applied simultaneously, the evaluation of the effectiveness of each of the approaches is made difficult, as is the evaluation of the overall progress of the therapy. Monroe (48) warns, for example, that a dramatic response to drug therapy is not in itself sufficient indication that psychotherapy should be reduced or ended. And for many patients it becomes necessary to reduce tension by psychotherapy or behavioral methods first before medication can become effective.

The ideal drug treatment for seizure has not yet been discovered, according to Merritt (45). Drugs now used appear to act diffusely upon the whole cortex, depressing its activity. Ideally, an anti-convulsant medication would selectively inhibit only those neurones that are discharging excessively, with little or no effect on normal neurone areas. Despite this imperfection the armamentarium of anti-convulsants has increased since the early part of this century with more refined selectivity for *grand mal, petit mal,* and psychomotor seizures. Optimal success in the drug treatment of seizures depends upon the neurologist's precise understanding of the types of epilepsy and the properties of the various drugs (37). While Phenobarital, introduced in 1912, and Dilantin, reported effective in 1938, probably remain the most generally used anti-convulsants, the newer drugs are finding an increasing role in selective therapy.

Anti-convulsant medications are usually needed over a long term. Their use is indicated for several months to several years, the latter time span being more often necessary. When the epileptic phenomena have disappeared, reduction of dosage is accomplished gradually. Frequently, a variety of anti-convulsant agents must be used in combination for effective seizure control. Toxic effects are possible but rare. To guard against these, and to assure that dosages and combinations of drugs are expertly determined, the patient should be under the care of a physician experienced with the disease, especially subictal phenomena.

The phenothiazine family of tranquilizers is cited by Monroe (48) as contraindicated in suspected epilepsy because of their potentiating action in seizure cases, in lowering seizure threshold and increasing seizure frequency. This quality indicates that the phenothiazines may also increase frequency and intensity of episodic behavioral disorders associated with epilepsy. When phenothiazines appear necessary in an episodic behavioral disturbance it is wise to combine them with an "anti-convulsant or benzodiazepine," such as Valium or Librium. Two cases at a rehabilitation center support this approach. In one, the patient became more disturbed when given phenothiazines and improved when they were removed. In the other the patient improved when an anti-convulsant was added to his regimen.

Episodic depressive reactions, Monroe finds, tend to respond poorly to anti-depressant medication, but may remit dramatically with the benzodiazepines, the anti-convulsants, or a combination of the two. The ultimate diagnosis in sub-ictal states is often dependent upon the effect of drug therapy, i.e., does the patient improve in response to anti-convulsant medication? Then indeed a seizure disorder is the diagnosis. Placebo effect can be ruled out by the failure of tranquilizers to produce beneficial changes. However, not all anti-convulsants work equally well in all types of epilepsy or in all cases of the same type of epilepsy, and often the neurologist must empirically adjust both dosages and types of medication until an effective combination for the individual patient is achieved. Monroe (48) warns that the attempt at a therapeutic diagnosis may result in false negative findings, unless careful attention is given to both dosage levels and length of the trial. He is also especially concerned that the pursuit of medical control of the seizure may overlook the motivational and dynamic aspects of the patient's state that require psychotherapy as well as medicine.

A single case has been reported (52) in which desensitization significantly reduced frequency and intensity of seizures from a base rate of 58 gross body movements to 10 barely noticable facial tics after anti-convulsant medication had failed to benefit the patient. While the study was weak in that the effort to find an appropriate medication was neither energetic nor thorough, the point of interest is that seizures in this patient were touched-off by emotional stress, a precipitant rather frequent among epileptic patients.

The effectiveness of EEG biofeedback training has been studied for over a decade in animals by Sterman (68). He found a specific EEG rhythm in the sensorimotor cortex (12 to 14 cycles per second) of voluntarily sedentary, relaxed cats. He then established that a similar rhythm existed in man and could be encouraged by EEG biofeedback techniques. He reports success with four epileptic patients whose seizures could not be controlled by anti-convulsant medications. All patients received three biofeedback training sessions per week with machines that gave both visual and auditory signals whenever the patient produced the desired sensorimotor rhythm. The patients were able to produce the rhythm at will after one month of training. A pronounced reduction in both frequency and intensity of seizures and improvement in EEG patterns was obtained after three months of training.

Sterman acknowledges that the biofeedback technique itself may not be the determining factor in reducing seizures. The technique fosters and teaches relaxation and internalization and involves the patient in his own treatment.

Hypnosis is reported also to help induce relaxation and diminish seizure frequency and intensity (21).

The behavioral modification techniques promise to become a valuable adjunct in the treatment of epileptics, especially for those whose seizures appear to be initiated by or intensified by stress, who do not respond to medication even at toxic levels or who respond only to toxic plasma levels of medication.

Because of the high priority given to seizure control, one is tempted to paraphrase A. E. Housman comparing malt and Milton and say the Dilantin does more than Freud can for temporal-lobe or sub-ictal epilepsy. But the sad truth is that these patients need both, and misdiagnosis often keeps both from them. The victim of temporal-lobe epilepsy may no longer experience hallucinations or blackouts when the required dosage of anti-convulsant medication is administered, but attendant problems of anxiety, withdrawal, sensitivity, and impaired social relations will remain and those are within the province of psychotherapy. And in many, perhaps most, cases medication alone may not be sufficient either to control seizures or for those patients who exhibit both seizure and behavioral problems.

The experience of covert seizure phenomena—those that do not become obvious—impairs the sense of body integrity, sharpens fears of vulnerability, lowers confidence, impedes independent action, and leads to fear of intimacy in relationships. Persons so afflicted are unable to establish autonomy, and require protracted dependency. Their conflict is intensely painful; their cerebral dysfunction heightens their dependency while making them dread the closeness that dependency involves. The patient may cling to the parents or a mate, while railing against over-protectiveness. The parents may apply more pressure for independence than the patient can tolerate. The patient may persist in a destructive relationship with a single person because that person accepts his dependency and is aware of and not repelled by the seizure manifestations. Intimacy fears and dependency-autonomy conflicts are the usual foci in psychotherapy of the epileptic patient. The fears and conflicts often must be interpreted to the patient so that he comes to understand them as concomitants of the cerebral pathology. Such explanations may provide the motivation the patient requires to embark upon a re-education program rather than to seek the resolution of some vague or non-existent intrapsychic conflict.

Psychotherapy often should focus upon the reality of the seizure behavior, helping the patient to break through denial to accept the fact of his disorder, to understand its manifestations and to facilitate cooperation with medication and relaxation regimens.

Causes and precipitants are identified and the patient is helped to avoid them or to develop more effective means of mitigating them. The seizure patient tends to increase stress by attempting to fight off the seizure and its manifestations and so increases the probability of the seizure occurrence and it intensity. Increasing relaxation by accepting the seizure can have a minimizing effect.

Where anxiety is associated with the seizure experience and threatens ego disruption, the patient is helped to ask for help, for companionship.

Monroe (48) has written most extensively about the psychotherapy of severe episodic behavioral disorders. His observations are equally applicable to most instances of the more moderated disturbances.

The therapist's expectations about outcome profoundly influence the actual outcome. So if the therapist is pessimistic about amelioration of organically related emotional problems and believes that the patient cannot improve, the outcome predictably tends in that direction. Prognosis is more favorable as the patient's behavior and adjustment in intervals between episodes is normal. Keeping this interval-behavior in mind helps the therapist establish a more optimistic expectation.

Some patients who view their emotional problem as organically caused may have insufficient superego and psychotherapy may have to first make the behavior ego-alien, and then increase the patient's feelings of responsibility for the behavior. Obviously, this is likely to increase anxiety. Monroe attempts to minimize this consequence by focusing upon the patient's needs rather than his narcissism, by creating an atmosphere of acceptance of the patient's needs as normal and justified, that it is proper to feel hostility, anxiety, dependency. Without identifying the patient's intensity of needs as pathological. he encourages substitute or alternative gratifications. The approach combats resistance, presents the therapist as an ally rather than a critic, and at the same time encourages alienation from maladaptive behavior. In harmony with this approach, the patient is not terminated if he flouts the usual rules of psychotherapy to the extent that they are patterned after psychoanalytic procedures. The therapist looks for dyscontrol behavior within the therapeutic setting, overlooks minor ones at first so as not to arouse resistance or rationalization, and works with the more serious ones. Where drive control should be improved, specific psychopharmacological aids may be introduced, but where there is a strong psychodynamic motivation, insight into the drive and working through contribute to control. The patient is helped to understand why the expression of normally sublimated urges and impulses arouses anxiety in him. A capacity to express this level of drive is developed and thus avoids the build-up of affect, impulse, and tension that otherwise erupts as a dyscontrol act.

Where acting out is a major component of the patient's dyscontrol behavior, resisting manipulation may become important. In this approach, the therapist expresses concern for the patient's welfare but emphasizes that the patient's self-concern should be greater than the therapist's concern for him. Monroe prefers the pupil-teacher model, as in music, indicating that only through hard work and practice will the patient improve, that new learning through re-education is their joint goal. The patient's acceptance of this approach may be impaired by a simultaneous medication regimen. Reliance upon the drug as a magical cure may diminish the patient's tolerance for the longer and harder pull of psychotherapy. Or a patient may feel that the use of drugs means that the therapist is seeking a short cut out of disinterest in the patient. The re-education process is emphasized, in which the role of drugs as a facilitator of re-learning in their ability to diminish the intensity of interfering affects that overwhelm cognition is made clear.

The therapist must also be alert to the twin dangers of drug habituation and rejection of drugs. Intense orality is a frequent concomitant of some seizure patients; and with them the deleterious effect on progress of inconsiderate drug use is stressed. With those patients who refuse to take the drugs Monroe recommends focusing upon the sense of childish rebellion and the guilty, obsequious manner with which the transgression may be reported. In my experience drug refusal may occur for a variety of reasons: the patient may experience alarming alterations of self-image as a result of idiosyncratic drug effects; he may feel that the drug is not being effective; he may have always been resistant to any drug ingestion; he may be phobic about medications.

Finally, Monroe warns that the psychotherapist of the dyscontrol patient must possess an "unusual degree of equanimity and self-confidence" to tolerate the larger risk that his patent's dyscontrol behavior will evoke criticism of the therapist in the community and from the patient's family and friends. Severely pathological dyscontrol behavior by the patient may damage the therapist's reputation; the therapist who needs to play it safe cannot treat this type of patient.

The seemingly inexplicable eruptive, bizarre behavior of many seizure patients may arouse anxiety in the therapist that compels him back into the security of established psychodynamic interpretations, however ineffective they may be, or arouse a policeman-like vigilance and reprimanding attitude about the patient's behavior and his excessive reliance upon or his rejection of medication. So, while striving for therapeutic success, the therapist must accept the reality of possible failure and continuously examine his own behavior and his countertransference tendencies. A stance of therapeutic flexibility must include a willingness to depart from the usual one-to-one relationship to include joint and family sessions where interrelational stresses are contributing, and to muster adjunctive therapeutic means—vocational, educative, rehabilitative, and environmental (65).

CASE ILLUSTRATIONS

Temporal-lobe epilepsy and the subictal states are the great mimics among neuropsychological disorders. They resemble anxiety, hysteria, depression, and schizophrenia, indeed an array of emotional and behavioral disorders; these depend upon the pre-existing personality of the patient, the functional area of the brain where the "firing" occurs, and the speed at which excitation spreads in the brain tissue.

Such conditions are therefore those most likely to be of concern in a psychotherapeutic practice. They are, in my experience, the most frequently encountered of the equivocal neurological conditions. For this reason the extensive case material presented illustrates the varieties of manifestations, to alert the clinician to the mimicry and to the need for diagnostic skepticism.

1. *A seemingly schizophrenic girl is found to have symptoms strongly suggestive of temporal-lobe epilepsy, which responds to anti-convulsant medication despite negative EEG readings, so that a therapeutic diagnosis is obtained.*

K., a seventeen-year-old girl, was referred by a psychiatrist friend of her parents, after being in treatment for about a year with a psychiatrist, who recently told her parents that K. was schizophrenic, suicidal, and homicidal. He had arrived at a final diagnosis of Ambulatory Paranoid Schizophrenic. The referring psychiatrist doubted this diagnosis, but believed that the girl was severely schizoid.

She is the younger of fraternal twin girls. When one year old, she underwent exploratory surgery for stomach cancer. Her parents were told that the prognosis was hopeless, and thereafter she underwent intensive x-ray treatments. For seven years she visited hospitals frequently for tests and checkups. She has been considered cured for the past 10 years.

At first meeting, K. seemed very shy, sweet in manner, unusually poetic and literary in her references and style of speech. She was about to be graduated from high school and had been accepted at a local college. But school had become impossible for her. Social relations had been very difficult for her all of her life. She felt that she was not in tune with the life style of her classmates. She had always been able to attract boys, however. She was close to, dependent upon, and ambivalent about her twin sister, who was both supportive of her and irritated with her. An older brother was away from the home and married. He had made several serious sexual proposals to K., which, while she was tempted to accept, she had declined. Her father was described as a sweet, compliant man, who allowed the mother to dominate. The mother was obviously a severely acting out individual; with the knowledge of all the children and the husband she had been having an affair. K. denied that she had any feelings about this. The father had ulcers; the mother had had hypoglycemia and endocrine imbalances. K. described her as tense and labile. In the past she would scream and hit K. at the slightest provocation. Since successful treatment for the hypoglycemia, her mother was calmer, more loving and supportive.

K. complained of crushing depressions and episodes that we came to call "Blue Meanies." These involved feelings of uncertainty about who and what she was. She would feel removed from the present moment, that she was powerless and would remain so for the rest of her life. Then came tremendous anxiety in which she was fearful of being alone. She had given up smoking marijuana and using aspirin, because both were associated, she believed, with these strange events, although they often happened independently of their use.

K. complained that she had not been able to read for several years, that she was unable to concentrate upon a book, that she became irritable and restless when she tried to read.

K. had used Dexamyl with beneficial results, but its effect was no longer apparent. A physician had prescribed Ambar, a combination of amphetamines and barbiturates. This was now her magic drug; it kept her from going into these strange episodes. After taking it, she feared the diminution of its effect as presaging the onset of an episode. Her intake of this drug was slowly and steadily increasing.

These Wechsler Adult Intelligence Scale (WAIS) "scale" scores were obtained during the diagnostic work-up:

Information	14	Digit Symbol	14
Comprehension	11	Picture Completion	11
Arithmetic	7	Block Design	12
Similarities	13	Object Assembly	5
Digit Span	10		
Vocabulary	16		

(Picture Arrangement was not administered because of time pressure.)

A striking feature is the disparity between the scale score of 5 for Object Assembly and 14 for Information. The average scale score for the major verbal functions is 13, for attention-memory functions it is 10, for perceptual-analytic ones it is nine. This is a relatively moderate spread, thus only moderately suspicious of organicity. The Object Assembly-Information disparity was alerting, however, to the possibility of a perceptual-analytic impairment, most evident where she was called upon to integrate parts into a whole without a guide. A moderate impairment of attention-memory is also suggested. Nothing else in the psychological examination that included the Rorschach, the Thematic Apperception Test, the Bender Visual Motor Gestalt Test, and the Human-Figure Drawings was suggestive of organicity, other than this WAIS-scale score examination.

All too apparent was depression, focused in a great rage that her body had been violated, that she was vulnerable to attacks, that she was frightened, and in turn enormously infuriated. Her view of the world, of relationships between people, of her own vulnerability is perhaps best portrayed in her response to Rorschach Card X: "Sort of like a war." Object relations were obviously severely disturbed. There was no test evidence of a thought disorder or of impaired reality perception and testing.

Very early in the therapeutic relationship, it was possible to get a detailed account from K. of her experience in a "Blue Meanie": "I got a deep sinking feeling; my heart dropped to my toes, then I felt a slow series of explosions, but they were not orderly, they were disorganized. I'm into it in a flash; then I'm in a different state of mind; I'm a different kind of person. At the height of this, not before, it's sort of convulsive feeling, not a panic, but very slowed down, moving is slow. My head and eye movements are all very slow. But with the slowness I feel convulsive inside. I will stagger if I walk. My body seems to drain out and into my hands; they tingle, mostly the fingers and the palms. Then I feel that I'm sick and that I may die. I don't come out of it as fast as I go into it, but sometimes I do come out of it fast and I feel that I'm K. again, and I'm so happy that I could kiss the floor."

Neurological Findings

The report from the neurologist stated in part: "Neurological examination reveals a small, quiet, somewhat withdrawn, and defensive individual. Spontaneous motor activity well performed, gait and station normal, muscle status appears intact except that the patellar DTRs are symmetrically and markedly hyperactive. Cerebellar system is intact. Sensory system is intact; cranial nerves intact.

"The electroencephalogram . . . reveals a normal recording.

"The history of episodes of unfamiliarity, unreality, distorted percepts, and anxiety is strongly suggestive of temporal-lobe abnormality. To be sure, this could be of psychological origin, but in view of being a twin, the age of onset and periodicity of the episodes, her sensitivity to alcohol, dexidrin (sic!), etc., and the hyperactive patellar DTRs, I feel these may very well be temporal-lobe seizures due to transient cerebral anoxia at birth. It would have been helpful had the EEG shown some abnormalities. The normal EEG is not of any value, as a number of abnormalities has been recorded from the hippocampal regions with depth electrodes which have failed to show up on scalp recordings. I would definitely recommend treating this patient as suffering Temporal-Lobe Seizures and put her on Dilantin O.1 b.i.d. for a three-month trial period."

Relatively large doses of both Dilantin and Dexedrine were necessary to bring these phenomena under control. K.'s intake of Dilantin was increased to 400 mgs., a moderately heavy dose, the Dexedrine to

30 mgs. The seizures have ceased. K. has been successfully employed as a legal secretary for more than two years. She reads with great pleasure. Her social relations are still very disturbed, depression remains. These two major problems are the focus of continued psychotherapy.

2. *Auditory and olfactory hallucinations, lapses, and automatic behavior in a school boy lead to positive neurological and EEG findings.*

F., 12, is referred by his school. Information accompanying the referral is that the parents and a younger sister are in therapy, that F. tends to withdraw, that he appears not to trust his parents, that he feels ganged-up on by other students, and that his academic work is good. A recommendation concerning advisability of psychotherapy is requested.

F. is a charming, open, sociable, observant, reactive lad. He acknowledged that he at times became sad and attributed it to being bullied by older boys in the school. This he said was his only problem. He stated explicitly that matters were "just great," at home.

There appeared to have been considerable improvement in intellectual functioning and integration since F. was tested three years earlier. The most significant change had occurred in Comprehension in which he moved from an original scale score of nine to one of 15, now achieving a prorated I.Q. of 131 in this function. His abilities in concept formation, abstract thinking, and in arithmetic processes were excellent. As a consequence of the general improvement, his I.Q. scores had improved seven points on the Verbal Scale, 13 points on the Performance Scale and 11 points on the Full Scale. There was still some Verbal specialization over the Performance Scale, but this differential had decreased moderately in the intervening years.

A possible visual dysfunction was suggested as F. began to work on the Digit Symbol subtest. He perceived the numeral 1 as 7. He tended to overlook errors for quite some time, but did scan his work before he gave up on it, often finding the error and correcting it. F. did better when he was permitted to make a conceptualization entirely within his mind, without the need for achieving congruence with an external model or stimulus. He did better, for example, with the assembly of familiar objects at a prorated I.Q. of 128 than he did with Block Design at a prorated I.Q. of 114, where he must conform with a printed card. The same observation applied to the Bender

Visual Motor Gestalt drawings where he did somewhat better on reproduction from memory than he did on direct copy.

His poorest function appeared to be in attention and memory for recent auditory material. Despite a dogged, perseverating effort to succeed in this latter test, his work for him was relatively poor at a prorated I.Q. of 113.

His Bender Visual Motor Gestalt drawings suggested a cerebral dysfunction. There were distortions, he employed circles for dots, he perseverated in drawing the figures, the figures collided with each other, and there was generally poor management of the space allocated for the drawings.

In similar fashion, the body image appeared to be immature and poorly developed.

F. operated under a moderate degree of visible tension: he hummed, sang and exclaimed, "Oh dear" almost continuously as he worked.

A conflict in relationship to his father appeared to be central to his personality development. He portrayed the father as a brave, aggressive, domineering man, and told how his father scared off a burglar by snapping cartridges into a revolver for which the father has a license. F. seemed to anticipate severe physical punishment from his father, anticipating that his father might deal with him as unequivocally, dramatically and as harshly as he dealt with the would-be burglar. He had a strong wish to rebel against the father, but the danger involved was apparently great enough to abort whatever rebellious feelings he generated. He was left, however, with hostile feelings towards his father which caused him a great deal of trouble. They led to placatory behavior at times, but have also led to the development of considerable passive-aggressive, negativistic behavior.

With this there was a feeling on F.'s part that he is persecuted, so he was extremely sensitive to the possibility that he was being bullied. He became depressed rather easily. He had developed a capacity for denying that he felt bad, was in danger or that he was troubled.

There was evidence of an intense degree of emotional responsiveness in F. which contributed to his conflict since it put him in the danger of impulsively defying authority, so he tended to withdraw to protect himself from both external and internal dangers.

Basically, his relationships with people were good and had potentiality for development. He identified with people and had a wish to be with them; there was nothing schizoid or characterologically withdrawn about this lad.

The intense affect noted may have had an emotional basis, but it also may have been related to possible seizure phenomena which were elicited on interviewing. F. described himself as clumsy and unathletic; he rather often fell down steps and bumped into things. His earliest memory was of falling down the stairs when he was four years of age. He said he was not hurt but he was very much shaken by the experience. He occasionally heard high pitched sounds. He may have experienced phosphenes (flashing lights which appear to pass the side of his face in a dark room). He reported severe headaches, which were responsive to moderate medication. He got dizzy rather frequently but without loss of consciousness. He reported automatic behavior, and told of one experience, when having last remembered himself in the grape arbor of his home, he became aware of suddenly being in front of the television set in the house, and not recalling how he had gotten there. He reported what may be blackouts, an inability to respond when called, when he must be sharply nudged by someone's elbow. He experienced what may have been altered states of consciousness in which he was awake, yet in a dreamlike state so intense that he had to be pushed to be brought out of it, not responding to the calling of his name. He described something like convulsive feelings in the abdomen. He was extremely sensitive to noise, finding that even his favorite music becomes noisy and unpleasant on occasion. He described sensitivity to smell, that the pleasant odor of his favorite food will suddenly "smell like skunk." He said, "I seem to be dreaming when the steak smells like skunk, and as soon as I stop, it smells better and I am able to eat it." Interviewing failed to elicit any data suggestive of a traumatic or febrile event in his life. It was advised that the parents and the pediatrician be queried for possible etiological events.

Neurological Investigation

The psychological test data and the accompanying interview material suggested that a neurological exploration was advisable. Among the material sent to the psychologist was an electroencephalogram report performed a few months before and interpreted as being within normal limits for the age of the child. However, a sleep recording was not reported, and such a reading was considered important. In addition, a clinical assessment of behavioral and cerebral functions was recommended as part of the diagnostic work-up. Once the neurological probabilities were clarified, the advisability of psychotherapy for **F.** could be considered.

Neurological consultation was obtained, with the following report:

"On questioning, the patient stated that he had 'trances.' At intervals of two to four weeks, he has episodes which last from seconds to minutes, during which he performs purposive behavior for which he is later amnesic. He has somewhat more frequent, briefer episodes, during which the alteration in consciousness is only partial. 'It is like daydreaming.' Towards the end of these briefer episodes, he may experience an intensification or distortion of normal perception. He specifically relates episodes in which substances which normally smell very pleasant to him appear to have an extremely unpleasant repellent odor, and states that immediately after he experiences this sensation the seizure terminates.

"The patient's mother stated that he was the older of two children, born at term in a normal spontaneous delivery. There were no complications of pregnancy or delivery. His birth weight was 8 pounds, 7 ounces. He showed no abnormalities as a newborn child.

"He has had no serious illnesses. No head injury. No convulsions. His growth and development were all within normal limits, and he was speaking clearly by the age of one year.

"He does not make many physical complaints, rarely has headaches, or abdominal pain. His vision is normal with glasses. He has been described as being somewhat clumsy.

"The family history includes one paternal uncle who is said to have had some kind of convulsive episodes, which were believed to be post-traumatic.

"On examination he was alert, oriented, and cooperative. The mental status was entirely normal. Speech was clear and coherent. No evidence of aphasia.

"The cranial-nerve functions were intact.

"Strength and coordination were normal. There were no abnormal involuntary movements.

"Deep and cutaneous sensation was normal. The deep tendon reflexes were active and equal. Flexor plantar responses.

"The electroencephalogram was abnormal, showing non-focal paroxysmal characteristics.

"There is a clear-cut clinical history of psychomotor seizures, and this clinical diagnosis is confirmed, to some extent, by the abnormal-ities seen in the EEG.

"A trial at medication with Dilantin, 100 milligrams, two to three times daily is indicated. If the episodes persist, other medications may be tried."

3. *A man married to an epileptic woman begins to manifest seizure behavior. Pronounced feminine identification suggests an hysterical basis, while other phenomena indicate a true seizure disorder. Finally, a positive EEG is obtained and the seizures stop when he is treated with Dilantin.*

J., 43, was referred for vocational rehabilitation following a series of very short psychiatric hospitalizations. His diagnosis was said to be Latent Schizophrenia, with Depression. When 22, the patient mar-ried a young woman with whom he was very much in love, and whom he laughingly called his twin because they physically resembled each other. He became increasingly dependent and depressed. His wife re-lated that he would sit with head bowed and cry for hours, and that he stopped having sex with her. Much time elapsed before she became aware that he was seriously depressed and not rejecting her. The wife was epileptic and had many seizures before they were controlled.

The agency psychologist reported:

"The patient is a nice looking man in a somewhat poetic, artistic style. He has an appealing charisma. He seems sad and burdened; his responses often are accompanied by expressions of labor, as if he must overcome a difficulty in order to assert himself. One is impressed immediately with the idea that he has a problem in assertion or a strong orientation toward passivity.

"The intelligence-test material indicates that he is of superior level intellectual potentiality; this is evidenced by the prorated I.Q. of 141 he obtains in ability to conceptualize: Information is at a pro-rated I.Q. of 123, Comprehension shows a marked impairment; it was here that his difficulty in expressing himself emerged. There is suspi-cion of a thought disorder, but it is not quite manifest; it is more implied. There is a deficit also in attention-memory: he obtains a prorated I.Q. of 100 in Digit Span and 105 in Digit Symbol. Per-ceptual-analytic functions are also impaired: Picture Completion is at a prorated I.Q. of 92. The suggestion here is primarily of impairment of reality perception and testing, but again this is only a soft sign.

"The Bender is not much help in making a differential diagnosis. It tends primarily to indicate that perceptual-analytic functions are intact. It does point to a moderate degree of obsessiveness, but this is not a predominant feature.

"The Thematic Apperception Test stories are highly revealing. The difficulties of assertion and aggression are quite evident. A latent homosexual trend of considerable weight is also evident. Confused sexual identification is clear; he seems to long to be a woman, to be as graceful, as beautiful, as attractive as he thinks women are. The consequence, however, is threatening to him. He is depressed both by his wish to be a woman and by the fact that he cannot permit himself to be so. He makes it clear that the woman in some ways is a castrated human being; he wishes to elevate her to his position or lower himself to hers. So he says for the frankly sexual card: 'Why do you expose your body to me? I wish to tune into your mind also. I try to see you as an equal to me, as a person in the world. That's how I wish to identify myself with you at the outset.'

"Early memories indicate a rather obscure medical history in childhood which may have early damaged the body-image ego. He recalls childhood dreams of recurrent nature which indicate a passive identification. A recent dream is of a person having a seizure; the seizure stops and another person comes into view carrying a human body.

"He considers his best trait now to be a feeling of freedom and awareness; he is not as preoccupied with himself as he used to be. He relates the onset of this freedom to a specific moment in January, 1967. He was at a union hiring hall; he had gone to the coffee shop and suddenly began to feel tremors in his body. Words came to him as signs and symbols: 'receptor, eyes, sun, ears.' He says it was like a revelation; he felt 'high' and good. He called his psychotherapist who told him he ought to sign himself into a hospital. He told him that it was a good feeling, that he would call him again that night. Later he did; he felt good, he said, but strange. Again his therapist said sign in, and he did. He indicates this experience was like a transformation.

"He experiences strong tingling sensations in the right arm. He also reports what he calls an aura, and says it is like a spell. He says 'I am aware of what is going on. It is not a dulling sensation, but it does overshadow my full consciousness. I can be sitting here and talking to you; I can see you and I can hear you, but I have to bear with this feeling. People tell me my eyes twitch also when this happens. My daughter has seen this happen to me.'

"He then indicates that his wife had *grand mal* epilepsy, until it was controlled by medication and is now a *petit mal*.

"There is a need for differential diagnosis. The phenomena indicated could be on either or both a psychogenic or neurological basis. It would be important to evaluate the neurological before relying solely upon the psychogenic. The psychogenic basis would seem to involve his passive, feminine identification and his wish to be a female, to experience what she does sexually. He appears to equate the female orgastic experience with an epileptic seizure. This in itself suggests a thought disorder of a psychotic nature. Depression is also very real and will have to be accounted for, but he does not seem to be in great danger of suicide because of his excellent object relatedness and his ability to seek help when he needs it."

An agency psychiatrist then saw the patient and concluded that the patient was delusional:

"J. reported having had some kind of experience during his sleep two nights ago and also during his time at the shop yesterday, apparently became ill, was trembling, his lips turned blue, though he was conscious and aware of what was happening and subsequently, on the way to the hospital, had several episodes of vomiting. Nevertheless, after that, he apparently felt well and when examined at K. Hospital, nothing could be found that was out of order.

"In discussing what transpired with this man, he related similar concerns about what might have happened to him through the night on two different occasions. This had been reported to the people who are taking care of him and they had gotten an EEG. He claims that that was normal. It became clear as he spoke about his symptoms that he clearly had delusional ideas about their meaning and their significance and also related the beginning of some of his unusual bodily experiences to about a year ago, when he had a rather unpleasant experience with his wife. At that time, he had gone to her apartment, refused to leave, and had to be forcibly ejected by the police.

"In going over his description of symptoms rather carefully, I cannot elicit any real evidence of seizure. This man has experienced other people's seizures, particularly those of his wife, who is epileptic, and clearly makes all kinds of delusional connections, and one cannot help but feel that there is some dynamic involved here which precipitates something akin to a seizure in him. He certainly does not view what happens to him as a seizure.

"He is oriented and cooperative and speaks quite freely. However, as one gets farther and farther into the discussion with him, it becomes clear that he is quite delusional. He has many notions about soul, freedom, his body, that these things are manifestations of his freedom and the like. It is rather difficult to follow, although he is firmly convinced of them. I have no doubt that this man is schizophrenic."

A second psychiatrist concluded that the patient was "anhedonic," but kept open the differential diagnosis between a functional and an organic aberration.

A third psychiatrist viewed the clinical picture somewhat differently and insisted upon additional neurological investigation:

"The current question is whether the patient could possibly have a seizure disorder. Apparently, the patient periodically has episodes in which he feels his eyes are twitching and has paraesthesias in his fingers. He also gets a funny warm sensation in his lower abdomen and genitals. He has never lost consciousness nor has he seen the room going around. However, he occasionally has spots in front of his eyes, but there are no other visual phenomena.

"The patient has no depressions at present, although he occasionally gets depressed for a few hours at the time. He feels good when he is with his friends and generally feels fairly well. He sleeps well and has good and bad dreams. A recent dream is one in which there were two human forms, a larger one witnessing the smaller one having a seizure. He says that he was both the observer and the person having the seizure. Patient also says that these episodes of seizure-like nature may be related to his being upset by seeing grief, sadness, and despair in the eyes and gestures of other people, particularly the people he has in the group therapy sessions with him.

"There has been an EEG, awake only, which has been read as normal.

"I think that we cannot rule out the possibility of the patient having a seizure disorder, despite the fact that his wife had one and there may be some identification with her and the fact that he has rather bizarre thinking and some concrete ideation which would indicate a schizophrenic process. I think what we should do is ask for a repeated EEG both awake and asleep. I think we should then try him on a trial of Dilantin for two months and see how he responds to this. Following that, I would either add or substitute phenothiazines such as Prolixin or Stelazine in combination with an anti-depressant if necessary. I think that the sequence of medication should be anti-convulsant and then a phenothiazine. I think the first order of business is to get a sleep EEG and then try medication regardless of the outcome."

Two weeks later this psychiatrist again reported:

"J. was seen today an a semi-emergency basis. Apparently last night while sitting in a launderette, the patient experienced a warm feeling in the lower part of his abdomen and genitals and a tingling sensation in his right hand. He also had a funny sensation in his head. He then could not continue reading and had difficulty concentrating. He also bit his tongue during this episode. I would suspect this is again a minor seizure, characteristic of what I think is the patient's seizure disorder."

Neurological Findings

"J. is still being followed in Neurology Clinic at X Hospital. The doctors there are not certain that his episodes are true seizures, but they recommend that he continue to take Dilantin, and that he not operate any potentially dangerous machinery at the present time.

"Although J. had an abnormal sleep EEG, his neurological examination, skull x-rays, and brain scan were all normal. Thus, there is no evidence of progressive neurological disease at present. He will continue to be reevaluated in this respect at intervals in Neurology Clinic.

"In addition to Dilantin 100 mgs. t.i.d., J. currently takes Mellaril 100 mgs. at bedtime."

One month later the psychiatrist offered a summary report indicating that the seizure phenomena have ceased, that the patient is no longer depressed, although he experiences loneliness. A tendency to a thought disorder of mild degree is noted.

CASE VIGNETTES

The summarized cases that follow illustrate further the variety of the problems in differential diagnosis once the diagnostician is aware that a symptom or syndrome may arise from more than a single cause. While the data here will seem inconclusive and one will be left wondering, "What is this?" this sense of diagnostic bewilderment is more desirable when the patient's condition is an ambiguous one than is a false diagnostic certainty.

Anxiety or Epilepsy?

A referring psychiatrist insisted that the patient suffered from "free floating" anxiety and prescribed Librium. Her background had been extremely traumatic, with mentally-ill parents and institutionalization for her at an early age. Psychodiagnostic assessment identified the anxiety and depression, but also a marked perceptual confusion that required differential diagnosis. Both a history and symptomatology of neurological significance were obtained. She had suffered two head injuries, at ages five and eleven, that resulted in unconsciousness. On one occasion she suddenly and inexplicably struck a companion. Severe headaches were a frequent occurrence and were becoming worse. She experienced blackouts, dizziness, nausea, blurring of vision, tingling in the fingers, altered states of consciousness, and a prescient feeling that something terrible was going to happen to her—not a visitation from the outside but within her. The referring psychiatrist rejected the "psychological" findings. However, he acquiesced in obtaining neurological consultation when the agency psychiatrist concluded after his examination, "The clinical picture psychiatrically is that of emotional instability which is probably secondary to her cerebral dysfunction and probably secondary to familial dysfunction." The patient responded quickly to anti-convulsant medication, her social worker reported, feeling vastly better, finding employment that enabled her to leave the welfare rolls, and establishing a promising relationship with a man.

*   *   *

A 17-year-old youth suffered an intensification of anxiety after the ending of a homosexual love affair, during which his academic performance had improved. After the affair ended, he became anxious and depressed and his work deteriorated. Psychodynamic roots of both homosexuality and anxiety were visible in a phallically competitive attitude to his deceased father and a view of women as deformed and grotesque. Intensity of affect and impulsivity were indicated in an account of fire-setting when he was six or seven. When pushed to do something—by a teacher, parents, a boss, a friend—he became tense, random and "flightly." As he becomes anxious he begins to hyperventilate; if this continues he faints. Intellectually, he functioned uniformly at a rather high level, with signs that were he less anxious he would function at an even higher level. No dysfunctions suggestive of a cerebral dysfunction were observed. He had undergone surgery twice: an eye operation when six and a tonsilectomy at an unrecalled age (both of possible dynamic import). Occasionally he experiences ringing sounds, numbness in one toe, and easily aroused anger. Neurological signs were so equivocal that the diagnosis of Anxiety Neurosis was favored and reliance placed upon psychotherapy.

*   *   *

A woman of 27 is referred for psychodiagnostic assessment to help determine if her career difficulties are the result of anxiety, which is clear, or a thought disorder, which is suspected. She cannot maintain concentration upon a task because of anxiety, fails to complete her assignments, loses jobs or isn't promoted. Her therapist is concerned that a borderline thought disorder is producing her anxiety; the thought disorder is suspected because of curious use of words and odd expressions.

No evidence of a thought disorder was found on testing. Extraordinarily high verbal skills resulted in a Verbal I.Q. of 140. Despite her reputed difficulty in maintaining concentration, all the subtests of the attention triad—Arithmetic, Digit Span, and Digit Symbol—were well performed, with scale scores of 17, 15, and 19 respectively. However, she complained of fatigue on the Digit Symbol subtest, which she completed before time ran out. Against these high levels, an impairment in spatial visualization was found, with Block Design at a scale score of 12, Object Assembly at 10. Even when given an opportunity to see that her construction was erroneous on Block Design, she failed to do so. She had great difficulty for a person of her verbal level in explaining the meaning of "He shouted the warning." Difficulty in accepting a feminine identification was indicated. Intense affective experiences were reacted to with disgust, and fear that she would be abandoned. As expected, an intensely conflictual relationship with the mother was depicted.

In addition to fatiguing on Digit Symbol, semantic difficulties with an unusual statement, and marked constructional difficulty, she reported that even when tired she could not rest because of hyperkinesis, and that eye movement caused lassitude, forgetting, and restlessness. She has difficulty answering questions because she is uncertain of their meaning. She frequently loses balance, stumbles, bumps into things. She sees double, her vision blurs, and when tired her eyes seem to cross. She hears ringing sounds, and experiences sizzling-like sensations in the right hand only, especially in the index finger. She describes episodes that may be blackouts, automatic behavior, and aura-like experiences that fill her with dread.

She likens the latter to explosive feelings that never erupt. She is compelled to stop and rest until the feeling passes. She becomes irritated and enraged without cause. When 16 she had measles, with a very high fever and her vision was poor for two weeks thereafter.

Neurological examination was recommended; continuation of psychotherapy was deemed advisable.

* * *

An established history of seizures until the age of 12 was discounted in the patient, now 35, when he could not remain at work because of anxiety. His parents and siblings were all high-school graduates but he had been unable to remain in school beyond his 13th year. Evidence for a psychogenic base to his disturbance could not be obtained. An attention impairment was apparent in the average scale score (WISC) of 2.5 in these functions, in contrast to 5.5 in both verbal and perceptual-analytic functions, both of which, however, were adversely affected by a memory deficit. Specifically oriented interviewing elicited the circumstances that precede his bouts of anxiety: he first begins to get dizzy, the environment appears to turn and tilt. He sees double and is made tense by moving lights, and has "jumping feelings" in his finger tips. An EEG was requested. and a "left temporal slow wave focus" was found.

Psychosis or Epilepsy?

A 26-year-old mother of three young children born out-of-wedlock suffered severe depression after being deserted by her common-law husband. She hallucinated voices telling her to kill herself, although she was able to resist their instructions. An examining psychiatrist noted that no gross delusions were observed, and that while the patient was depressed, her judgment was reasonably good. Diagnostically, he considered her a chronic schizophrenic who was not a suicidal risk. Medications—Mellaril and Tofranil—were not relieving her depression significantly, and she had discontinued the use of Mellaril because of the adverse side effects.

Subsequent observation brought out a number of possible paroxysmal phenomena. She reported several experiences of fainting, during each of which she was unconscious for a relatively long time. She suffered severe frontal headaches accompanied by nausea, unrelieved by aspirin. Objects around her and the floor often appeared to tilt, making her hold on to keep from falling down. She saw colors when she knew that colored objects were not present. At the workshop where she was involved in a rehabilitation program, she experienced dizziness but had not complained to anyone. The patient was aware of feeling unreasonable rage and stated that her rage was inappropriate. She reported paraesthesias in both fingers and toes. Despite medication and availability of psychotherapeutic services she was terrified at night, hearing voices that tell her to kill herself. She was afraid to sleep, saying, "I need a friend to stay with me during the night."

Psychiatric and psychological consultants agreed that the patient did not appear to be a schizophrenic personality, but rather was essentially a primitive, dependent girl who might be suffering seizure phenomena that should be investigated.

*   *   *

A 27-year-old woman is referred to a vocation-training agency from a state mental hospital with a diagnosis of Schizophrenia, chronic undifferentiated type. Ambitious and perceptive, she had suffered enormous damage to her self-esteem for many years because of a learning difficulty, having been put in a class for retarded children. She became depressed. The family culture appears to have been restricted and punitive. Both her vocabulary and grammatical usage suggested that she was at least of above average intellectual ability. This impression was somewhat substantiated when she achieved a prorated I.Q. of 105 in the Similarity subtest of the WAIS. However, no other function came close to that level. She was severely impaired in the Verbal area, with Information and Comprehension scores falling in the mental-defective level. Recognition of essential details was poor, the assembly of familiar objects was moderately good. She complained of poor peripheral motor control, which appeared in the Digit Symbol subtest.

Concentration and memory were poor, with a prorated I.Q. of 64 in the Digit Span subtest.

This patient presented a diagnostic conflict. She reported hallucinatory experiences in childhood which could have had a cultural determinant. It had been her custom to fall asleep in a rocking chair on the porch before going to bed, and so what she described may have been hypnogogic phenomena. In one, a ghost came after her, but her mother and godmother "both saw the ghost," pulled her into the house, and saved her.

Recently, while on a subway train, while thinking about the unfairness and critical attitudes of her first husband and his mother, she suddenly felt drained of energy and strength; she could speak only at a slow pace and volume, and she felt she could walk only at a very slow pace. She was convinced that she was losing her mind. Interviewing around neurological phenomena indicated that she experienced occasional blurring of the vision and dizziness (for example, she cannot play with her children because if she turns her body one complete 360 degree turn she becomes dizzy), floor tilting, a whistling sound in the left ear only and excessive clumsiness.

*   *   *

A 44-year-old woman entered a psychiatric hospital after one of her two sons was convicted on a narcotics charge. It became known that she had been experiencing auditory hallucinations for at least 15 years, but had never sought psychiatric help before this. She reported that a brain tumor had been suspected at one time, and that she had recently undergone a hysterectomy. She belonged to a spiritualist group with which she spent a great deal of time. Her diagnosis was Schizophrenic Reaction with depressive features. When seen at a rehabilitation center after the hospitalization, the patient appeared to be alert, responsive, and socially competent. She did not impress as being schizophrenic in the usual ways associated with that term. She was hypochondriacal, and complained immediately of sweating, then revealed that she had high blood pressure, which she stated fluctuated a great deal. She reported numbness in the extremities, she fainted or had been close to fainting often, she experienced tilting sensation when lying in bed, severe headaches, and blurred vision. Moving lights produced momentary blackouts. She reported what might be altered states of consciousness which incorporated an aura phenomena. She said that she had "feelings of nervousness inside me and I am upset as if

I had been hit by a car." She described an episode in which she saw a car coming from a place she knew a car could not be coming from, yet it seemed real to her. She crossed the street, this time to see a car coming along the street, and had a vision of its running into her. She knows that these are visions, that they are not real, and feels that they are an omen of bad things to come. Most interesting were experiences of automatic writing, even though writing is difficult for her and was the skill hardest for her to learn. In one episode she wrote several pages automatically and was aware of fatigue in her wrist when she became conscious of what had been going on.

*   *   *

Following the break-up of an affair, a 25-year-old woman withdrew into isolation. After a year and a half she sought help because she feared increasing deterioration and that she was "losing my mind." She began to take amphetamines, first as a diet pill, but became dependent upon them for any functioning at all. Without the amphetamines she would lie in bed and "just feel dead"; with them she at least was able to move around. She had an inner panicky feeling, a nameless dread. She was afraid to go out, but more afraid to be alone. The diagnostic problem appeared to be differentiation between depression or the severe anxiety of a schizophrenic type of break. Specific interviewing, however, revealed a possible complication of the diagnostic picture by neurological features.

She had been told that during infancy she suffered a head injury in a fall down a flight of steps. At the age of 11 there was another head injury with loss of consciousness. Between the ages of 12 and 19 she was frequently beaten on the head by her brutal father, but does not recall whether she lost consciousness. She suffered migraine headaches at the age of 12. These were extremely tense frontal temporal headaches, associated with nausea, at times with spots in front of the eyes, and blocking of various parts of the visual field. Moving lights upset her and she frequently saw lights flashing past the side of her eyes in a dark room. She had itchiness and tingling in her finger tips which she tried to shake off. She was dizzy almost every day; the dizziness lasted for a short time, came on suddenly and ended suddenly, so that she always regained consciousness by the time she hit the floor. When fatigued she experienced altered states of consciousness: "I am awake, yet I'm not. I know where I am. I know I am having a dream. I'm seeing these things happen, but it's very much like watching them from the outside. I get a sense of fright. They start and end suddenly too."

An electroencephalogram was normal, except that a sleep recording could not be obtained. The neurologist felt that the history indicated the presence of a mixed seizure disorder with kinetic and psycho-motor seizures. The normal EEG, he believed, did not rule out this diagnosis, particularly because the sleep record could not be obtained.

Hysteria or Epilepsy?

A 21-year-old woman was referred by a community mental health center for vocational training. She was seeking a divorce from her drug-addicted husband by whom she had two children. She had never been hospitalized, but several times had been treated at hospitals on an emergency basis for "hysterical attacks." On one occasion she found herself sitting outside of a hospital, kicking the dashboard of her car. The police took her into the hospital, she was medicated and released. Another time she "just flipped out" in the ladies room of a restaurant, and again was taken to the hospital by the police who found her screaming and pulling her hair. She was discharged after a few hours. The agency psychiatrist considered an organic factor secondary to a head injury with unconsciousness sustained when she was 15 in an automobile accident. However, he considered that her symptoms of amnesia might also represent a hysterical dissociated state not unusual in an infantile hysterical personality.

The agency psychologist detected an expressive difficulty that re-sembled an aphasia, in which she could not comprehend the meaning of language and was not able to control the production of speech. She showed a verbal deficit on the WAIS with a pronounced specialization in the perceptual-analytic area, achieving a prorated I.Q. of 132 in Object Assembly in contrast to 89 in Information and 83 in Com-prehension. She described automatic behavior, in which she found herself in places without recalling how she got there. She had black-outs in the presence of people who called her but she didn't hear them, or was unable to respond; she heard ringing in her ears. She felt herself to be extremely clumsy and she described aura-like feelings that made her fear she was going to die.

* * *

A 14-year-old boy, hyperactive, had bursts of fury in which he hit and screamed. He would strike his mother and sister and break valuable objects. Recently he had been able to control his outbursts some-what by "bashing pillows." He was extremely bright (Verbal I.Q. 150; Performance I.Q. 138; Full Scale I.Q. 149). The history suggested the possibility of over-stimulation as a child, which created fear of physical vulnerability. While being examined by a psychologist, he fell out of his chair onto the floor, saying that he had tripped on his own foot; however, he had not ventured to rise, but had been lean-ing forward, resting his elbow on his knee. He moved constantly, jerking a hand or foot, asking if he could get up, and strolling about the room. A speech push was noted. He was suspected of having a verbal expressive dysphasia. This was hard to be explicit about, except that he often had trouble finding the word he needed. He acknowl-edged frequent experiences of dizziness, particularly when he rose quickly. Moving lights irritated him and he often became angry with-out reason. Nothing more of neurological implication was obtained, but the data justified concern about a differential diagnosis between a neurological process and a hysterical state in this adolescent boy.

*   *   *

An 18-year-old girl was taken to an emergency ward when she be-came paralyzed and could not walk. She had fainted a number of times. This was attributed to anemia, for which she was under the care of a private physician. She always had had learning difficulties and was in classes for mentally retarded children. A psychiatrist had given her that diagnosis. On interviewing at a rehabilitation agency she was observed to be a lovely girl with an engaging, direct manner, pleasant and personable. Her social competence and employed vocabu-lary exceeded the levels of psychological test scores. These ranged from a high prorated I.Q. of 85 on ability to conceptualize to a low of 49 on Digit Span, the recall of auditory material.

She reported two injuries to the head on the same day when she was about 12 years of age. In one a bottle fell on her head from the fifth floor; in the other she was hit on the head by a bottle which supposedly fell from the top of a door. She said that she was uncon-scious for about 15 minutes after one of these accidents and suffered lacerations of the scalp. Thereafter she experienced severe headaches and dizziness. She fainted rather often; the most recent episode oc-curred several days before the interview. She described it in this man-ner, "If they rush me to eat, I get cramps in my stomach and then I faint." She experienced definitive tingling sensations in the hand. She also had episodes in which the floor tilted. She saw what seemed to be colored lights. The girl was allowed to help with housework but not with cooking because her mother feared she would burn herself. She was not allowed to bring friends into the home because the family distrusted the environment in which they lived. The only socialization she was permitted was with relatives. Diagnostically, there was need to differentiate between a possible hysterical reaction to a restricted, moralistic upbringing and a post-traumatic epilepsy.

Depression or Epilepsy?

A 35-year-old married woman was seen for vocational evaluation following hospitalization for an attempted suicide. She had been divorced for 11 years. In recent years she had become increasingly depressed, feeling less important to her children. She had had several outbursts of rage which were followed by periods of dizziness and later by inability to recall what had happened. In an interview with the agency's psychiatrist, the patient described episodes or vertigo in which the room went round and in which she saw spots. On occasion she feared that she would faint. She had numbness in her finger when her hand had not fallen asleep and severe periodic headaches not relieved by any medication. The psychiatrist considered it advisable to try to establish the neurological condition and medicate it, before attempting to evaluate the severity of the depression.

Fugue State or Epilepsy?

A lovely young girl, not quite 16, was seen for psychodiagnostic assessment as part of her application to a therapeutic school. She reported rather unusual experiences while driving a car, looking at moving lights, or listening to music. At such times she might go into a dream-like state from which she could not extricate herself. She acknowledged that she was a hazard when she drove. For the moment there was no concern because the state in which she now resided did not permit her to drive, but it would become a matter of concern soon when she became of age. She was a very anxious girl and still required a light in the room in order to sleep. Her parents were divorced when she was three, and she saw her father for the first time in nine years several months before the examination. There was indication that she had been and remained subject to periods of depression. There was much denial surrounding these periods and the intensity of the depression was difficult to evaluate. She described what she called hysterical attacks, in which she was easily hurt, put under strain, and became "very emotional about everything." She suffered a slight concussion when she was eight, when dragged by a horse. Consideration had to be given to the states she described. They might be fugue states, they could be altered states of consciousness associated with epileptic phenomena, they could reflect the denied depression which might find an outlet in a disguised suicidal gesture. They could also represent preoccupation with intense affects hidden behind the denial.

High Blood Pressure or Epilepsy?

A 33-year-old woman referred for vocational rehabilitation reported an almost incredible medical history: a knee operation for an injury she suffered by slipping resulted in a permanent gait handicap; three other surgical experiences, one for the removal of a uterine tumor, two for a pilinoidal cyst; she was in a car accident at an unspecified age and bore a large scar on the upper right forehead. Four other large scars were visible on both arms which could have been the result of a failure to suture a wound properly or an untreated infection in wounds that had been sutured. She had high blood pressure and complained of headaches that did not respond to medication, and of clumsiness, and dizziness. These symptoms might be associated with the high blood pressure. It was suggested that she was accident prone, either because of a cerebral dysfunction which causes dizziness and poor motor control, or the high blood pressure which caused her to faint and to miscue perceptually. Another alternative could have been the inward deflection of fury in a masochistic reaction.

*   *   *

A 40-year-old woman was referred to vocational rehabilitation agency with a diagnosis of hypertension and emotional disturbance. She reported that she had fainted a number of times, but that she had not told anybody about these experiences. She became upset and experienced nausea when she encounterd inability to do somthing that she knew she could do, as when she would be doing arithmetic. She experienced blurring and double vision. She had experiences of the floor tilting so that she had to hold on to sustain an upright position, citing that it happened that very morning and she had had to get off the subway. She experienced tingling sensations "like pins sticking" in both feet and hands, and what appeared to be severe states of altered consciousness. Diagnostically, it was considered necessary to attempt to determine whether her symptoms were anxiety phenomena, were associated with her high blood pressure, or were manifestations of seizure episodes.

Diabetes or Epilepsy?

A 43-year-old economically deprived woman presented a variety of medical and psychiatric problems. She was diabetic, suffered weakness in the lower extremities and dizziness. She took Orinase. She was blind in the right eye from cataracts, which because of her diabetic condition had not been removed surgically. She had arthritis and severe stomach cramps, particularly around her menses. She complained of dizziness for a good part of her life, accompanied by headaches; she denied fainting. She had some hearing difficulty. Her manner was belligerent, hostile, questioning, and sneering. Her associations appeared to be loose. There was some evidence of concretization of thought processes. A number of diagnostic questions were suggested. Some of the symptoms—the dizziness, weakness in the lower extremities, and auditory and visual problems—could be secondary complications of the diabetes. Her inappropriateness and poor tolerance for new situations suggested that an endocrine imbalance related to the menstrual cycle might produce a transient psychotic state. Finally there was the possibility of a seizure-like disorder.

*   *   *

These difficult situations are typical. Few indeed are pure instances of diagnostic categories; all deserve to have all possibilities weighed.

BIBLIOGRAPHY

1. *Alvarez, W. C.:* Nerves in Collision. New York: Pyramid House, 1972.
2. *Ames, F. R.:* Self-induction in photosensitive epilepsy. Brain, 94:4, 1971.
3. *Assael, M. I.:* Petit mal status without impairment of consciousness. Dis. Nerv. Syst., 33:8, 1972.
4. *Babb, R. B.* and *Eckman, P. B.:* Abdominal epilepsy. J.A.M.A. 222:1, 1972.
5. *Ball, J. R. B.:* A case of hair fetishism, transvestism, and organic cerebral disorders. Acta Psychiatrica Scandinavica, 44, 1968.
6. *Beaussart, M.:* Epilepsy and heredity. Revue de Neuropsychiatric Infantile et d'Hygiene Mentale de l'Engance, 19:6, 1971.
7. *Blumer, D.:* Hypersexual episodes in temporal lobe epilepsy. Amer. J. Psychiat., 126:8, 1970.

8. *Bruens, J. H.:* Psychoses in epilepsy. Psychiatria, Neurologia, Neurochirurgia, 74:2, 1971.

9. *Burgemeister, B. B.:* Psychological Techniques in Neurological Diagnosis. New York: Hoeber Med. Div., Harper and Row, 1962.

10. *Chen, Rong-Chi* and *Forster, M.:* Cursive epilepsy and gelastic epilepsy. Neurology, 23:10, 1973.

11. *Chess, S.:* An Introduction to Child Psychiatry, 2nd Edition. New York: Grune and Stratton, 1969.

12. *Chien, Ching-Piao* and *Keegan, D.:* Diazepam as an oral long-term anticonvulsant for epileptic mental patients. Dis. Nerv. Syst., 339-2, 1972.

13. *Currier, R. D. et al.:* Sexual seizures. Arch Neurol., 25:3, 1971.

14. *Dallos, V.* and *Heathfield, K.:* Iatrogenic epilepsy due to anti-depressant drugs. Brit. Med. J., 4, 1969.

15. *Dodrill, C. B.* and *Troupin, A. S.:* Effects of repeated administrations of a comprehensive neuropsychological battery among chronic epileptics. J. Nerv. Ment. Dis., 161:3, 1975.

16. *Dodrill, C. B.* and *Wilkus, R. J.:* Relationships between intelligence and electroencephalographic epileptiform activity in adult epileptics. Neurology, 26:6, 1976.

17. *Dodrill, C. B.* and *Wilkus, R. J.:* Neuropsychological correlates of the electroencephalogram in epileptics: II. The waking posterior rhythm and its interaction with epileptiform activity. Epilepsia, 17:1, 1976.

18. *Erwin, C. W. et al.:* Lithium carbonate and convulsive disorders. Arch. Gen. Psychiat., 28:5, 1973.

19. *Flor-Henry, P.:* Schizophrenic-like reactions and affective psychoses associated with temporal lobe epilepsy. Amer. J. Psychiat., 126:3, 1969.

20. *Friis, M. L.,* and *Lund, M.:* Stress convulsions. Arch. Neurol., 31:3, 1974.

21. *Gardner, G. G.:* Use of hypnosis for psychogenic epilepsy in a child. Amer. J. Clin. Hypnosis, 13:3, 1973.

22. *Geller, M.* and *Geller, A.:* Brief amnestic effects of spike-wave discharges. Neurology, 20:11, 1970.

23. *Gibbs, F. A.* and *Gibbs, E. L.:* Borderland of epilepsy. J. Neuropsychiat., 4, 1963.

24. *Gibbs, E. L. et al.:* Psychomotor epilepsy. Arch. Neurol. Psychiat., 60:4, 1948.

25. *Gilligan, B. S.:* Primary reading epilepsy. Med. J. Australia, 1:20, 1969.

26. *Goldensohn, E. S.:* Seizures and convulsive disorders. *In* B. B. Wolman (Ed.): Handbook of Clinical Psychology. New York: McGraw-Hill, 1965.

27. *Graham, P.* and *Rutter, M.:* Organic brain dysfunction and child psychiatric disorders. Brit. J. Med., 3, 1968.

28. *Guerrero-Figueroa, R. et al.:* Electroencephalographic study of Diazepam on patients with diagnosis of episodic behavioral disorders. J. Clin. Pharm. and J. New Drugs, 10:1, 1970.

29. *Grunderson, C. H. et al.:* Sleep deprivation seizures. Neurology, 23:7, 1973.

30. *Hughes, J.* and *Cayaffa, J. J.:* Seizures following burns of the skin: I. Review of the literature. Dis. Nerv. Syst., 34:5, 1973.

31. *Ikonomoff, S. I.:* Anti-cholinesterase drugs and epileptic seizures. Brit. J. Psychiat., 117, 1970.

32. *Ives, A.:* Learning difficulties in children with epilepsy. Brit. J. Disorders of Communication, 5:1, 1970.

33. *Johnson, S. M.* and *Lewis, J. A.:* The hysterical seizure. Amer. J. EEG Technology, 16:1, 1976.

34. *Jonas, A. D.:* The emergence of epileptic equivalents in the era of tranquillizers. Int. J. Neuropsychiat., 3:1, 1967.

35. *Jonas, A. D.:* The subictal state. Bol. Assoc. P. Rico, 59:3, 1967.

36. *Klove, H.* and *Matthews, C. G.:* Neuropsychological studies of patients with epilepsy. *In* R. M. Reitan and L. A. Davidson (Eds.): Clinical Neuropsychology: Current Status and Applications. Washington, D. C.: Winston, 1974.

37. *Kutt, H.* and *Louis, S.:* Anticonvulsant drugs: Pathophysiological and pharmacological aspects. Drugs, 4, 1972.

38. *Lawall, J.:* Psychiatric presentations of seizure disorders. Amer. J. Psychiat. 133, 1976.

39. *Lewis, J. A.:* Violence and epilepsy, J.A.M.A., 232:11, 1975.

40. *Lilienfeld, A. M.* and *Pasamanick, B.:* The association of maternal and fetal factors with the development of cerebral palsy and epilepsy. Am. J. Obst. Gynec., 70, 1955.

41. *Lilienfeld, A. M.* and *Pasamanick, B.:* Association of maternal and fetal factors with the development of epilepsy. 1. Abnormalities in the prenatal and perinatal periods. J.A.M.A., 155, 1954.

42. *Malcolm, M. T.:* Temporal lobe epilepsy due to drug withdrawal. Brit. J. Addiction, 67:4, 1972.

43. *Marinacci, A. A.* and *Von Hagen, K. O.:* Alcohol and temporal lobe dysfunction: Some of its psychomotor equivalents. Behavioral Neuropsychiat., 3, 1972.

44. *Mark, V. H.* and *Ervin, F. R.:* Violence and the Brain. New York: Harper and Row, 1970.

45. *Merritt, H. H.:* The treatment of convulsive disorders. Med. Clin. N. Amer., 56, 1972.

46. *Millichap, J. G.:* Drug therapy: Drug treatment of convulsive disorders. N. E. J. Med., 286:9, 1972.

47. *Mirsky, A. F.:* Neuropsychological bases of schizophrenia. Annual Rev. Psychol., 20, 1969.

48. *Monroe, R. R.:* Episodic Behavioral Disorders: A Psychodynamic and Neurophysiologic Analysis. Cambridge, Mass.: Harvard Univ. Press, 1970.

49. *Niedermeyer, E. et al.:* Classical hysterical seizures facilitated by anticonvulsant toxicity. Psychiatrica Clinica, 3:2, 1970.

50. *Novak, J. et al.:* Petit mal status in adults. Dis. Nerv. Syst., 32. 1971.

51. *O'Donohoe, N. V.:* Abdominal epilepsy. Develop. Med. Child Neurol., 13:6, 1971.

52. *Parrino, J.:* Reduction of seizures by desensitization. J. Behav. Ther. Exp. Psychiat., 2, 1971.

53. *Pinto, R.:* A case of movement epilepsy with agoraphobia treated successfully by flooding. Brit. J. Psychiat., 121:562, 1972.

54. *Pond, D. A.:* The psychological disorders of epileptic patients. Psychiatria, Neurologia, Neurochirurgia, 74:2, 1971.

55. *Pond, D. A.:* The schizophrenic-like psychoses of epilepsy: Discussion. Proc. Royal Soc. Med., 55, 1962.

56. *Rake, F.:* Diagnostiche Problems bei der unterscheidung von hysteuschen und epileptischen Anfallen. Nervenartz, 41:9, 1970.

57. *Rodin, E. A.:* The Prognosis of Patients with Epilepsy. Springfield, Ill.: Charles C. Thomas, 1968.

58. *Rodin, E. A. et al.:* Differences between patients with temporal lobe seizures and those with other forms of epileptic attacks. Epilepsia, 17:3, 1976.

59. *Rowan, A. J. et al.:* Is reading epilepsy inherited? J. Neurol. Neurosurgery Psychiat., 33:4, 1970.

60. *Schmeck, Jr., H. M.:* Depths of brain probed for sources of violence. New York Times, Dec. 27, 1970.

61. *Schwartz, M. L.* and *Dennerll, R. D.:* Neuropsychologic assessment of children without and with questionable epileptogenic dysfunction. Percept. Motor Skills, 30:1, 1970.

62. *Sherwin, I.:* Temporal lobe epilepsy: Neurological and behavioral aspects. Ann. Rev. Med., 27, 1976.
63. *Silverstein, M. et al.:* Recall of verbal material in temporal lobe epilepsy and schizophrenia. Dis. Nerv. Syst., 34:5, 1973.
64. *Slater, E. and Beard, A. W.:* The schizophrenic-like psychoses of epilepsy. Brit. J. Psychiatry, 109, 1963, a and b.
65. *Small, L.:* The Briefer Psychotherapies, 2nd Edition. New York: Brunner/Mazel, 1979.
66. *Standage, K. F.:* The etiology of hysterical seizures. Can. Psychiat. Assoc., 20:1, 1975.
67. *Stensman, R. and Ursing, B.:* Epilepsy precipitated by hot water immersion. Neurology, 21:5, 1971.
68. *Sterman, M. B.:* Neurophysiologic and clinical studies of sensorimotor EEG biofeedback training: Some effects on epilepsy. Seminars in Psychiatry, 5:4, 1973.
69. *Sterman, M. B. and Friar, L.:* Suppression of seizures in an epileptic following sensorimotor EEG feedback training. Electroencephalography and Clinical Neurophysiology, 33, 1972.
70. *Stores, G.:* Studies of attention and seizure disorders. Devel. Med. Child Neurol., 15:3, 1973.
71. *Taylor, D. C.:* "It," or the ghost in the temporal lobe. Devel. Med. Child Neurology, 13:6, 1971.
72. *Theaman, M.:* The performance of post-traumatics, post-traumatic epileptics, and idiopathic epileptics on psychological tests. Doctoral dissertation. New York University, School of Education, 1960.
73. *Trotter, S.:* Biofeedback helps epileptics control seizures. APA Monitor, 4:12, 1973.
74. *Tutton, J. C.:* New treatment for old neurologic disease: Status epilepticus treatment with diazepam. N.Y.S.J. Med., 70:19, 1970.
75. *Walker, A. E.:* The libidinous temporal lobe. Schweizer Archiv fur Neurologie, Neurochirugie und Psychiatrie, 11:2, 1972.
76. *Waxman, S. G. and Geschwind, N.:* The interictal behavior syndrome of temporal lobe epilepsy. Arch. Gen. Psychiat., 32, 1975.
77. *Wells, E.:* Transient ictal psychosis. Arch Gen. Psychiat., 32:9, 1975.
78. *Whitten, J. R.:* Psychical seizures. Amer. J. Psychiat., 126:4, 1969.
79. *Yuill, G. M.:* The production of epileptiform electroencephalographic discharges by psychological factors. Amer. J. Clin. Hypnosis, 14:3, 1972.

CHAPTER 4

Aphasia and Dysphasia

"This is a tape of a brouse to make buke deprold in the auria." (Response of patient diagnosed as having Posterior Aphasia to the query, "What do you use a pen for?") (4).

"Because . . . Why? In the State the people have agreed and the law handles what they are money-wise, you know." (Response of patient with a diagnosis of Minimal Cerebral Dysfunction and Dull Normal Intelligence to the query, "Why does the State require people to get a licence in order to be married?" This patient achieved a prorated I.Q. of 118 on the Similarities subtest of the WAIS.)

SPEECH AND PSYCHOTHERAPY

Psychotherapy, the talking therapy, centers upon spoken language for the communication essential to the process. Body language, play, art or written productions are all ancillary to spoken language. The therapist is trained to be alert to the intrusion of defense mechanisms upon the character, quality and content of the patient's speech. Does the patient mean what he says? Say what he means? Does he understand what the therapist says? Means? (The therapist must presume that he himself is without language dysfunction.)

The therapist is trained to use the content, character, and quality of language production by a patient to determine the diagnosis of his symptoms and the selection of a treatment approach. Extremely limited vocabulary, phonetic and grammatical errors, concreteness of thinking, and limited ability for abstractions are associated with mental retardation. Over-elaboration, emphasis upon minor details, uncer-

138

tainty of accuracy and over-inclusiveness are associated with obsessional thinking. Semantic errors, grammatical disorganization, and elision of unrelated or incompatible ideas (contamination) are linked with psychotic states; as thought disorders they are identified with schizophrenia.

But the therapist is not always trained to ask whether these language impairments may be organic rather than emotional in origin. Nor does the therapist often ask to what extent the impairments represent a fusion of the two—in fact, the more likely situation. Just as hallucinations incline many therapists almost automatically to diagnose schizophrenia without considering a seizure disorder (See Chapter 3), so disorganized speech may appear so bizarre or loosely associated as to evoke the same automatic diagnosis. We interpret thought from speech, and from thought the level of some aspects of ego development. The clinician knows well that schizophrenia is manifested in disturbances of thought and language along with disorders of judgment, reality perception and testing, and relationships with people. Loose associations, primary-process thinking, bizarre ideation, compelled thinking, over-ideational thinking, all appear frequently in the schizophrenic and in borderline schizophrenic disorders. The psychotherapist should recognize equally well that organically caused impairment of or loss of language functions is likely to produce emotional disturbances, that behavioral and emotional problems appear that are part of, and also go beyond, the language impairment itself. These emotional problems may arise from the patient's response to the limitations imposed upon his language functions, or, more directly, from damage to cerebral tissue. The emotional problems associated with schizophrenia and those arising from organically disrupted language are often similar. The language disturbances that appear in both schizophrenia and some kinds of brain damage are also similar in many respects. Chapman (8) found that young schizophrenic patients experienced changes in speech, attention, memory, perception, and motility long before the schizophrenia became overt. His clinical data suggested that schizophrenia is an organic psychosis related to aphasia. Central here is not the issue of etiology of schizophrenia (perhaps the most important current issue in psychiatry), but rather the obvious fact that the two disorders may be confused; aphasia may be diagnosed as schizophrenia.

The psychotherapist is rarely confronted with the dramatic interruptions of language function produced by extrinsically or intrinsically traumatic events, such as a penetrating head wound or a stroke. These losses of function are extremes of aphasia. We will be concerned in this chapter with dysphasia, those relatively moderate *impairments* of function, rather than total losses or severe impairment. We will consider those impairments that are so small that we do not ordinarily suspect organicity. We think instead of peculiarities of thought and seek their psychodynamic explanation. The peculiarities of language by which they are sometimes manifested may at first encounter impress us as serious psychodynamic disturbances.

Normal functioning is often best illuminated by study of severe pathology of the functions, so we will look first at aphasia and its several manifestations.

APHASIA

Loss of language functions is chiefly correlated with lesions of the cortex. The lesions may occur in different anatomical locations. Losses can be associated with areas fairly specifically and may appear in response to a variety of events. While functional disorders—catatonia, for example—may result in loss of language, these causes are relatively minor. More important are organic changes in brain tissue produced by intrinsic or extrinsic factors. These include occlusions of blood vessels that destroy neurons and interrupt established pathways, tumors, physiological disruptions, toxemias, anoxias, severe febrile episodes, penetrating wounds of the skull. Thrombosis, the rapid occlusion of a blood vessel appears to be the major cause of aphasia (14). More than 400,000 cases of stroke occur each year in the United States (26).

Behavioral changes—losses of muscle, sensory, language functions— accompany the destruction of neuronal tissue, and emotional reactions appear in response to the behavioral changes. These striking and definite changes appear with dramatic suddenness. In a moment the victim is no longer able to speak, read, walk, move an arm or a leg, or comprehend what is said to him.

Ongoing studies of the behavioral changes and their anatomical correlates have produced an enormous and not altogether uniform nomenclature and many sets of classification systems. Wyke (39) warns that because language itself is so complex and defies classification, its disorganization also defies classification.

Broca and Wernicke led off this semantic debate over a century ago.

In 1865 Broca associated the loss of speech motor functions, or *motor aphasia,* with damage to a portion of the frontal lobe just anterior to the lower third of the motor cortex. This area appeared to mediate articulate speech, involving coordination of buccal, lingual, laryngeal, palatal and diaphragmatic muscles (1). Auditory comprehension of language, reading (but not aloud), writing, and intelligence remained intact. The patient has few words, speech is often limited to a few perseverative responses, to some exclamations and profanities. The patient usually cannot write and is acutely aware of his dysfunctions (1). Nearly a decade later, Wernicke identified *sensory aphasia,* associated with the destruction of a specific verbal auditory center at the foot of the first left temporal convolution. Lesions of this area resulted in loss of *comprehension* of speech and defects in writing ability. Well-educated patients may continue to read, while the less-educated patient tends to be alexic. If Broca's area is intact the patient can speak, but his speech is disordered because his comprehension is severely impaired (30). This speech would be fluid, words would be abundant, but disconnected and meaningless. The patient does not understand spoken language, and cannot follow directions. Writing, like speech, may be abundant but disconnected. The patient is not too aware of his language difficulties (1).

Wernicke reasoned that motor aphasia and sensory aphasia were separate, discrete syndromes, a reasoning based upon Meynert's contention that motor functions are localized anteriorly in each hemisphere, sensory functions more posteriorly. This localization, he further concluded, explained why hemiplegia frequently accompanied motor aphasia and was not present in sensory aphasia.

He then elaborated a third aphasia syndrome, *conduction aphasia,* produced by a lesion that interrupted the connection between the motor and sensory areas, both of which remained intact. Speech is present but paraphasic; comprehension is intact. In *global aphasia* both motor and sensory areas are destroyed, both speech and comprehension are lost, and severe hemiplegia is usual.

Over the following decades efforts at a more descriptive terminology and nomenclature continued. Broca's *motor aphasia* has been replaced in some lexicons by *anterior aphasia, expressive aphasia, non-fluent aphasia,* or *agrammatism.* Alternatives to Wernicke's *sensory aphasia* appear as *posterior aphasia, receptive aphasia, fluent aphasia,* or *paragrammatism.* Other systems are based either upon rates of speech and word frequency (17), or upon linguistic analyses.

Major differences continue to this day about the major hypotheses associating certain behaviors with specific anatomical loci. Geschwind (14) reports repeated confirmation of these links. Others reject both the types of aphasia described and the anatomical localization of the speech functions lost.

One of the objectors, Smith (30), reminds us that the limited so-called pure aphasia rarely occurs. He observes that claims of the existence of a state in which some intact language components persist in the presence of loss or impairment of other components are based upon *clinical* studies only and that these claims are refuted by every study that uses objective measures of all language components. Standardized tests of speech, writing, reading, and comprehension permit measures of the severity of loss in each function. Broca's and Wernicke's hypotheses, his criticism continues, were derived from "highly subjective assessments of language functions" and "meager neuropathologic studies of a few aged patients." Wernicke's clinical testing, he comments, shifted technically from one patient to another.

Moreover, Smith (31) contests the neat anatomical localization of two aphasia, one motor, the other sensory, noting the lack of precision in defining the primary variable in neuropsychological study—the lesion producing the observed behavioral change. The effects of lesions vary according to location, size, extent, nature (whether evolving or resolving) and their influence upon both adjacent and remote brain structures.

Linguistic approaches have brought more refined methods to the study of aphasia, particularly to its speech aspects. These study phonemic, morphemic, syntactic, and grammatic losses, changes, and impairments. They derive hypotheses concerning the development of speech that seem to parallel those in embryology, where ontogeny can be seen to recapitulate phylogeny. A major linguistic theory describes a regressive process in phonological breakdown in aphasia that is the reverse of the developmental process in the child's acquisition of language (24). The type of aphasia does not alter this pattern of regression. Spreen (32) cites an hypothesis by A. Pick, a German linguist, that speech is generated from *nonverbal content* through *thought* to *language,* the final step being the selection of words. Hence *word-finding* difficulties seem to be the most frequently observed of language difficulties and the one likely to persist the longest. Schuell and Jenkins (27) had earlier established that the predominant errors made by aphasics are associative in nature (chair = table); rhyming error (chair

= stair) are much less frequent, while unrelated errors (chair = apple) are extremely rare. Spreen notes further that even in jargon speech, aspects of melody, rhythm, intonation and sometimes grammatical structure are preserved. In this scheme of regression, words with strong associative meaning tend to be more easily substituted than others, and, in accordance with Kurt Goldstein's concepts, the use of abstract words is more impaired than is the use of concrete words. Spreen concludes that there is no true loss of vocabulary in aphasia, but rather a decrease in the use of low-frequency words which are those acquired later in the development of speech and language. Language acquired later in life tends to be more severely impaired in aphasia. True of both normal persons and aphasics is a difficulty in naming that varies according to the age when the word was acquired, so that the aphasic is making an error that is made by normal persons, only much more frequently. Difficulty of comprehension relates inversely to the frequency of use of a word. Words learned earlier are used more often. Nouns are relatively infrequent in normal speech and Spreen reasons that their greater difficulty for aphasics (anomia) reflects the general rules of frequency and usage. Hence while all types of words are lost in aphasia, loss of nouns is more impressive because they occur less frequently in language. Many now argue that the classification of aphasia should employ linguistic criteria, that the aphasias be classified by the qualitative and quantitative features of expressive speech alone. This does not imply that comprehension difficulties are not present; it focuses on the manifest aspects of the disability, and avoids the almost insurmountable problem of diagnosing a *comprehension* disorder accompanied by apraxia that prevents the patient from indicating what he does in fact comprehend (24).

Disorders and Terminology in Aphasia

There follows a glossary of common terms applied to various aphasic disorders. Note that neither the terms nor their definitions relate to the degree of severity of a disorder. However, the terms have been established to describe severe losses and impairments. Nonetheless, knowledge of them is helpful to the psychotherapist because the disorders may appear in lesser degree in patients not identified as aphasic.

Impairments of perceptions, the *agnosias,* have tremendous implications for language development (12). The agnosias must be separated from impairments or dysfunctions of the peripheral sense organ itself.

Acoustic agnosia is a defect in the comprehension of the sound of language, that is, of the phonemic system. Errors in speech-sound discrimination increase as the differences between sounds decrease. For example, t and p are more difficult to discriminate than k and r. In *auditory agnosia* there is impaired recognition of *sounds* or combinations of sounds, without regard for ability to discriminate between them. There may be loss of ability to comprehend speech, or nonsymbolic sounds such as mechanical or animal noises, or human nonlinguistic sounds such as sneezing or coughing. *Visual agnosia* encompasses impaired visual recognition and may separately relate to objects, representations, geometric forms, colors, words, or letters.

Alexia is a disorder in the comprehension of written symbols. Tactile, or haptic, *agnosia* includes impairments in recognition through touch and may separately relate to objects, sizes, shapes, textures, and locations on the body.

In some aphasias there are impairments of the voluntary movements necessary for speech or writing. *Articulating apraxia,* impairment of voluntary control of the speech-producing apparatus, is most apparent when the patient must perform an imaginary, hypothetical or pretended act. So-called propositional speech is impaired, while reflex, involuntary speech is not. When a person sneezes, the patient is able reflexively to say "God bless you," but is unable to respond to the question, "What do you say when a person sneezes?" (18).

Agraphia is a disorder of writing. It may appear in all writing or only in particular aspects such as the writing of nominal words, in the use of faulty grammar, or in the omission of words that indicate the relationship between parts of a sentence.

Some disorders affect both or either spoken and written language. *Anomia,* or word-finding, difficulty, has been discussed above in connection with the loss of command over nouns. But the difficulty can involve any part of speech, as well. The patient tries to use a substitute: a synonym, an operational phrase, or a word in the same class. The patient will talk around the word, seeking perhaps to define it. The efforts at finding a substitute may require another specific word he cannot find and produce, and so the cycle of search and frustration intensifies. Benson (4) cautions that while word-finding difficulty may occur in severe anxiety states, depression, and catatonic schizophrenia, it is virtually ubiquitous in aphasia and should be an alerting sign to the psychotherapist. *Agrammatism* includes impairments not of vocabulary but of syntax, that is, errors in the systematic use of words in sentences in written and spoken language. *Acalculia* is a disturbance of arithmetic; it may be an actual inability to use the arithmetic process or an anomia for writing or saying the symbols used in arithmetic.

Other manifestations of speech impairment may not affect written language, or may be difficult to detect there. *Dysprosody* is a disorder of the accent, cadence, rhythm, and intonation of speech. In *paraphasia* a required word is replaced by an erroneous one that bears some relationship to the correct word. The relationship, writes Eisenson (12), may be a phonemic similarity ("The car sped swiftly" becomes "The car spit sweetly") or associational ("flower" is spoken as "flose," combining *fl* and *rose*). *Neologisms* may be a form of paraphasia, as in "flose," or if not readily apparent as such, may seem to be "nonwords." *Perseverations* are the continued repetition of a word or phrase (or gesture or action). The utterance, appropriately evoked in one situation, continues to be made in another context that makes it inappropriate. Or the original usage may be inappropriate to its context and continue to be so. The aphasic patient tends to perseverate when anxious, when situations change suddenly, when fatigued, or when placed in a new or difficult context (12). *Jargon* is an outpouring, a profusion of speech, much of it incomprehensible to the auditor, though not necessarily to the speaker. The patient seems unaware that he is not speaking satisfactorily. His speech tends to be more fluent and fluid than is normal speech. Eisenson (12) observes that regular phoneme and morphene substitutions can often be identified in jargon speech that suggests an underlying though not necessarily comprehensible meaning. The patient with this disorder, writes Benson (4), speaks with an air of being understood. While he cannot monitor his own speech output and cannot understand spoken language, the visual modality of communication enables him to imitate and obey gestures. In Benson's experience this patient is often erroneously diagnosed as a "word-salad" schizophrenic because of his bizarre verbal output and the absence in him of neurological signs. Complete *mutism* never occurs in aphasia; the aphasic patient can always make sounds: grunts, groans, whispering, whistle-like noises, for example. *Echolalia,* the repetition of a word or sound just made by another person, is rare in aphasia. A form of verbal perseveration, it is presumed to result from the isolation of the speech mechanism from the rest of the cortex. The patient repeats without modification what is said to him. An entire sentence, an end phrase, or a word may be repeated several times.

Destructive lesions in some specific areas of the brain produce aphasias that are routinely *transient,* an effect that may result from lesions in other areas when they too are transient and non-destructive.

Childhood (or *developmental*) *aphasia* is assumed to arise from an auditory agnosia; the child can hear but cannot understand. The seat of the disorder is believed to be an auditory-perceptual dysfunction within the brain, not the result of sensory, motor, intellectual, or social impairment (9, 13). Unless properly diagnosed, a child with aphasia may be placed in a school for the deaf, losing the opportunity for the special training that could develop his remaining speech and language potential. The aphasic child may come to reject sound, to ignore it, as if he considered it a useless stimulus. A small group of such children become mute; some very infrequently verbalize; some develop jargon speech in an effort at communication, accompanied by gestures and expressions that are complex and appropriate; some employ a jargon interspersed with intelligible words or phrases ("sit on" for "chair," "knife" for "fork"); others may be echolalic, repeating words without meaning (9).

The number of young children so affected is not small; Cantwell and Baker (7) report that about 5 percent of the children first starting school speak so poorly that strangers have difficulty understanding them.

Children whose aphasia arises from known lesions of the brain manifest both expressive and receptive disorders of language according to the nature and site of the lesions, and the stage of language development achieved at the time the lesion was suffered. Potential for recovery, as we will see, is greater among children than adults, and greater among younger than older children.

Hemispheric Dominance for Language and Recoverability

The preponderance of evidence indicates that the left cerebral hemisphere in the right-handed person is most frequently dominant for language. Experimental studies support this clinical impression, which is based upon the comparative tabulation of the incidence of aphasia in patients with right-hemisphere and left-hemisphere lesions.

The experimental studies are predicated upon the contralateral relationship between handedness and cerebral hemisphere dominance. Right-handed persons more frequently develop both language disturbances and right-side paralysis from lesions in the left hemisphere. Only two percent of right-handed people with lesions limited to the right hemisphere develop aphasia, and only 10 percent of right-handed people developed aphasia when sodium amylobarbitone was injected into the right carotid artery (39). This relationship between hemispheric dominance for language and handedness has been found to be more marked in the right-handed than in the left-handed person.

The experimental and clinical findings for the left-handed person are far less structured. In the left-handed, aphasia is more likely after either right- or left-side lesions (30). Thus language functions appear to be controlled, atypically, by the right hemisphere in a small percentage of right-handed people and in a considerably larger percentage of left-handed people.

The important facts here are those that support two concepts: lateral dominance for language and bilateral representation of language. Bilateral representation of language is more often observed in left-handed persons. These observations underwrite both the predictability of language disruption with dominant-sided lesions and the potentiality for the minor hemisphere to assume language functions. With patients in whom the interhemispheric connections have been surgically severed (commissurotomy) or in whom the dominant hemisphere has been surgically removed (hemispherectomy), studies of language have shown that the non-dominant hemisphere has some function or capacity for comprehension of verbal material (30, 39).

This language capability in the minor hemisphere plus the known ability of neighboring cortical areas to assume disrupted functions (20) appear to explain certain observed recoveries from aphasia that occur either spontaneously or in response to rehabilitation efforts.

Some degree of spontaneous improvement from aphasia is a phenomenon much reported. Benton (5) observes that some patients improve over a long period of time, some remain unchanged for years, and some return to normal. Spontaneous improvement has been correlated by Vignola (34) with several factors. He reports more spontaneous improvement in receptive functions than expressive ones. A conflict of evidence concerning the opposite finding is reported by Smith (30). Vignola found more in the younger than the older patient, and more in those who receive longer periods of treatment. He observes that the latter finding may reflect a tendency to keep in therapy for longer periods those patients who show an early response to treatment, so that degree of initial spontaneous improvement and degree of early response to treatment may be the chief prognostic factors.

Reviewing the spontaneous recovery process, Culton (11) notes that Head earlier believed some types of aphasia recovered more rapidly than others, while Eisenson and Wepman stress age and psychological adjustment, and Schuell stresses that physiological factors must be allowed to stabilize before a prognosis is possible.

An early rapid rate of improvement that then slows down is demonstrated in Culton's measures of eight language functions over time. Patients who recently became aphasic showed significant improvement within 30 days of study; those who had been aphasic for some time did not show such significant improvement.

"The condition of the entire brain and especially the status of the right hemisphere" are cited by Smith (30) as the major prognostic factor. Prognosis is less favorable where the brain is diffusely damaged, general health is poor, mental impairment is severe, or there is dementia. Severity of language disturbance alone is not a valid basis for prognosis. The persistence of nonlanguage reasoning ability tends to indicate that the right hemisphere is not damaged or only slightly so and can be trained, even in the patient who is left-hemisphere dominant for language.

DYSPHASIA

Relatively moderate language dysfunctions are probably present more frequently among psychotherapy patients than psychotherapists tend to recognize. While all of the forms of language impairment found among severely aphasic patients may appear in moderate degree, speech dysfunctions are those most likely to be remarked in the process of psychotherapy. Reading and writing problems may be identified in a good history or brought out spontaneously by the patient, but more readily observable are peculiarities of articulation and spoken language, word-finding difficulties, paraphasias ("Please: *P*refer me to a job"), and associative responses.

As indicated early in this chapter, they are likely to be diagnosed as indicative of serious emotional disturbances, thought disorders, obsessional or bizarre thinking, or mental retardation.

Diagnostic ambivalence is a frequent reaction, as evidenced by this observation by a pediatric psychiatrist about a young teenage lad referred with a diagnosis of aphasia of unknown etiology:

"His language dysfunction included both an articulation pattern and a thinking disorder characterized by clang associations and bizarre responses. There was a suggestion of hallucination but this was not clearly substantiated. His figure drawings showed a fairly good body concept which was not in keeping with the clinical interview and suggested a possibly better prognosis."

With many patients, a history of brain damage can be established and the etiology of the dysphasia assumed—a gunshot wound, a severe febrile episode, a concussion suffered in a fall or accident. But in many patients the etiology is buried in obscure, even unknown details and only be inferred or presumed. I have seen, for example, a young woman of 28 manifesting word-finding difficulty, who had received about 20 electric-shock treatment at the age of 19, soon followed by *grand mal* seizures for which no neurological base could be established. Another young woman with a suspected dysphasia dimly recalled high fevers with delirium in her youth and also reported that "when I was small, my cousin and I were going down the sliding board. I get the funniest feeling that I fell and I hit my head and was unconscience (sic!)." Careful history-taking often discloses perinatal experiences that may be implicated: maternal bleeding during gestation, premature birth, or a difficult labor.

Dysphasia arising early in life has several possible pathological effects. Communication with others becomes difficult. The child may become aversive and develop an apparent schizoid mode of relating. Self esteem is damaged and may restrict efforts at mastery even in areas that do not emphasize language. Responses of others to the dysphasic person are often affected and contribute to the sense of isolation. The plight of the dysphasic child or youth is poignantly epitomized in this statement by a 16-year-old lad: "My worst characteristic is that I have trouble expressing myself. I ask people if they understand; they say yes; then I ask them to do what I say, and when they do it, it comes out different from what I said. It comes out like something else."

Diagnosis of a dysphasia is made difficult by a history of acute psychotic episodes, severe depression, or apparent mental retardation. These more dramatic features obscure the dysphasic situation, which may be, as stated earlier, attributed to the psychopathology. A person with a history of 15 years of psychotherapy and poor social, sexual, and work adjustment is not likely to have his speech peculiarities given much attention.

Moreover, evaluation of the qualities of speech in a clinical setting is likely to be subjective.

A standardized test instrument becomes a valuable diagnostic adjunct for the psychotherapist, especially if the instrument is one widely used and well-known to therapists. The Wechsler tests of intelligence are precisely such devices.

They provide valuable insights into language peculiarities more than a cut above the subjective impressions of clinical interviewing. Though not designed as a test of aphasia, and not covering all of the language processes in an aphasia test battery, the Wechsler tests do require a variety of speech processes and also allow an estimate of general level of endowment against which the extent of a suspected specific dysfunction can be examined. For example, a patient with a Full-Scale I.Q. of 100 may obtain a prorated I.Q. of 125 in Similarities and only 89 in Comprehension, suggesting a much higher endowment level than the lower scores alone would indicate. Often higher-level endowment may be inferred by the ability in a specific subtest to respond accurately at a higher level than the patient's total score in that subtest would indicate, succeeding partially or entirely with more difficult items after failing easier ones.

Obviously, both receptive and expressive language ability is required by the tasks of the Wechsler scales. Particular difficulty in comprehending the spoken instructions may be a clue to a receptive disorder. Or the patient may seem not to have heard a word properly, or offer an associative or rhyming response. For example, *obstruct* was defined by a patient as meaning "to build, to wreck," suggesting that she linked the sound of *obstruct* with both *construct* and *destruct*.

Expressive difficulties are more readily apparent on the Wechsler scales. Word-finding difficulties are observable in responses to the Picture Completion subtest where the important missing part must be identified. The patient may point to the area from which the part is missing, attempt to describe it, seek a substitute word, or use gestures: for a violin bow one patient said "I don't know what to call it" while making sawing motions with one hand. Another said for an oarlock, "The thing that they use to hold the oar," while the stirrup of a saddle was identified as "where you put your feet." Of course, such word-finding difficulties are common and when only one or two occur during a subtest they are not necessarily diagnostic of anomia. Increased frequency, however, should arouse diagnostic suspicion.

The Comprehension subtest requires verbal expression of propositional thinking. The patient must explain that he would do so and so, for example, if such and such were the case. He must take the given facts, examine them in light of the question advanced, arrive at a conclusion to be expressed orally. A patient obtained an I.Q. equivalent of 89 in Comprehension in contrast to 118 on Similarities. To the Comprehension question about finding his way out of a forest in the daytime he said, "Look in the direction the sun is set in the area and how I'm set in the area, and the position of the sun, and find my way out." On the Similarities subtest where a single-word response is required rather than a propositional statement, he was able succinctly and accurately to state that north and west are directions, a table and chair are furniture.

Major differences may occur in levels of functioning between these two subtests, the one requiring propositional thinking revealed in rather extended verbal expressions, the other verbal concepts often expressible in a single word.

The Wechsler Scales also tap abstract verbal thinking with questions about the meaning of metaphoric expressions. *Shallow brooks are noisy* evoked this explanation from a young woman, "Oh well, shallow is without depth. People's speaking without thinking of what they're saying. Oh! I just can't bring out what I have in my mind. I know what I'm thinking but I can't bring it into words." For the same expression, a 43-year-old man with a vague history of lead poisoning in childhood said, "A little knowledge is a dangerous thing, a lot of bombasm, bombastic, dilettantism, a flash in the pan." In these somewhat chaotic efforts are evidences that the patients understand the question and that the receptive process is probably less impaired than the expressive, a situation particularly frustrating for the person.

The scales also present tasks that require visual, nonverbal reasoning. These, compared with Comprehension, allow comparison between verbal and arithmetical reasoning and between expressive and nonlanguage visual reasoning (Picture Arrangement).

A general difficulty in responding to projective techniques may also suggest a dysphasia in which the patient is unable to find the words, expressions, or even concepts to formulate his intention.

EMOTIONAL REACTIONS TO LOSS OF LANGUAGE

Many behavioral and emotional problems may appear with aphasia in adults that go beyond the specific problem of language disruption itself (35). These additional disturbances may arise directly from organic damage to cerebral tissue, from the individual's response to the language impairment, or, more significantly in children, from the reaction of others to the person's difficulties or peculiarities of communication.

The range of emotional reactions observed in aphasia are described by Benson (4). They may include: efforts to "crack through" the imposed language barrier; an attitude of surrender in which the patient avoids conversations and uses only the limited responses of which he is capable—yes and no; gestures; eruptions of anger of which the most violent are directed at people close to the patient; profound depression marked by frustration and feelings of impotence, helplessness, and hopelessness; catastrophic reactions described by Goldstein (15) characterized by overwhelming feelings of frustration, depression, and anger; and an attitude of unconcern accompanied sometimes by euphoria or paranoia, with comprehension defects, where the patient does not understand that he does not understand.

Specifically, Benson associates the extremes of the range with the anatomical location of the aphasia-producing lesion. Affective responses of depression, frustration, anger, and catastrophic reactions appear in patients who comprehend and have non-fluent speech; their lesions usually are in the posterior portion of the frontal lobe of the dominant hemisphere. Comprehension difficulties with fluent paraphasic speech and attitudes of unconcern, unawareness, denial, euphoria, and paranoia arise where lesions involve the posterior superior temporal lobe and the adjacent anterior parietal lobe of the dominant hemisphere. These locations respectively are congruent with anterior or Broca's motor aphasia and posterior or Wernicke's sensory aphasia. Smith (30) questions the frequency of the denial mechanisms—elation, euphoria, *la belle indifférence*—that indicate a lack of awareness of the seriousness of the patient's condition. These inappropriate reactions he finds tend to be associated with very extensive brain damage and with dementia.

Efforts at categorization may lead to oversimplification, both in one's view of the emotional reactions to and the possible anatomical locations of the causative lesions. Lesions are not likely to occur within such precise anatomical limitations. Moreover, the possible emotional reactions are likely to include regressions of all kinds, damage to self-esteem, feelings of isolation and loneliness, aversion, anticipation of failure, and the avoidance of efforts at achievement or ego-restriction. These responses are more likely to arise as the patient strives to recover; they affect adversely the very efforts needed to foster recovery. Smith emphasizes that the patient's ability to work through initial depression and accept the fact that there may be more permanent residues unless he works at rehabilitation is prognostically significant.

Moss (26), a clinical psychologist, has described his own struggles to recover from an aphasia that encompassed all language modalities, speech, reading, and writing. For two months he lost the ability to use words in his thinking, and he lost also the ability to dream. At first he did not experience even anxiety; this returned only as he made efforts to perform. Depression emerged only as he underwent hypnotherapy and began to recapture the past and integrate it with both the present and the future. He regards the depression as preferable to the intellectualized defenses penetrated by the catharsis he experienced with hypnotherapy.

That the emotional effects of aphasia are neither limited nor precise is evident in the reactions of children who suffer brain damage and aphasia. While there is an evident tendency for children with receptive disorders to develop "autistic-like impairment of social relations" and those with expressive disorders to be rejected by peers, Cantwell and Baker (7) overall find that children with speech and language disorders develop emotional disorders similar to those found in children of the same age in the general population. The longer the speech-language problem persists, the more likely is the development of emotional problems. These and other brain damaged children are at greater risk of emotional disorders, but of virtually any kind of emotional disorder. There is no "brain damage syndrome," conclude Cantwell and Baker; neuroses or anti-social behaviors are as likely to develop among them as is hyperkinesis.

In children these emotional reactions to aphasia influence the child's future; in adults the emotional past undoubtedly must affect the present response to aphasia, but we have no data to illuminate this process. While we have no specific knowledge of how people with past emotional problems react to the traumatic impact of aphasia, or of the reactions of people who have benefitted from psychotherapy before aphasia, all individual clinical experience indicates that the past person influences the present patient. Premorbid role and status must contribute to emotional reactions. Higher socio-economic status prior to aphasia is reported by Smith (30) to make the necessary downward adjustment more difficult.

TREATMENT

Without doubt the best psychotherapy for the aphasic patient is the recovery of lost or impaired language functions. Reeducation therefore has priority; initial improvement bolsters the patient's self-esteem and increases motivation for the longer and often arduous process to follow.

Confidence in anatomical localization of language functions tended earlier to discourage confidence in language therapy, according to Smith (30), and to limit its applications. He recalls that Wilson as early as 1927 commented that reeducation efforts were sufficient to cause surprise at their neglect. Wilson believed that the observed improvement in response to reeducation was fostered by the restitution of tissue damaged but not destroyed, the development of auxiliary mechanisms in undamaged areas, the fuller development of existing auxiliary mechanisms, the participation of both hemispheres in comprehension, and the potentiality of the right hemisphere for speech.

The remedial effort, Smith cautions, must be sustained; what seems a failure after 45 hours may become a success in 145 hours. And given the complexity of language and its disruptions, the varied patterns of response to varied lesions, there is need for careful definition and tailoring of the language therapy of each patient; it cannot be standardized. Goodkin (16) observes in the use of verbal operant conditioning that the behavioral technique of token reinforcement may serve well with a patient of lower education and socioeconomic level, but not with a patient of higher level, with whom verbal reinforcement is prefered provided comprehension is possible.

The patient's shifting levels of interest, motivation, and cooperation must be observed and in effect exploited. Wepman (35) has found that it is better to use the favorable periods to their possible optimum than to attempt to stimulate the patient during periods of disinterest or uncooperativeness.

Smith (30) has derived some useful observations on prognosis from a study employing standardized before and after measures. Stroke patients with an average of 395 hours of treatment were compared with 15 stroke patients who did not receive extensive therapy, and 13 traumatic lesion patients of lower mean age who did receive treatment. Significant improvement of language functions was recorded in treated patients (both stroke and traumatic lesions) in contrast to untreated ones. This reflects improvement beyond that expected from spontaneous recovery, improvement attributable to training. Hemiplegics benefited as much as non-hemiplegics, refuting a contrary expectation.

Age is not prognostic in this study. Although the older third showed more improvement initially, at the end of the study no difference between older and younger third was observed.

While limited education proved not to be an obstacle, the more educated group did better in reading and writing.

Duration of therapy was prognostically critical in the study reported by Smith. Those who received 500 to 1000 hours of therapy did better in all language functions than did those who received 125 to 250 hours. Early initiation of treatment after language loss was also favorably prognostic.

As might not be expected, those patients with the most severe impairment of language approximated the gains of the least impaired.

Behavioral reinforcement techniques are widely and fruitfully used in re-establishing language functions among the aphasic. Family members of the patient, usually the spouse, are often enlisted on the treatment team to provide continuity and repetition in the training and to combat extinction during intervals between sessions with professional therapists. Speech therapy in groups with similar types of aphasia helps counteract feelings of isolation and uniqueness and furnishes a bearable stimulus.

Impaired comprehension and speech are, of course, major obstacles to psychotherapy for the severely aphasic patient. Benson (4) advises that efforts at communication with the patient who appears to be unconcerned should be continued, but kept short to avoid overload, as well as, presumably, to avoid an increase of denial. In these brief efforts all forms of language are used: writing, speech, and gestures. Long rest periods are interspersed between very slow gradual increments of language stimulation. Tranquilizing medication may be necessary.

The depressed patient, Benson states, needs active supportive therapy, with attention given to concerns of the family and to business and employment obligations. Friends and work colleagues as well as family may be involved fruitfully in helping the patient to see that his world has not collapsed and that a place in it awaits him. Reiterated, structuring of the planned speech and physical therapies can combat the sense of helplessness and hopelessness that besets the aphasic patients. Repeated recognition of gains made also supports this process.

Psychotherapy becomes possible, although still difficult, with the moderately aphasic patient or with the patient somewhat recovered from a severe aphasia who has become what we may term dysphasic. Even with these patients the therapist must continually make certain that what is being said is comprehended, that what is intended is said. With some patients, the therapist will seem to be acquiring the patient's language. All forms of communication become important as adjuncts to speech: writing, pointing, gestures, mime, drawings, use of objects and toys, construction material.

Ability to communicate understanding of what the aphasic patient feels about his lot is essential in establishing rapport and unleashing energy-binding affects. The therapist must comprehend the rage and despair, the humiliation of helplessness, the frustration of muteness and immobility, the crushing depression of hopelessness, the enormous damage to self-esteem, the sense of isolation and fear of recurrence that the aphasic patient suffers. These affects are often buried not only in inability to communicate but also by denial and repression. Working through these defenses is a priority and a continuing focus. Moss (26), the psychologist already quoted who became aphasic, sought catharsis in hypnotherapy and reports the integrating effect upon his time sense and the cutting through of his intellectualized defenses the experience provided.

The therapist must be prepared to make large leaps into unconscious and primitive levels of both body-image and self-image, to identify with the distortion and the narcissistic injury that take place at these levels, in order to help the patient bring them to awareness and clarify them.

In speech recovery, certain plateaus are likely, paralleled by halted progress in re-establishing motor and sensory functions. Such intervals are likely to revive and intensify rage, depression, and denial; they require intensified psychotherapeutic effort. Longer intervals re-evoke pessimism. Finally, the patient is likely to be confronted with what seem irreversible impairments, those residues of dysfunction that do not change for the better. Hopelessness must be countered by helping the patient reconstruct his life and functioning around the reality of these persisting limitations. Some patients may need help in accepting a lower level of vocational functioning, or a more limited activity at the former level. Here again clarification and sharing of affects facilitate realistic acceptance.

Group psychotherapy, where possible, of recovering aphasic patients, couple or family therapy, vocational counseling, vocational rehabilitation, environmental manipulation, and supportive measures along with availability of allied professional persons are significant adjuncts to psychotherapy. While no research data are available to support this, it is reasonable to assume that the pre-aphasic personality of the patient very much determines what the tasks, course, and outcome of psychotherapy are likely to be. Persistence and assertiveness facilitate progress; passivity, dependence and depressive tendencies impede it. Masochism may place more value on impairment than on recovery. Impulsiveness and acting-out proclivities may disrupt progress and promote regression. Hypochondriasis is likely to emerge or fulminate. So the psychotherapist of the recovering aphasic patient must attempt to evaluate both the response to the aphasia and the prior personality. Interviewing of family members, friends, and colleagues will help, although the data thus obtained can be accepted only with caution.

CASE ILLUSTRATIONS

1. *Shot in the head, body and extremities seven times, a 34-year-old female high-school graduate seeks vocational retraining. One bullet remains in the brain.*

J. has shown steady improvement in the physical sense and in other respects since the trauma. She is now able to move about painfully but without a cane; her mental status is described, however, as "strange and changed from before"; there is a right homonynous hemianopsia. While she has good muscle strength, the deep tendon reflexes are increased on the left side with coolness of the ankle. Coordination is also impaired on the left side and there is a sensory decrement on the left side. The suggestion is therefore strong of greater injury to the right side of the brain. The psychologist's report follows.

"J. is a sweet, attractive, smiling woman with a mobile, expressive face. She is strongly motivated to do well. She does move painfully, but cooperates to the hilt. Former traces of High Average intellectual endowment, if not higher, are manifest in the fact that she operates across a wide range of difficulty in the vocabulary subtest, obtaining partial success with difficult words after having failed easier ones completely. Had she been able to function with complete success across the range of difficulty in which she now operates, she would have achieved a prorated I.Q. of 117, but she manifests the problems of an aphasia, impairment of expressive and comprehensive language. Her response for the word *cavern* is to spell it correctly and then say, 'I don't know';

terminate means, 'You're fired,' which shows comprehension of the meaning of the word but inability to define it expressively other than in a customary usage situation. *Winter* is defined as 'the time of the year when Christmas comes, and it snows and there are whole lot of things going on, and it gets cold.' *Repair* is defined as 'something that is bad and you have to call in; the pipes are bad so you have to call the plumber.'

"Aphasic difficulties are manifest throughout the verbal portion of the Wechsler in spite of the fact that this is where she does better. A thermometer is, 'It depends. You use it for—to try—for—to test out when you're having a fever.' Rubber comes from, 'I don't remember.' In response to the query, 'what to do with the sealed, addressed, and stamped envelope found in the street,' she repeats, 'Sealed. It is addressed. It has a new stamp.' She registered each of the component parts of the statement in terms of comprehension, then went on to say, 'I don't get that.' Asked why child-labor laws are necessary, she responds, 'Give it to me another way. I don't understand it.' The labor laws are defined for her and she goes on to say, 'The law makers figure a child would be responsible at a certain age.'

"Returning to the verbal area, ability for abstract thinking and verbal conceptualization are extremely impaired and she achieves zero in the Similarities subtest. Capacity for attention and concentration is somewhat better when the auditory modality is involved in contrast to the visual so that where she obtains a zero scale score in Digit Symbol, she achieves nine in Digit span (where she can retain seven digits forward but only two in reverse order) and six in Arithmetic.

"Her comprehension difficulties were also manifested to extraordinary degree during the Digit Symbol instructions where it took her an inordinately long time to catch on to what was expected of her. Part of this appeared to arise from the confusion created by what was, for her, the complicated visual field in which she had to shift between the guiding stimulus, the task itself, and then back again. Once she grasped the instructions, which took a long time, simple as they are, it was clear that she comprehended, but her pace was so painfully slow that she received a zero scale score, an unscorable total. The unscorable level was obtained in the recognition of essential details, also it seemed, because of the complicated visual field. In the assembly of familiar objects, her scale score averages out to a prorated I.Q. of 37. The perceptual-analytic impairment is pronounced.

"The dual administration of the Bender and the Heimburger-Reitan confirm the severe impairment in spatial relations, resulting in a pronounced constructional apraxia. Graphomotor control is moderately good, though painfully slow.

"J. indicates that she experiences blurred vision, dizziness, paresthesias in which the whole left side is involved, phosphenes, near-hallucinatory episodes, and altered states of consciousness. These occur more frequently when she neglects her medication which she says is Phenobarbital and Codeine. It is likely that she is subject to paroxyomal phenomena which are being treated with the Phenobarbital.

"She obviously has come a long way since her massive injuries and undoubtedly will make continued but slow progress with time."

2. *An equivocal diagnostic situation in which dysphasia or a thought disorder may be present in an adolescent reported to have been bizarre and assaultive.*

M. has had two psychiatric hospitalizations in three years. Preceding both he became bizarre, wildly waving his arms, threatening people, and was disorganized. It is said that he never hit anyone. He had a bad reaction to large doses of Thorazine, again becoming hyperactive and bizarre. He was then placed on Stelazine in smaller amounts.

The circumstances surrounding the precipitating events of each of his acute episodes are not made clear. For the present illness, it is said that for about two weeks prior to admission he became increasingly more disorganized, finally became assaultive toward his family. His first break came during his freshman year in college; he states that it was due to pressure from both school and his girl friend. That time, too, he became disorganized and assaultive, threatening to smash his father's face in.

M. is an attractive, charming lad, muscular and husky; he has somewhat of a chip-on-the-shoulder attitude about appointments and timing of appointments, but withal he is as indicated pleasant, seemingly relaxed, communicative.

Superior level potentialities are indicated in a prorated I.Q. of 138 in Comprehension and 126 in Information. However, there is a tendency toward over-concreteness manifested in a prorated I.Q. of 114 in Similarities. There is indication of an attention-memory deficit with Average to Low Average scores in this area. He has good spatial visualization ability, achieving a prorated I.Q. of 128 in Picture Completion and 114 in the assembly of familiar objects (Object Assembly).

When called upon to make extended verbal propositions, his responses suggest either an aphasia or a basic thought disorder marked by primary-process thinking. Some of his responses are listed here as illustrations: 1) Why should people pay taxes?: "To maintain the civil and political setup, the conveniences, the commodities for the people and the services." 2) What is the meaning of the expression, "Strike while the iron is hot?": "Do what you have to do in the quickest fashion; go when the opportunity is there; when it knocks on your door, you open the door and go through it." 3) If lost in a forest in the daytime, how would you find your way out? "If I knew the longitude and the latitude of the sun and what the time it was in Greenwich meridian, I would then know north, east, south, and west and I would get out if I had a sextant. That would make it easy." 4) Why does land in the city usually cost more than land in the country? "The more people there are to the square mile to go to business you establish on the block, it has the potential to receive wealth and patronage of hundreds of thousands more than in the country which is less per square acre." 5) Why does the state require a license for people to get married?: "The woman has to be eighteen; the man has to be twenty-one. If you don't have it before you go to church, they wouldn't have a record of the age and address of the people that help facilitate records of the City of New York and of government agencies in the state and of the federal government. You have to deal with the future." 6) What is the meaning of the expression "Shallow brooks are noisy?": "If I can make a simile to people, if you have nothing going for yourself, or you always stick your face in the mirror, you really don't have any good looks or other qualities, that person is trying to reassure himself and he makes a lot of noise about how good and fine he is."

His responses to projective queries and projective methods indicate that M. was a hyperactive, assaultive child, prone to destructiveness, easily frustrated. He expressed his frustrations in gross physical movements that often were violent. Thus, he acknowledges that his temper has always been his worst quality, that he pushed kids around, that he wrecked the apartment, that the worst thing he has ever done was hitting a girl in the mouth when he was nine or ten because she wanted him to give back her hat that he had taken from her.

There is indication of an over-ideational quality which suggests the possibility of a thought disorder. He recalls at the age of three or four, being impressed with the fact that food was related to life, the absence of it to death, when a teacher told a child that the child would die if he didn't eat.

He had an appendectomy in August, 1973; the appendix he says was perforated. He was told that his birth was difficult, that labor was induced. There is some possibility that the experience of the appendectomy contributed to his most recent acute episode.

It is difficult to arrive at an exclusive diagnsois. There is evidence of a long-established tendency toward hyperactivity, assaultiveness, and a quickly escalating temper. This could well be the product of the sadomasochistic environment in which he grew up. It could also be related to an unstructured neurological deficit, so that what appears to be a thought disorder might well be an aphasia. Supporting this possibility is his negative reaction to Thorazine in which instead of becoming sedated, he became more assaultive and more bizarre.

BIBLIOGRAPHY

1. *Ajax, E. T.:* The aphasic patient: a practical review. Dis. Ner. Syst., 34:4, 1973.
2. *Andreasen, N. J. C. et al.:* The significance of thought disorder in diagnostic evaluations. Comprehensive Psychiat., 15:1, 1974.
3. *Bender, L.* and *Faretra, S.:* The relationship between childhood schizophrenia and adult schizophrenia. *In* A. Kaplan (Ed.): Genetic Factors In Schizophrenia. Springfield, Ill.: Charles C. Thomas, 1972.
4. *Benson, D. F.:* Psychiatric aspects of aphasia. Brit. J. Psychiat., 123:576, 1973.
5. *Benton, A. L.* (Ed.): Behavioral Change in Cerebrovascular Disease. New York: Harper, 1970.
6. *Brookshire, R. H.:* Probability learning by aphasic subjects. J. Speech Hearing Res. 12:4, 1969.
7. *Cantwell, D.* and *Baker, L.:* Psychiatric disorder in children with speech and language retardation. Arch. Gen. Psychiat., 34:5, 1977.
8. *Chapman, J.:* The early symptoms of schizophrenia. Brit. J. Psychiat., 112, 1966.
9. *Chappell, G. E.:* Developmental aphasia revisited. J. Communic. Disorders, 3:3, 1970.
10. *Critchley, M.:* The neurology of psychotic speech. Brit. J. Psychiat., 110, 1964.
11. *Culton, G. L.:* Spontaneous recovery from aphasia. J. Speech Hearing Res. 12:4, 1969.
12. *Eisenson, J.:* Adult Aphasia: Assessment and Treatment. New York: Appleton-Century-Crofts, 1973.
13. *Eisenson, J.* and *Ingram, D.:* Childhood aphasia—an updated concept based upon recent research. Acta Symbolica, 3:2, 1972.
14. *Geschwind, N.:* Language disturbances in cerebrovascular disease. Presentation 4. *In* A. L. Benton (Ed.): Behavioral Changes in Cerebrovascular Disease. New York: Harper and Row, 1970.
15. *Goldstein, K.:* The Organism. New York: The American Book Publishers, 1939.
16. *Goodkin, R.:* The modification of verbal behavior in aphasic subjects. Mimeo. 1970.
17. *Howes, D. H.:* Application of the word-frequency concept to aphasia. *In* A. V. S.

DeReuck and M. O'Connor (Eds.): Disorders of Language. Boston: Little, Brown, 1964.

18. *Jackson, J. H.:* On the nature of the duality of the brain. *In* J. Taylor (Ed.): Selected Writings of John Hughlings Jackson. New York: Basic Books, 1958.

19. *Jones, L. V.* and *Wepman, J. M.:* Dimensions of language performance in aphasia. J. Speech Hearing Res., 4, 1961.

20. *Kinsbourne, M.:* The minor cerebral hemisphere. Arch. Neurol., 25:4, 1971.

21. *L'Abate, L. et al.:* Exploratory studies of receptive-expressive functions in children, Mimeo, undated.

22. *Leicester, J. et al.:* The nature of aphasic responses. Neuropsychologia, 9:2, 1971.

23. *Luria, A. R.:* Traumatic Aphasia. Paris, France: Mouton, 1970.

24. *MacMahon, M. K.:* Modern linguistics and aphasia. Brit. J. Disorders Communication, 7:1, 1972.

25. *Maher, B.:* The language of schizophrenia: A review and interpretation. Brit. J. Psychiat., 120, 1972.

26. *Moss, C. S.:* Rehabilitation from the viewpoint of an "aphasic psychologist." Rehab. Psychol., 22:2, 1975.

27. *Schuell, H.* and *Jenkins, J. J.:* Reduction of vocabulary in aphasia. Brain, 84, 1961.

28. *Schuell, H.* and *Nagar, K.:* Aphasia studies. Geriatrics, 24:10, 1969.

29. *Shapiro, T.* and *Fish, B.:* A method to study language deviation as an aspect of ego organization in young schizophrenic children. J. Amer. Acad. Child Psychiat., 8, 1969.

30. *Smith, A.:* Diagnosis, intelligence and rehabilitation of chronic aphasias. Ann Arbor, Michigan: Neuropsychology Dept., Univ. of Michigan, 1972.

31. *Smith, A.:* Appraising the neuropsychological literature. Bull. Int. Neuropsychological Soc., August, 1978.

32. *Spreen, O.:* Psycholinguistic aspects of aphasia. J. Speech Hearing Res., 11:3, 1968.

33. *Van Dongen, H. R.* and *Van Harskamp, F.:* The token test: a preliminary evaluation of a method to detect aphasia. Psychiat., Neurol., Neurochir. (Amsterdam), 75, 1972.

34. *Vignola, L. A.:* Evolution of aphasia and language rehabilitation: a retrospective exploratory study. Cortex, 1, 1965.

35. *Wepman, J. M.:* Recovery From Aphasia. New York: Ronald Press, 1951.

36. *Whitaker, H.* and *Whitaker, H. A.* (Eds.): Studies in Neurolinguistics, Vols. 1 and 2. New York: Academic Press, 1976.

37. *Wiig, E. H.* and *Smith, P.H.:* Aphasia performance on visual tracking program. Percept. Motor Skills, 35:2, 1972.

38. *Wilson, S. A. K.:* Aphasia. *In* H. A. Christian (Ed.): Oxford Medicine. New York: Oxford Univ. Press, 1927.

39. *Wyke, M.:* Dysphasia: A review of recent progress. Brit. Med. Bull., 27:3, 1971.

CHAPTER 5

Schizophrenia

This disorder or conglomerate of disorders continues to baffle psychiatry after more than a century of effort to identify its causes and to classify and treat its manifestations. The work of the last three decades bears witness to the commitment of the National Institute of Mental Health to unravel the mysteries of schizophrenia. Mosher, editor of the *Schizophrenia Bulletin*, notes that a "reliable diagnostic system has eluded psychiatry since the time of Kraepelin's first systematic efforts" (61). Equally elusive have been its causes, the verified identification of its etiologies.

Understanding etiology is ultimately essential to the diagnosis and treatment of any disorder or disease. For schizophrenia, the pragmatic pursuit of treatment has not been fully revealing. The success of the psychotropic drugs in shortening hospital stay, reducing hospital populations, even in preventing hospitalization, has contributed some interesting hypotheses but few incontrovertible explanations. Why, for example, do some patients diagnosed as schizophrenic become worse when treated with the phenothiazines? Could it not be that the cause of their disorder is different from that of other patients with similar symptoms?

Our failure to reduce the incidence increases the urgency of a search for effective preventive measures, validated by establishing the etiology or etiologies of the condition. The quest has taken investigators into psychosocial, genetic and organic explorations. The diverse deficits in schizophrenia suggest such divergent courses of exploration: illogical use of language, learning disabilities, apathy and poor motivation, disturbed sensory and perceptual acuity, disrupted conceptual process (61). Also observed are deficits in ego functions that affect reality sense,

163

judgment, thought processes, relationships with other people, impulse control, and defenses (6).

Identifying, describing, and classfying these deficits require knowledge of "language and communication, emotion, motivation, perception, cognition, and personality, as well as the neural and endocrine bases of behavior" (61). Their causes may rest in body chemistry, genetics, relationships or communication within the family, emotionally traumatic events, lack of social support, and cerebral pathology, or in combination thereof.

The search for a single-factor etiology in schizophrenia has often produced promising findings that were soon found to conflict with data from other lines of investigation. Supporting the genetic etiology in schizophrenia, for example, is the repeated finding that monozygotic (MZ) twins are three times more often concordant for schizophrenia than are dizygotic (DZ) twins. Campion and Tucker (19) caution that while significant and well-documented physiological and developmental differences are found between MZ and DZ twins, these are seldom accounted for in such genetic studies. For example, perinatal death is three times more frequent in MZ than DZ twins, temporal-lobe epilepsy ten times more frequent.

The efforts to sort out and identify causal factors are obstructed also by major diagnostic problems. Symptoms, the major basis of diagnosis, may vary from observation to observation in the same patient; certainly they vary from patient to patient. The signs and symptoms reported vary under the influence of the diagnostician's knowledge and bias (61). Mednick (57) finds contributing to the confusion the unreliability of childhood records, because of the differing vocabularies used by past observers, the ways in which the life pattern of the schizophrenic may influence the disorder, and the complicating effect upon the family of the schizophrenic member, an effect similar to the family impact of other serious illness as well.

The important psychotropic drugs have proved a mixed blessing. Investigators of auditory-evoked potential in schizophrenics, confronted with the highly variable data they find, observe ruefully that "Drugs provide one of the most ubiquitous complicating factors in schizophrenia research" (18).

Neurological and neuropsychological procedures also confront failures to separate the functional from the organic factors in schizophrenia. Standard neurological procedures, including the electroencephalogram, all too frequently produce false negative findings (See chapters on *Epilepsy* and *Neurodiagnostic Approaches*). Yet neuro-psychological research must depend upon neurological data for cor-roboration.

In short, investigations of single-factor etiologies in schizophrenia produce insights and suggestive hypotheses, but few solutions. They have tended to be blind alleys. Garmezy (30), reviewing many and varied studies of children at risk for schizophrenia, concludes "If they do nothing else, risk studies will point up the danger of imputing causation to a correlational statement." And he doubts that risk studies will "unlock the riddle of the etiology of schizophrenia."

These seemingly discouraging results and observations have a brighter, more optimistic consequence. They are moving us away from simplistic unitary hypotheses to increasingly multifactorial concepts, al-though there is yet no system that integrates the multiple causal factors now associated with schizophrenia (60, 73, 88, 90). The interplay be-tween factors is receiving more attention and more effort is made to incorporate multiple variables into research. Is there, for example, a genetic disposition to prenatal and neonatal difficulties? How do neu-rological deficits of slight degree subtly affect the psychological aspects of infant-mother interaction? Does schizophrenia in the mother affect the birth process in ways that result in such neurological deficits? Garmezy's study (30) of recently completed and on-going risk inves-tigations shows that the more recent studies have more sophisticated research designs, more complex variables, and a commitment to a lon-gitudinal prospective strategy for studying the developmental process, efforts that hold more promise.

For the psychotherapist the word is *caution*. The absence of a valid multiple-factor explanation of diagnosis, etiology, and treatment does not remove the requirement that all possible factors and their inter-action be considered for the individual patient. This chapter reviews major neurological elements in schizophrenia which the psychothera-pist may try to integrate with his psycho-social concepts. The equally significant genetic and other organic factors, including metabolism, endocrinology, and neurophysiology, are outside the scope of this book.

LANGUAGE DISORDER OR THOUGHT DISORDER?

The diagnosis of schizophrenia is often based largely upon the speech of the patient. An earlier chapter in this book—*Aphasia and Dys-phasia*—suggests that the dysphasic speech of some patients may be misdiagnosed as evidence of a thought disorder, of primary-process thinking. In diagnosing a thought disorder, the therapist assumes that the thought processes are disturbing and disordering both the content and structure of speech. In diagnosing a language disorder, the therapist entertains the possibility of either or both functional and organic etiologies: thought disorder, learning disabilities, infant-maternal relationships, deafness and aphasia among others. These diagnostic differences may be crucial to the course of treatment, a status that warrants their exploration here. Knowledge of these differences increases in importance for the therapist when we stress the well recognized central role of speech in the therapeutic process.

Classic Concepts of Thought Disorder in Schizophrenia

Bleuler (15) considered disorders of thought to be the primary symptom of schizophrenia. These disorders appeared as a *loss of continuity* of associations between thoughts and ideas, resulting in confusion; the loss of continuity arose either from pressure of thoughts attacking and fragmenting an idea, or from a blocking which interrupted the thought process.

Goldstein (36) emphasized *concreteness* of thought as a major symptom, which appeared also, as he observed, in people who suffered brain injury; in both he saw a loss of capability for abstraction. The schizophrenic additionally manifested peculiar individual *autistic ideas* in both speech and behavior. This conception was developed further in Kasanin's (45) idea of *physiognomic* thinking, which is related to the concept of failure to progress, or actual regression to an earlier state, as a result of psychopathology. Kasanin saw physiognomic thinking as the earliest stage in the development of thought, one in which a child projects himself into objects, which he thus animates. A subsequent stage is the development of concrete thinking; the final stage is abstract or categorical thinking. He postulated that the schizophrenic, either because he has failed to progress or has regressed, tends to show more of the first two stages in his thought processes.

Schilder's (78) concept of thought disorders also includes a developmental progression: Every thought progresses from the indefinite to the more definite forms before it becomes conscious. Pathological thoughts result from a premature closure of the developmental process; in effect, the failure to progress.

Filling the void produced by decathexis in schizophrenia and the repression of instincts is seen by Rycroft (77) as the mechanism whereby thought disturbances are created. This drive to fill the void may be the pressure which fragments an idea, in Bleuler's concept.

The *overinclusive tendency* in schizophrenic thinking is described by McGhie (53) as one arising from inability to maintain conceptual boundaries, and may be primarily a disorder of selective attention arising from the schizophrenic's preoccupation.

More descriptively, Mosher (61) identified the thought and language disturbances of the schizophrenic as characterized by *looseness of association, blocking, neologisms, clang associations,* and *irrelevant responses.*

The psychoanalytic view of the thought process is also a developmental theory, proceeding from primary-process thinking (hallucinatory gratification of a need when actual gratification is not possible) to secondary-process thinking (the idea or thought of ultimate gratification enables tolerance of the tension necessary to delay immediate gratification). Thus the primary process or hallucination is the precursor of thought, representing both idea and gratification. The primary process is regulated by the pleasure principle. The secondary process—delaying gratification by using thought—emerges as a result of the development of reality perception, which enables the individual to combat the hallucinatory mode of gratification. In some schizophrenics this may be the basis for regression to hallucinatory gratifications. In others it may explain their emphasis upon language, the development of obsessional thinking as a means of containing sexual and aggressive drives, in order to avoid decisiveness or overt behavior. The brain-damaged person may resort to obsessional thinking as the reassuringly repeated expression of residual competence in support of self-esteem.

A most thorough recent effort to delineate the nature of the thought process in schizophrenia, and to evaluate the process, led Bellak (7) and his colleagues to define the constituents of thought processes and attempt to apply them to the diagnosis of schizophrenia. The constituents of thought processes as they identify them are: 1) adaptiveness in memory, concentration, and attention; 2) ability to conceptualize, i.e., the use of abstract and concrete modes of thought in manners appropriate to the situation; 3) the primary-secondary process continuum.

They raise this significant diagnostic question: Is the presence of a thought disorder both a necessary and sufficient criterion for the diagnosis of schizophrenia? Their search for answers drew them to a consideration of the various etiologies that have been associated with thought disorders. These include: 1) organic conditions which range from the "hard" signs of pronounced aphasia to the "soft" signs of dyslexic language disturbances; 2) the "double-bind" parent who says one thing but means another, so that communications lose meaning for the individual; 3) poor boundaries between self and the external world; 4) the use of over-inclusion to decrease anxiety; 5) the secondary effect of disruption of some other ego function (for example: the disruption of the synthetic function by emotional pressures, the disruption of object relations, or the use of excessive denial). Bellak and his colleagues conclude that in the absence of organic conditions, a severe thought disorder *may be* a sufficient sign of schizophrenia, but not a necessary one for such a diagnosis. The similarities between language disturbances arising from organic brain damage and those appearing in the thought disorders of schizophrenia are stikingly similar; on the surface they often can not be distinguished from each other. Missing from their conclusion are the conditions that make a thought disorder a *sufficient* sign of schizophrenia.

Forty-two clinicians interpreting quotations from undiagnosed authors, interpretations of proverbs, the words of manics, and the words of schizophrenics found thought disorders less frequently in the schizophrenics (3). And Goldstein (35) long ago observed that loss of abstract verbal functioning in a thought disorder is similar to that in brain damage.

Language Disorder in Schizophrenia

The many efforts to differentiate schizophrenia from aphasia in both children and adults have not been successful. Dysphasia early in life is argued by Lyle (52) to result in a thought disorder that is elaborated in fantasy and expression as speech improves. The suggestion is that dysphasia is linked to difficulty in processing and decoding sensory data—especially heard speech—selectively or rapidly enough. This leads to a loss of the sensory data because of an overload of short-term memory, so that only fragmentary information is relayed to higher cognitive levels, thus giving rise to thought confusion. Childhood schizophrenia, while not fulfilling the criteria for the diagnosis of schizophrenia in adults, is considered to be "continuous" with that diagnosis and is regularly marked by retardation of speech and language. The role of speech disorder in autism, when efforts are made to separate it from childhood schizophrenia is even clearer and more generally accepted. Rutter (74, 75, 76) considers the language disorder in autism to be severe and extensive, constituting aphasia and being fundamental to the syndrome. In turn he relates prognosis to speech development and cognitive functioning. The development of "adequate" functioning is reported in two children after they acquired speech, where both mothers talked to their children "constantly and constructively" (29). The prominence of language problems in autism is supported by the experience of Wing and Wing (90), who call attention to other problems as well.

In adults the growing effort to distinguish between schizophrenic thought disorders and aphasic language disturbances is reflected in the work of Gerson et al., (31) using recorded interviews in which both open-ended and directed questions were asked. They identified six major differences and five undifferentiating factors. Appropriateness of response was not useful in the effort to differentiate 8 diagnosed posterior aphasics from 10 diagnosed schizophrenics during acute episodes. Echolalia was absent in both groups, while blocking, reiteration and persistent themes were marked in both. The schizophrenic patients produced persistent bizarre themes while the themes of the aphasics were disparate. The responses by schizophrenics to open-ended questions were longer (100 + words) than those of aphasics (20-30). The aphasics were more aware of and disturbed by their difficulties, used more non-verbal substitutes or pauses to elicit help, and more often substituted letters and words incorrectly. Vagueness of expression was present in both; that of the aphasics was attributed to anomia, that of the schizophrenics to blocking caused by shifts in attention.

This study highlights the serious difficulties concerning criteria in research efforts to separate organic from functional groups of patients. Aside from the small populations, the ruling out of brain damage in a group of patients with presumably functional disorders remains an unreliable procedure. Standard neurological procedures, used in this study, are not reliable nor valid indicators of the subtle degrees of cerebral dysfunctions that are presumed in the language disorder theory in schizophrenia (See Chapter 16).

For decades certain language symptoms have been considered diagnostic manifestations of schizophrenia: perseveration, echolalia, clang associations, mutism, but Benson (12) found perseveration—the continued repetition of words, sounds or gestures—in the brain-damaged patient, the mentally retarded, and the acutely psychotic one. Echolalia was rarely observed in aphasia and occasionally as a transient symptom in catatonic schizophrenia; it may, he observed, occur in persons with low-level mental ability, in states of clouded consciousness, in the early stages of normal speech development; it is frequent in childhood autism.

Mutism is a major feature of stupor states in both severe depression and catatonic schizophrenia, and extremely rare in the aphasic patient who can almost always make sounds. (One must consider, of course, that many aphasic patients become severely depressed.)

Anomia—word-finding difficulty—is virtually ubiquitous in aphasia and is generally considered an alerting sign of that disorder, yet it occurs in severe anxiety states, depressions, and catatonic schizophrenia (12).

So the diagnostic separation of language disorders associated with aphasia from thought disorders that are concomitants or corollaries of schizophrenia is difficult and uncertain. It appears that the two share basic symptoms; one cannot safely diagnose aphasia on the basis of anomia, the pauses of the aphasic are difficult to separate with reasonable certainty from the so-called thought blocking of the schizophrenic. And that too is the state of the diagnostic art with circumlocution, circumstantiality, echolalia, and perseveration. Both the neurological and psychiatric diagnoses are weakened by false-negative and false-positive findings. The instrumentation associated with neurological examinations shares this weakness. What we observe to be a thought disorder may be an aphasia, or the converse may be the case. At best the findings are suggestive: in some schizophrenics a language disorder contributes to thought disorder.

SCHIZOPHRENIA IN CHILDREN

Probably no greater conflict exists in psychology and psychiatry, no sharper contesting of theoretical views, than that which attends the question of the etiology of childhood schizophrenia. Chess (22) states that though often diagnosed, childhood schizophrenia is poorly understood, its etiology remains obscure, that a diversity of both syndromes and symptoms pictures is grouped under the rubric. Diagnostic terminology is also confused between autism and childhood schizophrenia. Both are defined essentially by narcissism, decathexis, withdrawal, with some effort to introduce a differentiating time element, autism presumably appearing during infancy, schizophrenia later in child-hood. These efforts also became confusing as is evident in Rutter's (73) attempt to distinguish between infantile autism, childhood schizophrenia, and the "disintegrating" psychoses. He found it neces-sary to add another, catch-all category "other psychoses of childhood."

Etiology and Diagnosis

Various assumed causes are implied in the varieties of description. Kanner (44) describes children who from infancy fail to respond in an appropriate affective manner to their environment and to the people in it. They particularly do not respond to the people who take care of them, and they tend to be more responsive to objects than to people generally. They may not learn to talk and in many ways may resemble retarded or aphasic children. He has labeled this condition, "primary infantile autism."

A type of childhood schizophrenia, the "symbiotic," has been de-scribed by Margaret Mahler (54). This child is extremely clinging, virtually melting into the mother's body and ego; he cannot differ-entiate between himself and his mother, and so is not able to form an independent entity nor to function as such.

The biological nature of schizophrenia is emphasized by Bender (10, 11), who holds that a biological difficulty is the basis for the primary symptoms of childhood schizophrenia. As the child attempts to deal with his difficulty, secondary symptoms develop, which become recognized as the manifest schizophrenia. In her view, the biological difficulties constitute a "lag in maturation," a persistence of the plas-ticity of the central nervous system characteristic of the embryonic state.

Genetic factors are implicated by the observations of the high rate of congruence among identical schizoid twins (42). Biochemical de-fects have been implicated by other investigators (8).

The presence of clear-cut neurological pathology in many children believed to be schizophrenic has been identified by Goldfarb (34). Convulsions as well as other neurological disorders that were not or-iginally noticed are now being discovered among these children. Cere-bral lesions have been found at autopsy in some cases (23).

Using the Gesell examination and standards, Fish (26) identified neurological abnormalities as early as the first month after birth in an infant who later developed schizophrenia. Fish does not believe that a fixed neurological defect appears during infancy among schizophrenic children, but rather a disorder which affects the timing and integration of their neurological maturation. She believes that this primitive neurological immaturity is the prologue of the more complex disorganization subsequently manifested in adult schizophrenics.

Clinical differences among schizophrenic children do not imply different etiological circumstances, according to Fish. Thus, lower I.Q.'s and greater evidence of neurological disability may represent more severe variants of childhood schizophrenia. Gradations of severity, she believes, are demonstrated by the fact that children will shift from more severe to less severe clinical pictures, and vice-versa. These gradations of severity, she believes, point to a continuum of schizophrenia *with* and *without* central-nervous-system involvement. The more severe the immaturity of neural integration, the less important environmental factors may be. Conversely, the less severe the impairment of neural integration and maturity the more important role environmental factors may play in the clinical picture of childhood schizophrenia.

The ultimate severity of impairment depends upon the time of emergence of the early neurological disturbance, the duration of this disturbance, and the role that the environment plays in counteracting or exacerbating the child's difficulties. Fish's observations are based upon study of the history of children with childhood schizophrenia, where she was able to identify significant deviants in early motor development in the histories of half the children with specific organic brain disease but also in a large number of schizophrenic children. She believes that disturbances of neurological functioning occur well before two years of age in many schizophrenic children.

Taft and Goldfarb (81) after studies of schizophrenic children at the Ittleson Center indicate that children with schizophrenia represent a highly diversified group, differing among themselves in "capacities, symptoms, defenses, psychosocial backgrounds, and factors contributing to the aberrant adaptation." Among this broad universe of children, they establish one group who have been traumatized and neurologically impaired during the reproductive process, whose neurological impairment is traceable to both pre- and perinatal factors. This neurological dysfunction appears to be more typical of boys than of girls in their schizophrenic group. Establishment of a neurological involvement in the schizophrenic child does not vitiate the influence of environmental factors, nor does it remove the need to comprehend the symptoms and characteristics of the individual child, to formulate an individualized treatment for him. The cerebral impairment, of course, limits the child's competence and effectiveness in adaptation. The responses of parents to the child's limited abilities can reinforce behavior which has come to be termed schizophrenic. A psychodynamic analysis of the schizophrenic child should detail the child's biological potentiality for ego development and expression, along with his individual psychosocial environment and its capacity for reinforcing or impairing his ego development. Brain damage alone does not explain the specific, unique, schizophrenic symptom of the individual child.

This view is questioned by Birch and Walker (14) and Gittleman and Birch (33). Through their research they have attempted to evaluate the major views concerning the etiology of childhood schizophrenia, which they identify as these:

1) Childhood schizophrenia derives from pathological interpersonal relationships in a destructive family or other social circumstance.

2) Organic factors are primarily responsible for the development of childhood schizophrenia, which is fundamentally a developmental defect deriving from neurological malfunctioning and therefore can be grouped with other forms of brain damage.

3) An intermediate view argues for a dual etiology, reasoning that an organic component is primary in the origins of some schizophrenic disorders, while other individuals are schizophrenic because of inadequacies in their environments.

4) Schizophrenia develops in a child who is physiologically deviant and therefore interacts ineffectively with environmental circumstances which place various stresses and demands upon the incompetent organism.

Birch and Walker (14) attempt to illuminate the question by comparing well-defined functions in schizophrenic children with those with "clear and independent evidence of central-nervous-system damage." They employ a function earlier identified by Bortner and Birch (16) who demonstrated that both adults and children who are brain damaged are able to discriminate the patterns of the Wechsler-Bellevue Block Design subtest even though they have failed to correctly reproduce that design. The subjects were one group of children with diagnoses of childhood schizophrenia, etiology unknown, and a second group with diagnoses of psychosis due to brain damage. The initial perceptual-motor performance of both groups was essentially similar, as was their age and I.Q. The impressive differential feature in performance here is the different effect of failure upon the two groups. Failure in the perceptual-motor portion of the task did not affect the ability of brain-damaged children subsequently to identify the designs. The schizophrenic children, however, were severely affected in their ability to recognize the designs after they had failed in the perceptual-motor portion of the test. The authors conclude: "If childhood schizophrenia is considered to be one consequence of prenatal and perinatal neurologic disturbance, it is a different one from that sustained by the brain-damaged children of this study. . . ."

Gittleman and Birch (33) conducted a detailed study of 97 children with a diagnosis of childhood schizophrenia. More than 50 percent of this group were of subnormal intelligence; low I.Q. correlated with clinical findings of neurological dysfunction; intellectual level remained remarkably stable over a period of years. I.Q. level and age of onset of clinical symptoms were positively correlated; both age of onset and I.Q. level were found to be good indicators of the subsequent course of the illness. Perinatal complications were excessively frequent, particularly so among those children with subnormal intelligence. The presence or absence of central-nervous-system pathology was not significant for parental psychopathology or rate of institutionalization for mental disorder in the families. Among the group follow-up, 25 percent had been rediagnosed as mentally subnormal and/or given a subsequent diagnosis consistent with chronic brain disorder. Pathology of the central nervous system was manifest in 80 percent of all the children, either upon direct examination or from the clinical history.

The authors believe their findings support the views that neurological damage is frequently encountered in children diagnosed as schizophrenic who are not institutionalized, and that many children first diagnosed as schizophrenic are rediagnosed as mentally deficient when they become older. The conclude that their findings justify questioning the role of parental influences in the genesis of schizophrenia, and that it is more parsimonious to view the observed characteristics of parents of schizophrenic children as stemming from the nature of their response to their disordered child, particularly from the difficulty of responding appropriately to such children. They believe also that their data do not support the argument for a psychogenic etiology or even for a continuum in which psychogenicity is interrelated with organic factors. Rather, they hold that children with psychosis differ from normal children from the time of earliest development, in the sense that their sensory and response systems are disordered in primary fashion.

The evidence implicating organic factors in childhood schizophrenia appears convincing. Pollin (68) found among twins that the schizophrenic sibs tended to be smaller, with clinical history that they had received less oxygen. Schizophrenic children were found to have had significantly more perinatal complications than their non-schizophrenic siblings by Rutt and Offord (72). Pollin also hypothesizes that soft neurological symptoms which affect adjustment and behavior, and the small size, participated in the development of response patterns from parents which in turn contributed to the development of psychopathology in the child.

A high incidence of EEG abnormalities is reported among childhood schizophrenics. White et al. (89) performed a double-blind study of both psychiatrically disturbed and normal children. Fifty-one percent of the psychiatric population (autistic or symbiotic childhood psychotics, chronic undifferentiated schizophrenics, non-psychotic children with severe acting-out behavior, and neurotic children) produced abnormal EEG records, while none of the children without psychiatric evidences produced such records. The EEG abnormalities were remarkably similar, both qualitatively and quantitatively, among the psychiatric population, except for the neurotic subgroup. Thirty-three percent of the psychiatric population produced abnormalities of irregular paroxysmal spiking and wave complexes. These complexes were slightly, though not significantly, more frequent in the autistic-symbiotic subgroup than in the chronic undifferentiated schizophrenics or the non-psychotic children with acting-out behavior disorders. The investigators believe that increasing the length of time devoted to the EEG sampling would have yielded even greater frequencies of the organic component in the psychiatrically disturbed children. Their data do not permit them to state whether the cerebral dysfunction for which evidence was obtained is of a primary character or is secondary to some other factor, such as the effect of anxiety upon body chemistry. They consider the use of sleep recordings important in this assessment and employed them in their study.

Ritvo (71) reports that the chief factor contributing to the incidence of EEG abnormalities in a population of psychiatrically hospitalized children is the presence of organic brain dysfunction. When children with known or probable organic brain dysfunction were eliminated, none of the clinical diagnoses correlated with significantly higher incidence of EEG abnormality. Ritvo finds that his clinical experience, observations and research all support the view that children diagnosed as schizophrenic, autistic, or psychotic in the symbiotic sense are suffering a unitary disease process: they cannot maintain perception at a stable level. As a result, incoming stimuli cause random overloading and underloading of the central nervous system. These symptoms are characterized by alternating states of facilitation and inhibition and, when seen operating together, constitute "the syndrome of perceptual inconstancy." The usual clinical EEG does not exhibit the neuropathological factors contributing to perceptual inconstancy; however, extensive, elaborate innovative techniques during varying states of consciousness are able to identify those children with perceptual inconstancy and those without it.

Auditory-visual integration was employed by Walker and Birch (85) to assess neurointegrative ability in schizophrenic children, i.e., their ability to integrate data input from two different sensory modalities. The schizophrenic children at each age were significantly inferior in integrative capability to normal children. Normal children display a pronounced linear increase of competence with age; the developmental trend among schizophrenic children is weak.

A special report on schizophrenia issued by the National Institute of Mental Health (63) supports the view that a neurological deficit contributes to schizophrenia in childhood. Mothers of schizophrenic children *with* neurological difficulties appear to be less seriously disturbed than do mothers of schizophrenic children who are neurologically normal (Goldfarb). Disturbed children generally, *without* neurological difficulties, the same study reports, tend to come from abnormal family situations, while those with neurological difficulties tend to come from well-adjusted families. Psychotic children were found to be more similar to brain-damaged children without psychosis than to normal children in electrical rhythm of the brain, learning patterns, intelligence levels, and biochemical factors (DeMyer). And the use of telemetered EEGs indicates that the brain-wave activity of autistic children is similar to that of premature babies (Ornitz).

Ritvo emphasizes the unitary disease concept, observing that autistic children come from all types of social, economic, and ethnic backgrounds, and that their parents constitute a wide array of psychological types. Against this background of social, cultural, and parental variation, he states that the children have similar disturbances of development, perception, mobility, speech and manner of relating.

The complicating factor of mental retardation in childhood schizophrenia is reviewed by Pollack (67). Intellectual abnormality and perceptual-motor impairments indicative of cerebral dysfunction, he found, occur more frequently in schizophrenic children than in those with other emotional disorders. Further, it is possible to divide schizophrenic children into those with intellectual retardation and those without. He reasons that neither childhood schizophrenia nor mental retardation is a distinct clinical entity, and that when a severe behavior disorder is found along with an intellectual deficit in a child, the altered behavior observed may be a reflection of cerebral dysfunction. Pollack concludes that stress upon either the retardation or the behavioral problems is more a function of the observer's values and orientation than of the child's inherent behavior.

Through the intricate web of evidence that sometimes is seemingly clear and suggestive, at other times conflicting and confusing, at least two statements may be made with reasonable confidence.

1) The impairments in autism or childhood schizophrenia, whatever nomenclature one chooses, are multiple, appearing in different combinations and in varying degrees of severity. Rimland (70) suggests autism is a condition of underarousal, childhood schizophrenia one of over-arousal. Ornitz and Ritvo (65) maintain that they are variants of same disease, Wing and Wing (90), acknowledging the prominence of language disorders in autism, cite the importance of other manifestations: poor posture control; visual-perceptual difficulties in which the tendency is to use peripheral rather than central vision; difficulty in copying skilled movements, in right-left and other directional orientations; the paradoxical combination of hyper- and hypo-sensitivity to auditory, visual, and haptic stimuli; and immaturity in aspects of physical development. They conclude that multiple impairments do not require necessarily the presumption of multiple etiologies, since different brain centers may be affected by the same lesion, the phenomenon of diaschisis. White (88) appears to posit a conflicting anatomical explanation, i.e., that similar symptoms and syndromes may be caused by different types, degrees, or levels of brain damage. The multiplicity of impairments make it impossible to determine if autism is one disease or several. Kanner's (43) 30-year follow-up of 11 autistic children first reported in 1943 epitomizes the present impossibility of this determination. While in contrast to the authors cited above, he saw many symptom similarities in the children originally, 30 years

later they ranged from "complete deterioration to occupational adequacy" combined with limited, but superficially smooth, social adjustments.

2) The varieties of disorders observed in schizophrenic children make impossible ascribing a single etiology to them, although it is reasonable to assume that one cause may evoke another, and that the two or more causes may interact synergistically. The child with auditory agnosia, for example, has great likelihood of developing aversive, schizoid, or schizophrenic behavior that may in turn elicit rejecting, avoiding behavior from others, particularly in the infant-mother relationship (21).

Several reviews of the various etiologies ascribed to autism have appeared in recent years. Mordock (60) cites five current hypotheses: 1) A psychogenic one à la Bettelheim in which the parents are indifferent to the child, who fears for his life and withdraws; 2) A predisposition of unknown origin to withdraw. The fact that many parents of autistic children have normal children is the basis of this hypothesis, which, of course, may be countered by the argument that the parents change from child to child and so their behavior changes. 3) A rare recessive gene. 4) Brain damage. 5) Perceptual inconsistency because of inability to regulate sensory input.

A severe and extensive deficit in language comprehension and with processing of information due to an obscure cause is the explanation of Rutter and Bartak (76). The intellectually impaired autistic child suggests brain damage; the more intelligent one contests this, they argue. (This view in turn is questioned by the many children with Full Scale I.Q.'s in the mentally-defective range who produce superior performances in some subtests and abysmally low ones in others. See Chapter 6, *Mental Retardation*). Social and behavioral disorders are considered by them to be secondary consequences.

Reviewing all extant known features of autism, Ornitz and Ritvo (64) conclude that no psychological-environmental factors of primary etiological significance can be identified. The disorder is attributed by them to a "neuropathophysiological" process that affects developmental rate, perception, language, cognition, intellectual development, and ability to relate.

Little wonder that Laufer and Gair (48) conclude a review of a decade of study in childhood psychosis and childhood schizophrenia with the conviction that the etiological factors are many and varied, and a return to the contention of Bender and Fish that physical and psychological factors interact and intertwine. They see increasing acceptance of this view in approaches to the study of childhood schizophrenia that are less dogmatic, less polemical, and more holistic. Bender, in an overview (9) observed that the varieties of schizophrenic children are too many to allow identification of a single cause of pathology, be it neurological, psychological, social or genetic. Research into the problem has become more sophisticated as its design attempts to deal with its many complex variables.

BRAIN DAMAGE AND SCHIZOPHRENIA

If brain damage is implicated as one of the major etiologies of schizophrenia—as indeed the data indicate it to be—then some questions follow: What causes the brain damage? Does the age of the individual when brain damage is incurred influence whether or not schizophrenia will develop? What are the evidences of brain damage in schizophrenia other than those already discussed? Can the brain damage in schizophrenia be localized? Again the reader is warned: Questions in schizophrenia are many, answers few.

Evidence of Brain Damage in Schizophrenia

Such evidence has been sought by the usual means: the gross signs of neurological disorder obtained in the classical neurological examination, the readings of the instruments of neurology (the EEG, echoencephalography, and recently the CAT, i.e., computerized axial tomography), some rare autopsy studies of gross and histological structures, and neuropsychological studies.

Fairly consistent findings are reported (62) of significantly more equivocal neurologic signs (sensory changes, motor power changes, and reflex changes) in patients than in controls. Conversely, psychopathology is positively correlated with signs of neurological disorder. This report by Mosher et al. includes a review of several other studies as well as their own work with twins. The review underscores the frequent observation that the gross neurologic signs are not usually detected in schizophrenia, except as they are the symptoms of a corollary neurologic disorder or disease, quite separate from the schizophrenia. Most often the neurologic signs, when found, are "soft" or "equivocal" (see Chapter 1), and easily overlooked by the psychiatrist or even by the neurologist whose focus is upon "hard" signs.

Arieti (4) states ". . . we are not in a position to deny any organic predisposing, constitutional factor . . . ," but acknowledges that the role of the central nervous system in schizophrenia is a most controversial subject. He suggests that more concrete neurological evidence is not obtainable because the neurological impairment may be a biochemical modification, which has its impact on the brain at a molecular level and is not detectable even with histological techniques. His speculation is supported by an extensive review of the literature (17) that found little specific evidence for histological pathology related to schizophrenia. The investigation of this line of evidence concludes that no change in any tissue of the body *including the brain* has been demonstrated to account for the chemical syndrome of schizophrenia.

"Soft" signs, then, constitute the more typical evidence of brain damage in schizophrenia. These soft signs are the same as those observed in minimal cerebral dysfunction, learning disabilities, Gerstmann's Syndrome, the equivocal epilepsies, and mental retardation, to name a few disorders that confound the neurologic diagnosis. It becomes impossible, therefore, to infer that these signs are manifestations of a specific neurological disorder that results in schizophrenia. The more compelling assumption is that of an interaction between brain damage of a minimal order and any or all of the other etiological factors (genetic, physiologic, and psycho-social).

Interaction of brain damage assumed from soft signs with the infant- or child-mother interaction is identifiable in Mednick's (57) study of the fates of children "at risk," that is, of the children of chronic and severely schizophrenic mothers who became schizophrenic and those children who did not. At the time of first observation all of the children admitted to the study were functioning normally. Eight years later, at ages ranging from 9 to 20, the first wave of breakdowns occurred; 27 of the high-risk group had become mentally ill. Compared with the group who continued to function normally they:

1) had lost their mothers to psychiatric hospitalization earlier;

2) were more disruptive in school;

3) "drifted" on word association tests as if by loose association in chains of responses unrelated to the stimulus word;

4) were electrodermally different in response to auditory stimuli in that they became more irritable as the speed of response increased, rather than showing ability to accommodate;

5) had experienced more complications of birth and pregnancy

(PBCs), such as anoxia, prematurity, prolonged labor, placenta and umbilical difficulties, illnesses of the mother during pregnancy, and breech births. A study related in purpose by Lobascher *et al.* (51) identified more birth and postnatal complications in autistic children than in controls. These data coincided with evidence of more disturbed parents, and more neurological and EEG abnormalities in the autistic children. Birch and Hertzig (13) observe that PBC's associated with childhood schizophrenia are linked to epilepsy, dyslexia, and mental retardation, and, as observed above, also to minimal cerebral dysfunction and Gerstmann's Syndrome.

This association of injury related to birth or pregnancy with the subsequent development of schizophrenia and other equivocal neurologic disorders does not allow the simplistic deduction that the early onset of the damage is the etiologically responsible factor. The evidence on recoverability from brain damage (see Chapter 18) is that generally a greater degree of recoverability or less permanent loss of function is associated with earlier age of damage because of the plasticity of the brain. Obviously, many subtle factors are operating that are not now observable, much less measurable: for example, the nature, size, and location of the PBC lesion. Early infancy and childhood factors may be generated by or interact with the PBC-caused brain damage: febrile episodes, traumas, toxemias, child-parent and child-family interactions. And the review of childhood psychoses suggests that the nature of the dysfunction produced by brain damage may have a differential effect on personality and emotional organization. Some, such as language disorders, may have a profound effect. Others, a dyscalculia, for example, surfacing later in the developmental process of personality organization and maturation, may produce moderate, not severe, learning disabilities, and so have relatively minor impact on the emotional integrity of the child.

Epilepsy and Schizophrenia

Neurological instrumentation has been deployed frequently in the search for a link, an association between brain damage and schizophrenia. As might be expected, the prevalence of "soft" signs in contrast to "hard" ones is generally accompanied by equivocal instrument findings. Echoencephalography, useful in detecting epilepsy, brain injuries, and various other types of intracranial pathology, was used by Holden *et al.* (41) in a study of schizophrenics. No brain differences were identifiable between chronic schizophrenics and controls. However, those schizophrenic patients considered responsive to therapy had smaller third-ventricle measurements than those judged to be resistant. These findings were equivocal, not significant.

The EEG is most frequently used in the pursuit of a schizophrenia-cerebral pathology link. A recent review of EEG studies (5) detected cortical EEG abnormalities in process schizophrenics but not in reactive schizophrenic patients. Subcortical studies utilizing activation by drugs (see Chapter 3) and depth electrodes are reported to detect abnormalities in both process and reactive types but in different areas: abnormalities were detected in the frontal lobes of process schizophrenics, and in the temporal lobes of the reactive schizophrenics.

The high incidence of the 14-and-6-per-second positive spike pattern on EEG reported in young schizophrenic patients may make this particular EEG sign of considerable importance. The pattern generally has been associated with symptoms such as aggressiveness, affective impulsivity, and driven behavior. It is hypothesized that the symptomatic picture in schizophrenic disorders is modified to a considerable extent when 14-and-6 spike pattern and the cerebral mechanisms which presumably underlie it are also present. This specific positive spike pattern is discussed as a syndrome in Chapter 8.

A likely association between epilepsy and schizophrenia has for some decades stimulated much EEG research. Commenting on the early symptoms of schizophrenia, Chapman (20) observes ". . . a close resemblance between some of the subjective experiences described by schizophrenic patients and the ictal phenomena of temporal-lobe epilepsy." Lyle (52) presents the interesting case of an autistic male who exhibited early speech difficulties which improved. In adolescence he began to experience seizures that were soon followed by a full-blown psychosis. Lyle hypothesizes that either 1) the early dysphasia resulted in a thought disorder that later was elaborated in fantasy and open expression as speech improved, and finally allowed the incorporation of frightening images and stimuli provoked by the epilepsy; or 2) neuropathy caused both the seizure disorder and the psychosis. Slater and Beard (80) speculate that: 1) schizophrenia and epilepsy may co-exist without common etiology; 2) the psychosis may be a reaction to the seizure disorder; or 3) both may arise from the same cause.

Whatever the speculation, an unusually high incidence of epileptic-like wave patterns (with negatively deflected spikes) has been reported (79) in the electroencephalograms obtained from schizophrenic patients. However, treatment of a group of schizophrenics with this pattern with anti-convulsant medication had no therapeutic effect. Thus the relationship of this EEG pattern in schizophrenia to that in actual epilepsy was left in doubt. Further work distinguished between the spike-and-wave discharges of epileptic and schizophrenic patients; they were found to vary in frequency, voltage, location, and response to hyperventilation. Studies of psychotic patients with temporal-lobe spike patterns, but without clear evidence of epilepsy, were compared with those of known epileptic patients and with those of other patients who demonstrated neither the temporal spike patterns nor clinical epilepsy. Both the known epileptic patients and the psychotic patients with temporal-lobe spike patterns exhibited aggressive, combative behavior, rage episodes, and paroxysmal symptoms in the form of blackouts and hallucinations. The controls who exhibited neither clinical epilepsy nor the temporal-lobe spike patterns were characterized by delusions and other classical psychiatric symptoms. Further studies associated EEG abnormality with destructiveness, assaultiveness, irritability, religiosity, impaired personal habits, increased psychomotor activity, flattened affect, impaired association, persecutory and somatic delusions, perseveration, vagueness, auditory hallucination, time disorientation, difficulty with recent recall, and headaches.

Shagass (79) sees these ideas emerging from a decade of research:

1) Schizophrenic states are related to a chronic state of cerebral overstimulation or hyperarousal.

2) Some epileptic states which involve disordered activity of the brain resemble schizophrenia. (These conditions probably involve a lesion which is biochemical. The data which lead to this conclusion may be interpreted, however, to state that epileptoid forms of brain activity modify the clinical manifestation of the schizophrenia.)

3) Process schizophrenics—those with poor prognosis—tend to show unusually normal and stable EEG patterns. (What may be operating here is an impairment of the access of stimuli to the structures which generate the electrical activity. The reduced response of these patients to drugs and to sensory stimulation may reflect a similar fact.)

4) In schizophrenic disorders the temporal and spatial organization of brain activity is impaired, so that information processing is also impaired.

Monroe (59), whose EEG activation investigation of episodic behavioral disorders is described in Chapter 3, proposes two types of schizophrenia: one is chronically persistent, the other intermittent and remitting, sometimes epileptoid in nature. The episodic dyscontrol behavior of the latter group, which may extend over a period of days or months, usually manifests autistic preoccupations, primary-process thinking, disturbed affect, ambivalence. Also present may be hypochondriacal preoccupations, manic delusions, disturbed associations, bizarre and concrete thinking, altered awareness, dream-like states, and partial memory loss. In remission, the patient may seem to be making a relatively normal adjustment. Some, however, may continue to demonstrate severe psychopathology. Essential to the suspicion of an ictal process are two elements: the precipitous onset of alteration in their state of consciousness and level of awareness, and the abruptness of remission. Monroe reports patients whose behavior was as described, who produced normal EEG base line recordings, but who after alphachloralose activation exhibited abnormalities of an epileptoid nature. Monroe cites Rodin as suggesting that this syndrome is "phenomenologically related to schizophrenia but etiologically to epilepsy."

To enhance the treatment of schizophrenic patients, Monroe urges extreme care in differential diagnosis. He recommends the use of EEG activation techniques as well as the search for certain suggestive psychodynamic factors. If it can be established by activated EEG that the psychotic behavior is an epileptoid, episodic response due to excessive neuronal discharge, then therapeutic interventions may be ordered accordingly, with greater reliance on somatic measures along with the use of psychotherapy as an adjunctive technique.

If the precipitating circumstances can be identified as having been overwhelming and the patient's response predominated by reduced awareness, the possibility increases that the response is predominantly a psychodynamically motivated, adaptive withdrawal into psychosis. If the response, no matter how overwhelming the precipitating circumstances were, was a dissociated state, an altered state of consciousness, or primary-process thinking, diagnostic consideration should include both the epileptoid and the motivational genesis. Both should be explored. If the precipitating circumstances do not appear to be overwhelming for the ordinary individual, but yet for the particular patient can be identified to symbolize a catastrophe, the probability of a psychodynamically motivated reaction increases. However, if the precipitating circumstances were both overtly and symbolically neutral, the probability of an epileptoid psychotic reaction increases.

Monroe's experience is that when the reaction is epileptoid in nature, the patient is more likely to realize that his action was extreme, to report a feeling of having been driven beyond his control in an attack or spell. He may ask for restraint or isolation, or otherwise beg for help. After the episode has passed, the patient is more likely to admit sickness, to talk about his symptoms, to seem more willing to accept hospitalization, even punishment. These patients experience less guilt and shame and consequently less denial than do the patients in whom a psychodynamically motivated attack can be identified. Their self-esteem maintains itself relatively, despite the nature of their behavior. (In my clinical experience, however, patients who suffer brain damage or neurological disorders including epilepsy can be deeply depressed about themselves. Some even interpret their condition as a punishment for something they have done.)

In contrast, the more the behavior can be seen to have a psychodynamic motivation, the more likely the patients are to renounce responsibility through rationalization or some other defense mechanism. They tend to have complete amnesia, to project, to see themselves as passive victims; if they accept responsibility they deny premeditation. In effect, Monroe holds that they experience unconsciously the intentions of their acts, which are unacceptable to the superego and require repression, denial, rejection, and undoing and rationalization.

Neuropsychological Correlates

Perplexing difficulties plague the efforts to differentiate schizophrenia from brain damage with the use of psychological tests. DeWolfe (24) suggests that in part the reason for unsatisfactory discrimination between the two groups with the use of the WAIS may be reliance upon "overall performance." Both groups of patients suffer impairment of intellectual functioning, so that overall indices may seem similar for both. Yet the real differences in impairment, which may appear only with analysis of the pattern of performance on subtests of the WAIS, may be obscured. He found (24, 25) that the relationship between Digit Span and Comprehension differentiated the two groups reasonably well. Chronic schizophrenic patients tended to have higher scores for Digit Span than for Comprehension, while the reverse was true for brain-damaged patients. Among the patients for whom the scale scores for the two subtests were equal, the comparison of Digit Span with Vocabulary was helpful in a further effort to discriminate: higher Digit Span than Vocabulary scores characterized the chronic schizophrenic, and the reverse relationship marked the brain-damaged patient. But in personal correspondence, DeWolfe warns that these differentiation criteria may prove less useful clinically than his results might promise, since a study by a colleague has yielded confirmation with one population but not with another.

These studies reveal some of the difficulties investigators have met in establishing the etiology and role of the cognitive disorders observed in the schizophrenic, in distinguishing them from those caused by brain damage, or establishing that they arise from the same cause. Does, for example, cognitive deficit precede the development of schizophrenic symptoms, accompany them, or result from them? Using three measures of cognitive functioning (Shipley-Hartford scores converted to WAIS I.Q.'s, Abstract and Concrete scores on the Gorham Proverbs Test), Martin (55) found levels of cognitive deficit consistent through morbid and post morbid phases. These findings seem to raise more questions than they answer.

A limitation often found in the design of neuropsychological investigations of schizophrenia is the use of a severely restricted test battery. Most rely upon scanning of only a few of the many and varied types and degrees of cognitive dysfunctions arising from the equally numerous and varied types, locations, and qualities of brain damage. Some further examples of these limited studies follow.

Lilliston (50) administered the Bender, the Memory for Designs Test, and the Trail-Making Test to 90 male schizophrenics. From their performance on this battery, three groups of 30 each were identified. Group A were not classified as brain damaged by any of the three tests; Group B were classified as brain damaged by one or two but not by all three of the tests, Group C were classified as brain damaged by all of the three tests. The Phillips Scale was used to identify the process-reactive dimension along a continuum. It was found to increase significantly from Group A to B to C.

In a later study Lilliston (49), using the same three tests, identified three levels of brain damage *probability* in schizophrenic patients. The low probability group manifested greater affect, anxiety, and reality contact. They were more reactive, more concerned with their own welfare. The high probability group were more disoriented and withdrawn, less communicative, moving slowly, showing little affect or concern about their own welfare, and presenting perceptual abnormalities. The mid-probability group displayed a "confused array of mixed symptomatology." One might well add that the array was confusing as well as confused. Missing, for example, from the tiny battery of tests employed, among other omissions from the standard neuropsychological battery, were tests of verbal conceptualization, comprehension, and expression; symbol processing, complex constructional tasks; attention-memory tasks. Also missing were tests of various modalities of reception and response that are incorporated in the standard battery.

These limitations of design appear to result from the pursuit of a single-variable hypotheses: 1) the cognitive deficit in schizophrenia is a language disorder, while 2) in brain damage it is spatial or attention-memory. Generally supporting these hypotheses have been certain studies producing evidence that dominant hemisphere damage is more frequently associated with schizophrenia than with affective disorders. Flor-Henry's study (27) of epileptic patients with psychosis compared with those without psychosis was a pathbreaker in this line of investigation. He found in a group of 50 epileptics without psychosis that the focus of the epilepsy was identified by EEG as lateralized in equal numbers in either cerebral hemisphere. Of patients with schizophrenia psychoses but *without* affective components, 43 percent had left-sided or dominant hemisphere foci; the remaining 47 percent had foci in both hemispheres. Of the total epileptic-psychotic group, only nine percent produced right-side foci; 44 percent of these were manic depressives, 18 percent were diagnosed as schizo-affective psychotics.

Related data were obtained by Taylor *et al.* (82) through the use of Reitan's modification of the Halstead-Wepman aphasia screening test that they report was able to differentiate patients with schizophrenic disorders from those with combined schizophrenic-affective ones. In a subsequent study (83) their schizophrenic subjects produced more aphasia errors than did patients with affective disorders. The errors of the latter group were attributable largely to non-dominant hemisphere dysfunction, while those of the schizophrenic group were equally suggestive of dominant and non-dominant dysfunctions.

Corroborative data are also reported by Gruzelier and Hammond (37), who obtained lower WAIS verbal scores (Similarities, Comprehension, Vocabulary) than spatial scores (Block Design, Object Assembly) in chronic schizophrenic patients when on placebo than when the same patients were administered chlorpromazine before and after the placebo. These findings plus the obtained bilateral asymmetries in absolute auditory thresholds, auditory discriminations of temporal duration, and electrodermal orienting responses suggested to the investigators that "the dominant hemisphere of schizophrenics displays 'weak' nervous-system dynamics."

The speech dominant hemisphere dysfunction hypothesis correlates with earlier reported findings of lateralized asymmetrics (2, 27, 28, 56, 66, 69) associating Wechsler-Bellvue Verbal Scale dysfunction with left-hemisphere pathology and Performance Scale impairments with right-hemisphere disorders. The findings do not so readily correlate with reports of pronounced psychomotor deficits in chronic schizophrenics (86, 87).

Apparently when broad-coverage batteries of tests are used to detect both dominant and non-dominant hemispheric dysfunctions, the so-called "hit" rate increases. The administration of the Halstead-Reitan battery to a group of 66 chronic schizophrenics by Klonoff et al. (47) found that 80 percent performed "at least at a mildly brain-damaged level." But the authors wisely cannot conclude with certainty that this consistent deficit is validly attributable to brain damage, although the suggestion is strong.

At best the neuropsychological test findings are suggestive, at worst confusing. Their use in psychiatric settings, other than for research, is seriously questioned by Heaton (39) because of their inability to differentiate brain-damaged patients from those with serious functional disorders. Chronic or process schizophrenics do produce neuropsychological test profiles resembling those of brain-damaged patients. But the variables that could account for this phenomenon are many and so intertwined that they challenge research designers to separate and control them. By definition, for example, the chronic schizophrenic tends to be older than the reactive or acute schizophrenic, so that whatever cerebral pathology is present cannot be said definitively to be a cause of the schizophrenia rather than a consequence of aging or of the schizophrenic process itself.

A major problem in differentiating schizophrenia from brain damage, or in evaluating the role of brain damage in schizophrenia, is the criterion problem, *the establishment of clear-cut populations:* schizophrenic patients without brain damage, and brain-damaged patients without schizophrenia. The latter group would appear easier to identify. But certainty that brain damage is absent is far less available to the researcher; neurological criteria may be obscure, because signs are equivocal, or undetectable, because assessment and measurement procedures are inadequate. To this uncertainty is added the limitation inherent in all psychological assessments that are restricted to only one or a few brain-behavior functions. Given the sparseness of information about localization within the brain of behavior functions and their alternate connections, any pursuit of a differentiation of concise, limited functions seems restricted to modest success at best. Some statistical differentiation may be achieved with some instruments with some groups, but the constant appearance of false-negatives and false-positives undermines the reliance of clinicians in the instruments.

Lateralization and Localization

In the preceding sections of this chapter are numerous references to findings that suggest that brain damage and schizophrenia are linked by pathology of the speech dominant left hemisphere. Recent studies of laterality using handedness, eyedness and footedness by Gur (38) also support a left-hemispheric dysfunction with schizophrenia and a right-hemispheric dysfunction with affective disorders.

Hypotheses also abound that seek more precisely to localize the site of brain pathology.

Arieti (4) believes that most schizophrenic symptoms arise in the cerebral cortex. He does not exclude extracortical pathology, but does eliminate the Brodman area, the strip region, the pre-motor area, the extra-pyramidal area, and Broca's area. He reasons that many of the symbolic functions which arouse anxiety take place in the temporal-occipital-parietal areas, which he abbreviates to "t.o.p." These are among the "silent areas," so named because their functions are not easily discerned. Discernible lesions in these areas do not necessarily produce definitive symptoms. Arieti suggests that the schizophrenic avoids use of these areas because they produce anxiety, and that disuse may extend to the point where actual atrophy sets in.

Interacting with the t.o.p. area is the pre-frontal lobe area, in which are represented those functions capable of arousing the most anxiety, according to Arieti. The schizophrenic persists in an effort to reduce these functions in order to reduce anxiety. The reductive function may be extended as well to other areas of the brain. Arieti believes that the schizophrenic uses his cortex as little as possible and thus comes to resemble the typical picture of the organic, seen in the terms of Goldstein's concept of impaired abstract functioning. Schizophrenia represents both negative symptoms, resulting from the decreased functioning of higher cortical levels, and positive symptoms, arising through the release of lower centers. The ultimate result is dysencephalization, a process similar to Hughling Jackson's disinhibition.

The temporal region is also implicated by an EEG study of 100 chronic schizophrenic patients compared with 100 normal persons made by Abenson (1). He suggests the temporal area as the locus of the unstable EEGs associated with his schizophrenic populations.

Data obtained by direct brain recordings have associated psychotic behavior with electrical discharges deep in various brain areas, especially in the septal region. These resemble convulsive discharges, but are of a localized nature and may be correlated with severe behavioral disturbance rather than with any of the states specifically classified as schizophrenia. Some corollary work on an immunological theory of schizophrenia has also been directed in recent years to the septal region (8).

Research on the ascending reticular activating system, termed ARAS, is surveyed by Mirsky (58) for its relevance to biological and neurological factors in schizophrenia. Mirsky points out that almost every major advance in biological science has been examined for its possible relevance to schizophrenia and other psychoses. But as he comments, much research on specific biological and central-nervous-system structures has contributed more to knowledge about biological and neurological functions than to understanding of schizophrenia. Mirsky finds the evidence arguing for two distinct types of brain pathology in schizophrenia: 1) the chronic, nuclear, or process type is longstanding, and may be associated with diffuse frontal-lobe damage, including tissue destruction in the ventral and orbital frontal areas, and related subcortical structures (this group is described as stuporous, blunted, withdrawn); 2) the episodic paranoidal group, in whom damage is usually found in the septal-hippocampal and temporal-lobe areas, although frontal damage occurs as well (this group is more likely to be described as having personality difficulties, to be aggressive, assaultive, fragmented, and bizarre.)

Gruzelier and Hammond (37) review the "strands of evidence" that suggest that schizophrenic symptomatology may be lateralized to the left-hemisphere temporal-limbic systems, evidence deriving from neuropharmacology, neurology, physiological psychology, developmental psychopathology, neurosurgery, and electroencephalography. The significance of these lateralization and localization hypotheses rests in the generally accepted dominance of the left hemisphere for speech, and the still not well-established role of the limbic system, of widespread but interconnected structures that appear to integrate cognitive functions with emotional tone, among other activities.

TREATMENT IMPLICATIONS

Schizophrenia, apparently, has no single etiological source. Bellak (6) has argued that the only real constant in schizophrenia is in its manifestations, its symptomatology as an expression of ego weakness, which represent the common outcome of a variety of pathological causes—familial, cultural, genetic, physiological, and neurological. In some individuals a single etiology will seem clear and unequivocal, in others two or more etiologies may be implicated, while in some persons etiology may be unfathomable.

For the psychotherapist the watchword must be "caution." An association between brain disorder and schizophrenia is found often enough to place neurological factors among the variables to be considered in the diagnosis of any person suspected of schizophrenia.

The similarity between schizophrenic symptoms and some of the phenomena associated with subictal states has been discussed here and in Chapter 3, as has the frequency with which victims of brain tumors first seek psychiatric help, sometimes to have their symptoms interpreted as dissociative states. Behavioral abnormalities in subacute encephalitis are often similar to those in hysteria, depression, catatonia, and paranoia (40). Aphasia which impairs use of and comprehension of language may drastically impede the development of normal relations and thought processes, until these become so prominent in the clinical picture as to convince the unwary clinician that the patient is suffering from a primary thinking disorder. Fluent aphasia, warns Geschwind (32), may be diagnosed as a psychosis because many clinicians are unaware that it may occur without a hemiplegia. The psychoanalytic concepts of primary and secondary levels of thought parallel Goldstein's concept of concrete and abstract levels of thought. The unwary psychotherapist with roots in analytic theory may mistake aphasic speech as evidence of a primary-thought process, hence of a psychosis. Bizarre speech and other behavior must not be unreasoningly accepted as evidence of a functional disorder and allowed to deflect neurological exploration. Effective treatment depends upon understanding by the clinician of the relationship between symptoms and *all* possible etiologies in the particular patient. In the clinical treatment of the individual, adherence to a unitary model of schizophrenia may lead the therapist to overlook the contributions from other sources and reduce the chances of adequate treatment of the particular patient.

Kernberg (46) makes this point cogently in discussing treatment of the schizophrenic child. She underscores the major value of considering the possibility that a case of schizophrenia has an organic component: "The diagnosis of an organic problem may effect the type of psychotherapy offered, the choice of the living and learning situation best suited for the particular child, and the type of casework with the parents." She offers guides to differential diagnosis between psychosis with and without brain dysfunction. The psychotic patient possesses a level of cognitive function that is potentially normal at minimum. She believes that psychotic and neurotic conditions which are secondary to a central-nervous-system impairment are in only the most superficial areas similar to a functional psychosis, like schizophrenia, or to a classical neurosis. She further believes that the complex symptom formation found in the psychotic or neurotic individual, which is based upon the psychic processes of condensation, displacement, and symbolization, are either markedly reduced or absent in the organically-damaged patient.

The child's language during a diagnostic interview is an important clue. Echolalia is found in both schizophrenic and brain-damaged children, but with some important qualitative differences possible. In the brain-damaged child, the echolalia is usually accompanied by perseveration, and often represents an adaptive effort to reinforce the verbal communication in his own mind. The schizophrenic child, however, erupts with echolalia at any moment, abruptly and often irrelevantly, and sometimes the echolalia may be understood as a response of automatic obedience to the environment or a way of binding aggression. The brain-damaged child's inability to shift is manifested in his perseveration in the use of words, regardless of their emotional connotation, whereas the psychotic child repeats phrases or words which have a strong emotional meaning for him. The mere presence of primary-process thinking in either the language or the behavior of the child is not likely to help in a differential diagnosis, Kernberg states, between the organic and functional disturbance.

Finally, the responsibility of the clinician to search for all possible causes is contained in her observation that the brain-damaged child most likely to develop a type of adjustment so resembling that of the autistic or schizophrenic child as to cause him to be diagnosed a childhood schizophrenic is the one who experiences reality in a deviant way, but who is intelligent enough in some areas to be sensitive to his limitations in other areas. Thus his impairments and efforts at adaptation are not understood by either parents or peers.

An opposite view held by Tinbergen (84) suggests strongly that the role of organic brain dysfunction in schizophrenia must not be overplayed to the exclusion of other etiologies. He regards the autistic child as "primarily" suffering an emotional disturbance, and that "most" of these children and their parents are victims of emotional stress. His experience is that "emotional" therapy has repeatedly produced an "explosive emergence of speech and other skills." Diminishing anxiety and restoring socialization are more effective treatments, he maintains, than speech therapy.

I would conclude that both, as well as other interventions, have selective value. Diagnosis of the individual patient requires the integration of many diverse factors that often defy such integration. So far the search for etiology has produced little to influence the treatment of the schizophrenic. The widespread use of the psychotropic drugs complicates both the effort at individual diagnoses and the research of diverse etiologies. We approach the treatment of the schizophrenic person with many insights and few solutions.

CASE ILLUSTRATIONS

Many of the cases in Chapter 3 on epilepsy also illustrate issues in the differential diagnosis between schizophrenia and brain damage—especially the indications of hallucinations and altered states of consciousness. The following four cases call attention to additional matters: the confusion in differentiating between childhood schizophrenia and brain damage; psychological-test evidence in a presumed schizophrenia of long standing; etiological data that point toward both diagnoses in the adult; and the behavioral effects of traumatic brain damage.

1. *Psychological-test evidence of brain damage in a 32-year-old man with more than 11 years of hospitalization for schizophrenia.*

B., a black man, was first hospitalized when he was 16 with a diagnosis of Dementia Praecox and treated with 59 Insulin-coma therapies and with Thorazine. He was rehospitalized when 18, this time with the diagnosis of Schizophrenia, Chronic Undifferentiated, and he remained hospitalized thereafter for more than 11 years. His psychotic father separated from the family when the patient was a small child and thereafter took no interest in the family, or any responsibility for it. His mother described the patient as a very nervous child, shy, quiet, with a great deal of difficulty in learning. In the fifth term of high school he complained of being picked on by students, and sexually abused by some of them. He became agitated, talked about dope and heroin; he believed that communists were following him and hallucinated his grandmother's voice calling him. He realized that none of these things were true, but said he had to be hospitalized because it was the only safe place for him. At his second hospitalization he had different feelings: that he was electrically charged, that there were chemicals missing in him, that he could not live in the community, and needed hospitalization. He reported that during his first hospitalization he had received a lobotomy, but diligent search failed to uncover any report of this surgery, nor could his mother confirm it. After release from the hospital he became a devoted member of a religious sect.

Now, in psychological assessment for vocational training, he received a prorated I.Q. of 129 in Comprehension and 117 in ability to conceptualize, indicative of Above Average to Superior intellectual ability. In his responses to these subtests there was no evidence of bizarre ideation or any disturbance of thought processes. Information, however, was extremely low, at a prorated I.Q. of 87; here he appeared to suffer from a memory difficulty and from inability to complete the associational network necessary to produce a response. He could name three presidents since 1900, but was tremendously puzzled in his search for a fourth. In contrast with his ability to conceptualize, he appeared to have a moderate perceptual-analytic deficit, achieving a prorated I.Q. of 107 in recognition of essential details and 101 in the assembly of familiar objects. It was not possible to say whether his difficulty in this area was due to a peripheral visual defect (which it did not appear to be), to a problem of peripheral motor control (which might have been the case since his handling of the pencil was rather poor), or to some central integrational impairment. In any case, it was apparent here that his rate of response was slow rather than that he had some failure in power. His most serious defect, and it was quite serious, was in attention-memory. This deficit was pronounced with both visual and auditory stimuli: he achieved a prorated I.Q. of 76 in Digit Span and 61 in Digit Symbol; on re-testing in the latter he was not able to increase his speed.

Administration of the Bender Gestalt with reproduction from memory produced rotation and separation of one figure. On reproduction from direct copy he performed much better. This suggested that memory difficulty more than anything made for his deficits.

He was able to draw the square-triangle-cross (Heimburger-Reitan), but demonstrated relatively poor peripheral motor control. He could name the square but spelled it "s-j something." He named the cross but could not spell it. He could repeat and explain the statement, "He shouted the warning," but could not write it, and said, "I can't read and I can't write." He then claimed that he knew how to read before entering school, but efforts to teach him to read "according to their ways" caused him to lose the skill in reading he had already acquired.

The deficit in attention and memory was reflected by an average scale score of five in these functions in contrast to the average scale score of 12 for verbal subtests. Perceptual-analytic deficits were moderate and appeared largely related to the attention-memory factor and poor peripheral motor control. There seemed to be an alexia and writing difficulty of long standing.

There was no evidence of mixed lateral dominance. He reported highly equivocal manifestations of blurred vision, dizziness, tilting, fainting experiences, tingling sensations, and numbness. He told of one episode several years before when he wanted to have a meal but wasn't sure if he had enough money for it. He had the meal anyway; when he was unable to pay, the manager of the restaurant hit him in the body. On the way home he blacked out and stood in one place for approximately six hours. He calls it a blackout, but it may have been a catatonic episode.

Responses to projective queries indicated a great deal of amnesia, which may have been active repression or attributable to memory loss. He appeared to have been over-stimulated sexually as a child. This may relate to the separation of the parents, the father's psychosis, and the mother's behavior toward him, or the behavior toward him of his older sisters. As he entered adolescence, he set fires, evidence that he was in a state of excitement and tension much of the time. He cannot say whether this was a pleasant or non-pleasant state, simply that it was a state. He cannot dichotomize good and bad things about his life; he can remember that he had pleasant times, but cannot recall the details.

There was no doubt that B. had had schizophrenic episodes which involved both catatonic and paranoid features. He appeared now to be in excellent remission. It seemed clear also that there were organic deficits that manifested themselves in writing and reading difficulties, and problems with attention and memory and in the perceptual-analytic visual-motor area. The etiology of the cerebral difficulties was not apparent from the material at hand, nor from any history that could be obtained.

2. *Etiological conditions suggest both the schizophrenic and the neurogenic in a 22-year-old man.*

This young man was referred for vocational training with a diagnosis of Paranoid Schizophrenia. The history indicated a maternal rubella in the first trimester, resulting in a plasia of the right ear. His mother was so horrified of the "monster" she bore that she would not pick him up or touch him for the first several weeks of his life. Thereafter she became overly and reactively attached to him. He underwent 10 operations, including plastic surgery, repair of an inguinal hernia, and a tonsillectomy. His parents were in constant conflict about his upbringing, his mother indulging him, his father attempting to set some controls. He had measles with very high fever at four, chickenpox and German measles when nine. He shared his mother's bed until the age of five. The family had a one-bedroom apartment; the father slept in the living room. He suffered nightmares; only when he was in the early teens did he get his own bedroom. Prior to his hospitalization he refused to bathe because he had delusions that bathing resulted in grotesque body and facial changes. He had both auditory and visual hallucinations, always related to his appearance. The hospital record noted a possible *petit mal* epilepsy and other congenital or postencephalic brain disease with cerebral dysfunction. All EEG's, however, were within normal limits, and no effort to treat the *petit mal* was undertaken. He completed high school while in the hospital. He appears to have been sexually precocious, reporting that he masturbated from the age of five but with no indication that this was accompanied by ejaculation. In his ideation there was considerable emphasis on incestuous and polymorphous perverse sexual activity. A psychological examination resulted in the following report:

"Intellectually he appears to be of innately Superior level intellectual ability, evidenced by the prorated I.Q. of 130 he obtains in ability to conceptualize and in Information. Comprehension is somewhat below this at a prorated I.Q. of 118. Nowhere in his verbal productions in the intelligence test is there evidence of bizarre ideation or of a thought disorder that would suggest schizophrenia. He has marked impairments in attention-memory and in perceptual-analytic functions. In the attention-memory area he achieves a prorated I.Q. of 95 on Digit Span and only 73 on Digit Symbol. In this latter test his finger work is slow, careless, poorly placed, and poorly formed, and strongly suggestive of a problem in peripheral motor control. The perceptual-analytic appears to be his greatest deficit. He achieves a prorated I.Q. of only 73 in Picture Completion, and drops to a low of 60 in the assembly of familiar objects. In this latter test, he is much perplexed by the absence of a guiding stimulus, and seemed unable to work his way out of a morass of confusion.

"The extent of his impairments is apparent from a comparison of the formal scoring. Performance I.Q. is 54 points lower than the Verbal. The major verbal functions produce an average scale score of 14; the attention-memory ones average to 7; and the perceptual-analytic ones to 4.5. These are marked differences, strongly suggestive of a cerebral dysfunction with a right hemisphere focus.

"Dual administration of the Bender Visual Motor Gestalt Test confirms both the perceptual-analytic and peripheral-motor control problem. There is also an indication of a hypomanic mood level, or an expansiveness that suggests an alternation with depression.

"The figure drawings show a distorted and deformed body image, but it is not possible to tell from them whether there has been any special impact upon his body image from his ear deformity and surgery. He seems to see the female as more deformed and vulnerable in a physical sense than the male. She is much more disconnected and disorganized. Again his handwriting shows the problem with peripheral motor control. His self-concept seems to revolve around a feeling of a large empty void.

"The figure drawings point to ongoing bizarre ideation around sexuality with much perverse material intruding itself upon his consciousness. He is in effect over-stimulated and overly-excitable, so that the mood elevation observed appears to be one of his major ego-deficits, mainly a difficulty with affect control. In this connection we should point out that he is hyperactive.

"Denial is very much evident, both of sexuality, which seems surprising considering the perversity of his productions, and also of aggressivity. It is clear that he perceives the world in an intensely sado-masochistic fashion, that it is dangerous and that he is subject to injury and extinction.

"The Rorschach gives no evidence at present of any bizarre psychotic ideation. Also, perceptual-analytic functions seem reasonably intact when he may offer an oral rather than a written response. Sexual idea-tion appears again and there is also evidence for an explosive affect expression.

"Responses to projective queries are remarkable. This lad, with a traumatic history of insecurity from infancy, offers as an early memory falling out of a crib. Anal features have been commented upon in the record, as well as aggressivity toward the father, and his childhood dream is remarkable regarding these dynamics. At the age of three, he dreamed that his father ran out of the house, fell down next to garbage cans, then was collected as garbage and thrown into the garbage truck. He acknowledges that he has a bad temper but also feels that he is patient. It is not possible to obtain clear-cut evidence of seizure phenomena, but he has fainted on a number of occasions; he reports rather frequent sudden, short blackouts, but says that since he has been taking vitamins this phenomenon has been helped. He has also suffered from blurred vision and nausea, and has creeping sensations, like tingling, along the arms.

"This lad obviously has multiple disabilities on both a psychogenic and neurological basis."

The interplay of several types of causative factors is clear, but the evidence for a neurologic condition is strong. One can only conjecture what his adjustment would be today if the neurogenic factors had received treatment consideration along with the psychogenic.

3. Nineteen years of documented history available for a 23-year-old girl reflect the difficulty of differentiating between a psychotic and neurological conditions.

A young woman was referred for vocational training by a state hos-pital, to which she had recently been admitted for staying away from home for six days. When only two and one-half years old, she had begun to run away from home and had been running away ever since. Any change in routine seemed to upset her. She had cystitis at about the age of four. At the age of six, neurological and electroencephalo-graphic examinations were conducted: the EEG was abnormal, with a right-occipital focus; the neurological examination was within normal limits. She was admitted to a residential treatment center when she was about 14 because she had temper tantrums, threw things, hit her mother, often lay on the floor and kicked her feet. When 21 she ran away from home with a man by whom she became pregnant, was sent to a psychiatric hospital, and had an abortion. The vocational-agency psychiatrist found no evidence of schizophrenia, though he acknowledged that such pathology could have been covered by medication.

The patient's first referral to a child guidance agency came when she was in kindergarten. She had seemed detached from the activities of the group, but was also a disturbing element, talking to herself, not following instructions, repeating what the teacher told her, and displaying marked negativism. She was described as a pretty child but with an expressionless face. A psychological examination at the time commented about her distractibility, short attention span, scatter, relatively good verbalization, and poor motor coordination for her age.

Two years later another psychological report commented on the patient's vacant facial expression and almost continuous blank smile. Her gait was somewhat uncertain and immature for a child of her age. She drooled, and out of the classroom produced a strange atypical verbalization which suggested themes of hostility toward her baby sister. Weak motor coordination was apparent. Yet, though not quite six, her vocabulary was at the level of an eight-year-old. The possibility of organic involvement was noted.

At this time a school psychiatrist concurred with the psychological report, commenting that the possibility of organic involvement seemed strong, though a childhood schizophrenia was not ruled out because of the birth of her sibling and the fact that the entire family slept in one bedroom. A neurological examination was suggested. The mother sought this through her own pediatrician. At this time, the abnormal right-occipital focus mentioned above was reported and Dilantin prescribed. The school psychologist made many recommendations, attempting to explain the patient's condition to teachers, and suggesting aids to them to help her academically.

Ten years later, on being referred for residential treatment, the patient was again seen by a psychologist whose final impression was ". . . Schizophrenia, Paranoid Type, marked by a strong thinking disorder. The testing showed no signs of the presence of organic brain damage." Just three years before, however, a psychiatrist had commented, "This patient falls into a group of children who present a diagnostic problem because of the coexistence of symptoms suggesting both organic and functional brain disease. I would suspect that the primary disease in this case is the organic, and that the functional, disorder has been nurtured by the exceedingly noxious mother-child relationship." This psychiatrist had placed the patient on Dexedrine, with beneficial results in combating her distractibility. The mother discontinued the Dexedrine.

Now 23, the patient was again seen in connection with her vocational training, by a psychologist who reported:

"The patient apparently was hospitalized twice in the past year, not, so far as can be told, for valid psychiatric reasons, but because her parents could not control her dating and sexual behavior. She was going out frequently, unable to work properly, and so lost her job as a key-punch operator.

"There is an extensive history with many psychologicals, many psychiatric reports, and evidence that a neurological condition was suspected as contributory, but was thought to be minimal. The record shows a good deal of consideration given to a differential diagnosis.

"L. is a rather strange girl in the sense that she is both attractive and yet odd looking. She is rather tall and slender, with lovely figure and skin, but there is an odd way in which she looks at one as if she is not really quite there. Her language is the least bit odd, in the sense that she has trouble focusing, as if there is a moderate aphasia. She has a kind of flat, matter-of-fact way of speaking. Perhaps most disturbing about her speech were the suggestions of high-level intelligence that came through, and yet were almost never fulfilled. Thus her response for identifying the Book of Genesis is, 'It's the signs of the first people on earth; it's a religious book; it is the Bible; it's the history of religion.'

"She is hyperkinetic from the waist down. Her legs are in almost constant motion, either swinging together in the midline or one leg swinging out from the midline and back again.

"Unfortunately, only overall I.Q. scores are reported in the extensive material from past testing; these generally place her at the low end of the Average range, though on occasion the Full Scale I.Q. fell into the Borderline Mentally Defective level.

"We obtain some prorated subtest I.Q.'s today in the Borderline Mental Defective level; these indicate that there is a profound impairment in perceptual-analytic tasks (with a prorated I.Q. of only 73 in

Object Assembly) and great difficulty in concentration and attention. She achieves a prorated I.Q. of only 77 in Digit Span and 80 in finger dexterities (Digit Symbol) and she is not able to increase her speed at all on retesting; in fact, she drops a little bit behind. Yet, she obtains a prorated I.Q. of 112 in ability to conceptualize verbally, 106 in Comprehension and 101 in Information. The suggestion is rather strong that these are evidences of brain damage, that attention, concentration, and perceptual-analytic functions are impaired. In addition, there is some impairment of general abstract thinking, so that her innate level of intelligence was probably at the Superior level. Thus, she is able to say for the meaning of 'shallow brooks are noisy': "Things that are shallow make noise, you know, people who talk too much." It is clear that she has the concept but she is not able to bring it into sharp focus, nor does she often have the words she needs in order to formulate a concept. Recognition of essential details is rather good, with a prorated I.Q. of 93.

"The Bender Visual Motor Gestalt Test suggests that the attention-memory function is the most impaired, and that this function is largely responsible for the perceptual-analytic deficit noted. There is also some peripheral motor control problem.

"There is no evidence of seizure phenomena. She occasionally has a ringing in her right ear, but that is the only thing that could be elicited. Of course, as noted, there is the hyperkinesis of the legs, particularly. Projective techniques fail to elicit evidence of a thought disorder or of a psychotic process at the present time. It is clear that she was very disturbed, frightened, and severely phobic as a child. She is very dependent, very concretely in need of affection and very concerned if she thinks that people do not like her. She probably is open to sexual advances because of the concrete need for affection and love. She also has a strong wish for independence and competence. She is well-motivated, and certainly she has some good residual skills. Like so many brain-damaged people, she fatigues rather rapidly in the performance of motor operations."

4. *A severe head injury results in profound behavioral changes.*

When 10 years old, C. was hit by a car and sustained a severe skull fracture. From that time on, she displayed temper tantrums and had great difficulty getting along with both parents and two younger brothers. She had increasing difficulty in school, and occasionally had auditory and visual hallucinations. When she was 15, in the midst of a violent family argument, the parents called the police, who took C. to a city psychiatric hospital from which she was transferred to a state hospital, remaining there until she was 18. When she returned home, there were no difficulties between C. and her parents at first, but six months after her release she began to argue more and more with them. These quarrels increased in severity and frequency and led to her current hospitalization. Very little history could be obtained. Her birth was said to have been normal. It was reported that she sat alone at four months, walked and talked when she was one and one-half years of age. Prior to the accident, she had been a good student with many friends. The hospital referred her for vocational training with a diagnosis of Chronic Undifferentiated Schizophrenia. She was being medicated with Mellaril, but complained that the drug made her dizzy and was not helping her. Despite these complaints, her psychiatrist continued with that medication.

The vocational agency psychiatrist reported, "I think the patient does not have a schizophrenic process. I think she has organic brain damage and requires a thorough work-up. She may have had a psychotic acute reaction in response to severe stress precipitated by the environment's reaction to the signs and symptoms of organic brain disease. For example, I think that her tantrums, some of the social disability, her learning disabilities, and possibly some hallucinatory episodes were direct consequences of brain damage. I believe that the environment reacted in a hostile way which in turn caused social breakdown syndromes and further symptomatology on a functional basis."

The agency's psychologist reported:

"C. is a painfully thin girl with a lopsided face; she is full breasted and obviously sexually interested. She has a bright, alert manner that bespeaks an intellectual endowment that was High Average. It would be helpful to check on her school records prior to the injury to get some sort of baseline. She says that she was doing very well in school prior to the accident.

"Most of our time together was spent in efforts to assess intellectual functioning in order to determine the presence and extent of cerebral damage. The intelligence test data suggest extensive damage, with greater dysfunction in the left hemisphere than in the right. Right-sided in all hand, eye and foot tests, she has an aphasia in which she is able to use words correctly and define them in a functional sense, but not in a more abstract way. Her ability to conceptualize and think abstractly is severely impaired, as evidenced by the prorated I.Q. of 61 she obtains in Similarities. Information is poor at a prorated I.Q. of 79, and Comprehension at a prorated I.Q. of 73 reflects the perplexity and confusion under which she labors. The tendency to think by concrete associations, rather than to be able to abstract the situation, is observed in her meaning for the expression 'Strike while the iron is hot.' She says, 'One should be careful if they are using the iron.' She has a moderate degree of ability to attend to and retain material when the stimulus is aural.

"Poor peripheral motor control lowers performance on finger dexterities to a prorated I.Q. of 68. Apart from her showing on this subtest, she appears to be more intact in the perceptual-analytic and visuomotor area than the verbal. She achieves a prorated I.Q. of 81 in Picture Completion and a prorated I.Q. of 107 in Block Design, in which she is able to do all but the last of ten items. She shows insight and capacity in this area. Picture Arrangement and Object Assembly at a prorated I.Q. of 94 are moderate. If we assume that her former level was High Average, then the data indicate a moderate deficit in the perceptual-analytic area and major deficits in the verbal, semantic, abstract, and attention-memory areas.

"C. experiences tilting sensations, dizziness, tingling, and numbness in her limbs, feet, and hands, and severe headaches. She experiences the environment darkening and lightening, her vision blurs, she suffers nausea. She has frightening experiences in which colors seem to change and sides of the room switch; she becomes almost panicky when this happens.

"Evidences of a harsh family background with severe deprivation have produced a sado-masochistic view of object relations. Material from this pathological background seems to be intertwined with cerebral stimulation, very likely resulting from damaged tissue, to form frightening mental experiences resulting in behavior that could be either psychotic or the result of a post-traumatic seizure disorder.

"Reliance upon a diagnosis of Schizophrenia would require a careful neurological assessment, coupled with determination of her pre-traumatic intellectual status through educational records prior to the head injury.

"This conclusion is supported by the dual administration of the Bender Visual Motor Gestalt Test, which elicited evidence of difficulty in maintaining Gestalt, collisions, partial rotations, and more evidence of poor peripheral motor control. The Rorschach produced no evidence of psychotic ideation. Her stereotyped response pattern may be indicative of a regressive type of personality, but equally could be attributed to the perceptual difficulties of a brain-damaged individual who resorts to protective repetition of what she finds possible to do.

"A good deal of C.'s behavior is inappropriate. She suddenly utters statements that have no bearing on what is going on with her or with the other person with whom she is engaged. As an illustration, at one point she exclaimed: 'I would like to meet Senator Kennedy in person, because he is such a wonderful person.' "

BIBLIOGRAPHY

1. *Abenson, M. H.:* EEGs in chronic schizophrenia. Brit. J. Psychiat., 116, 1970.
2. *Anderson, A.:* The effect of laterality localization of brain damage on Wechsler-Bellevue indices of deterioration. J. Clin. Psychol., 6, 1950.
3. *Andreasen, N. J. C., et al.:* The significance of thought disorder in diagnostic evaluations. Comprehensive Psychiat., 15:1, 1974.
4. *Arieti, S.:* Interpretation of Schizophrenia. New York: Robert Brunner, 1955.
5. *Belford, B.:* Electrophysiological basis for a dichotomy in schizophrenia. Psychological Reports, 39:2, 1976.
6. *Bellak, L.* (Ed.): Schizophrenia: A Review of the Syndrome. New York: Logos Press, 1958.
7. *Bellak, L., et al.:* Ego Functions in Schizophrenia, Neurotics, and Normals. New York: John Wiley and Sons, 1973.
8. *Bellak, L.* and *Loeb, L.* (Eds.): The Schizophrenic Syndrome. New York: Grune and Stratton, 1969.
9. *Bender, L.:* Alpha and omega of childhood schizophrenia. J. Autism Child. Schiz., 1:2, 1971.
10. *Bender, L.:* A longitudinal study of schizophrenic children with autism. Hospital Community Psychiat., 20:8, 1969.
11. *Bender, L.:* Childhood schizophrenia: A review. Int. J. Psychiat., 5, 1968.
12. *Benson, D. F.:* Psychiatric aspects of aphasia. Brit. J. Psychiat., 123, 1973.
13. *Birch, H. G.* and *Hertzig, M. E.:* Etiology of schizophrenia: An overview of the relation of development of atypical behavior. *In* J. Romano (Ed.): The Origins of Schizophrenia. New York: Excerpta Medica, 1967.
14. *Birch, H. G.* and *Walker, H. A.:* Perceptual and perceptual-motor dissociation: Studies in schizophrenic and brain-damaged psychotic children. Arch. Gen. Psychiat., 14, 1966.
15. *Bleuler, E.:* Dementia Praecox or the Group of Schizophrenias. (First published in 1911). New York: International Universities Press, 1950.
16. *Bortner, M.* and *Birch, H. G.:* Patterns of intellectual ability in emotionally disturbed and brain-damaged children. J. Spec. Ed., 3:4, 1969.
17. *Brill, N. Q.:* General biological studies. *In* L. Bellak and L. Loeb (Eds.): The Schizophrenic Syndrome. New York: Grune and Stratton, 1969.
18. *Callaway, E., et al.:* Auditory evoked potential variability in schizophrenia. Electroencephalography Clin. Neurophysiol., 29:5, 1970.
19. *Campion, E.* and *Tucker, G.:* A note on twin studies, schizophrenia and neurological impairment. Arch. Gen. Psychiat., 29:4, 1973.

20. *Chapman, J.:* The early symptoms of schizophrenia. Brit. J. Psychiat., 112, 1966.
21. *Chappel, G. E.:* Developmental aphasia revisited. J. Communication Disorders, 3, 1970.
22. *Chess, S.:* An Introduction to Child Psychiatry, 2nd ed., New York: Grune and Stratton, 1969.
23. *Creak, M.:* Childhood psychosis: A review of 100 cases. Brit. J. Psychiat., 109, 1963.
24. *DeWolfe, A. S.:* Differentiation of schizophrenia and brain damage with the WAIS. J. Clin. Psychol., 27:2, 1971.
25. *DeWolfe, A. S., et al.:* Intellectual deficit in schizophrenia and brain damage. J. Consult. Clin. Psychol., 36:2, 1971.
26. *Fish, B.:* Study of motor development in infancy and its relation to psychiatric functioning. Amer. J. Psychiat., 117, 1961.
27. *Flor-Henry, P.:* Psychoses and temporal lobe epilepsy: A controlled investigation. Epilepsia, 10, 1969.
28. *Flor-Henry, P., et al.:* The neuropsychological correlates of the functional psychoses. Psychiat. Clin. Psychol., 3:34, 1975.
29. *Gajzago, C. and Prior, M.:* Two cases of "recovery" in Kanner syndrome. Arch. Gen. Psychiat., 31:2, 1974.
30. *Garmezy, N.:* Children at risk: The search for the antecedents of schizophrenia. Part II: Ongoing research programs, issues, and intervention. Schizophrenia Bull., 9, 1974.
31. *Gerson, S. N., et al.:* Diagnosis: Schizophrenia versus posterior aphasia. Amer. J. Psychiat., 134:9, 1977.
32. *Geschwind, N.:* Current concepts: Aphasia. N. E. J. Med., 284, 1971.
33. *Gittleman, N. and Birch, H. G.:* Childhood schizophrenia: Intellectual and neurological status, perinatal risk, prognosis and family pathology. Arch. G. Psychiat., 17, 1967.
34. *Goldfarb, W.:* Childhood Schizophrenia. Cambridge, Mass.: Harvard University Press, 1961.
35. *Goldstein, K.:* Methodological approach to the study of schizophrenic thought disorder. *In* J. S. Kasanin (Ed.): Language and Thought in Schizophrenia. Berkeley: University of California Press, 1944.
36. *Goldstein, K.:* The Organism. New York: American Book Co., 1939.
37. *Gruzelier, J. and Hammond, N.:* Schizophrenia: A dominant hemisphere disorder? Res. Communications Psychol. Psychiat. Behav., 1:1, 1976.
38. *Gur, R. E.:* Motoric laterality imbalance in schizophrenia. Arch. Gen. Psychiat., 34, 1977.
39. *Heaton, R. K.:* The validity of neuropsychological evaluations in psychiatric settings. Clin. Psychologist, 29:2, 1976.
40. *Himmelhoch, J., et al.:* Sub-acute encephalitis: Behavioral and neurological aspects. Brit. J. Psychiat., 116, 1970.
41. *Holden, J. M., et al.:* Electroencephalographic patterns in schizophrenia: Relationship to therapy resistance. Biological Psychiat., 6:2, 1973.
42. *Kallman, F. J. and Roth, B.:* Genetic aspects of preadolescent schizophrenia. Amer. J. Psychiat., 112, 1956.
43. *Kanner, L.:* Follow-up studies of eleven autistic children originally reported in 1943. J. Autism Child. Schiz., 1:2, 1971.
44. *Kanner, L.:* Problems of nosology and psychodynamics of early infantile autism. Amer. J. Orthopsychiat., 19, 1949.
45. *Kasanin, J.:* The disturbance of conceptual thinking in schizophrenia. *In* J. Kasanin (Ed.): Language and Thought in Schizophrenia. New York: Norton, 1964.

46. *Kernberg, P. F.:* The problem of organicity in the child: Notes on some diagnostic techniques in the evaluation of children. J. Amer. Acad. Child Psychiat., 8:3, 1969.
47. *Klonoff, H., et al.:* Neuropsychological patterns in chronic schizophrenia. J. Ner. Ment. Dis., 150:4, 1970.
48. *Laufer, M. W.* and *Gair, D. S.:* Childhood schizophrenia. *In* L. Bellak and L. Loeb (Eds.): The Schizophrenic Syndrome. New York: Grune and Stratton, 1969.
49. *Lilliston, L.:* Schizophrenic symptomatology as a function of probability of brain damage. J. Abnorm. Psychol., 82:3, 1973.
50. *Lilliston, L.:* Tests of cerebral damage and the process-reactive dimension. J. Clin. Psychol., 26:2, 1970.
51. *Lobascher, M. E., et al.:* Childhood autism: An investigation of etiological factors in twenty-five cases. Brit. J. Psychiat., 117-540, 1970.
52. *Lyle, J. G.:* Cognitive dysfunction in childhood and adult psychosis. Brit. J. Med. Psychol., 44:1, 1971.
53. *McGhie, A.:* Psychological studies of schizophrenia. Brit. J. Med. Psychol., 39, 1966.
54. *Mahler, M.:* On child psychosis and schizophrenia: Autistic and symbiotic infantile psychosis. Psychoanalytic Study of the Child. New York: International Universities Press, 1952.
55. *Martin, P. J.:* Impairment and prediction of cognitive functioning in schizophrenia. Res. Communications Psychol., Psychiat., Behavior, 1:4, 1976.
56. *Matthews, C.* and *Reitan, R. M.:* Correlations of Wechsler-Bellevue subtest means in lateralized and non-lateralized brain damaged groups. Percep. Motor Skills, 19, 1964.
57. *Mednick, S.:* Birth defects and schizophrenia. Psychology Today, April, 1971.
58. *Mirsky, A. F.:* Neuropsychological bases of schizophrenia. Ann. Rev. Psychol., 20, 1969.
59. *Monroe, R. R.:* Episodic Behavioral Disorders: A Psychodynamic and Neurophysiologic Analysis. Cambridge, Mass.: Harvard University Press, 1970.
60. *Mordock, J. B.:* Recent innovations in teaching the autistic child. Devereux Schools Forum, 6:1, 1970.
61. *Mosher, L. R., et al.:* Special report: Schizophrenia, 1972. Schiz. Bull., 7, 1973.
62. *Mosher, L. R., et al.:* Identical twins discordant for schizophrenia: Neurologic findings. Arch. Gen. Psychiat., 24:5, 1971.
63. *Mosher, L. R.* and *Feinsilver, D.:* Special Report on Schizophrenia. (Mimeo). Washington: National Institute of Mental Health, 1971.
64. *Ornitz, E. M.* and *Ritvo, E. R.:* The syndrome of autism: A critical review. Amer. J. Psychiat., 133:6, 1976.
65. *Ornitz, E. M.* and *Ritvo, E. R.:* Perceptual inconstancy in early infantile autism. Arch. Gen. Psychiat., 18, 1968.
66. *Parsons, O. A., et al.:* Different psychological effects of lateralized brain damage. J. Consult. Psychol., 33, 1969.
67. *Pollack, M.:* Brain damage, mental retardation and childhood schizophrenia. Amer. J. Psychiat., 115, 1958.
68. *Pollin, W., et al.:* Life history differences in identical twins discordant for schizophrenia. Amer. J. Orthopsychiat., 36, 1966.
69. *Reitan, R. M.:* Certain differential effects of left and right cerebral lesions in human adults. J. Comp. Physiol. Psychol., 48, 1955.
70. *Rimland, B.:* Infantile Autism. New York: Appleton-Century-Crofts, 1964.
71. *Ritvo, E. R., et al.:* Correlation of psychiatric diagnosis and EEG findings: A

double-blind study of 184 hospitalized children. Amer. J. Psychiat., 126:7, 1970.

72. *Rutt, C. N.* and *Offord, D. R.:* Prenatal and perinatal complications in childhood schizophrenics and their siblings. J. Nerv. Ment. Dis., 152:5, 1971.

73. *Rutter, M.:* Childhood schizophrenia reconsidered. J. Autism Childhood Schiz., 2:4, 1972.

74. *Rutter, M.:* Behavioral and cognitive characteristics. *In* J. K. Wing (Ed.): Early Childhood Autism. Oxford: Pergamon Press, 1966.

75. *Rutter, M.:* Influence of organic and emotional factors on origins, nature and outcome of childhood psychosis. Dev. Med. Child Neurol., 7, 1956.

76. *Rutter, M.* and *Bartak, L.:* Causes of infantile autism: Some considerations from recent research. J. Autism Childhood Schiz., 1:1, 1971.

77. *Rycroft, C.:* An observation of the defensive function of schizophrenic thinking and delusion formation. Int. J. Psycho-Anal., 43, 1962.

78. *Schilder, P.:* Medical Psychology. New York: International Universities Press, 1973.

79. *Shagass, C.:* Neurophysiological studies. *In* L. Bellak and L. Loeb (Eds.): The Schizophrenic Syndrome. New York: Grune and Stratton, 1969.

80. *Slater, E.* and *Beard, A. W.:* The schizophrenic-like psychoses of epilepsy. Brit. J. Psychiat., 109 a and b, 1963.

81. *Taft, L. T.* and *Goldfarb, W.:* Prenatal and perinatal factors in childhood schizophrenia. Develop. Med. Child Neurol., 6, 1964.

82. *Taylor, M. A., et al.:* Neuropsychological test performances in affective disorder and schizophrenia. Mimeo., 1976.

83. *Taylor, M. A., et al.:* Manic-depressive illness and schizophrenia: A partial validation of research diagnostic criteria utilizing neuropsychological testing. Compreh. Psychiat., 16:1, 1975.

84. *Tinbergen, N.:* Ethology and stress diseases. Science, 185, 1974.

85. *Walker, H. A.* and *Birch, H. G.:* Neurointegrative deficiency in schizophrenic children. J. Nerv. Ment. Dis., 151:2, 1970.

86. *Weaver, L. A.:* Psychomotor performance of clinically differentiated chronic schizophrenics. Percept. Motor Skills, 12, 1961.

87. *Weaver, L. A.* and *Brooks, G. W.:* The use of psychomotor tests in predicting the potential of chronic schizophrenics. J. Neuropsychiat., 5, 1963.

88. *White, L.:* Organic factors and psychophysiology in childhood schizophrenia. Psychological Bull., 81:4, 1974.

89. *White, P. T., et al.:* EEG abnormalities in early childhood schizophrenia: A double blind study of psychiatrically disturbed and normal children during promazine sedation. Amer. J. Psychiat., 120, 1964.

90. *Wing, L.* and *Wing, J. K.:* Multiple impairments in early childhood autism. J. Autism Childhood Schiz., 1:3, 1971.

CHAPTER 6

Mental Retardation

Mental retardation, a serious designation, should be arrived at only with the greatest care, after a series of considerations in differential diagnosis. It is a serious label because it implies irreversibility. Further, it often consigns the child so labeled to responses from those around him based on a stereotype of the most gravely limited mentally retarded individual. Most seriously, the designation may delay or obstruct introduction of the very services known to make a difference for the better: careful diagnosis of the individual's assets and impairments and a consistent, appropriate program of treatment and special training.

The very definitions of mental retardation are controversial. Differences center around which functions or abilities should be included in defining mental retardation. Should the definition include the level of abstract thinking? The amount of information? Or spatial ability? Or should it, instead, represent an overall global estimate of intellectual functioning? Another question is whether etiology should be included in the definition, since the term itself is merely descriptive and non-explanatory. Is the mental retardation primary, or secondary to some other disorder? Some workers distinguish between the mental defective and the mentally retarded. The distinction made by the use of these two terms can be considerable; the "defective" appellation may imply a more fixed condition with poorer prognosis than is the lot of the mentally "retarded." But both in present usage are less than precise.

ETIOLOGY

The discussion of etiology in mental retardation is even more heatedly controversial than is the effort to establish definitions, even when

208

an effort is made toward scientific discourse. Beneath open-mindedness, deliberation, and impartiality there appears all of the bias and all of the rage that has marked "nature-nurture" controversies. At issue are the roles of genetics, brain damage, familial, and cultural forces in the determination of mental retardation. Protagonists have much with which to fuel their fires: among the approximately six million persons in the United States now diagnosed as mentally retarded, nearly 200 causal factors have been identified, but etiology can be established for only about 25 percent of them (13).

Simple or *primary* mental retardation is considered to be the result of a constitutional lag in development, rather than the result of a disease process. Presumably it derives from either an incomplete growth of brain cells or an impairment of the neural mechanisms of association and integration. A combination of these two factors, of course, is possible. Usually it is impossible to establish whether the so-called primary mental retardation is genetically or idiopathically determined. An exception now is Down's Syndrome in which chromosomal aberration has been established (2).

Secondary mental retardation is retardation that is believed to be determined by organic rather than genetic factors. It may arise from infections or injury during gestation or the birth process. Mental retardation is one of the major consequences of congenital rubella, for example (5). It may be the result of chronically degenerative disease processes. Among the types recognized are those associated with microcephaly, hydrocephaly, post-encephalitic syndromes, paralysis, epilepsy, cerebral palsy, sclerosis, meningitis, congenital syphilis, and endocrine dysfunctions. Clusters of symptoms into syndromes are frequently observed; for example, mental retardation and schizophrenia or cerebral palsy may occur in the same child. And obviously pathological processes do not invariably produce mental retardation; a child with cerebral palsy may be intellectually brilliant.

Cultural-familial etiology is most frequently diagnosed among the mentally retarded. Physicians tend to pay little attention to this group, focusing instead upon the genetic, physiological, and neuropathological determinants. The category is based upon the belief that forces making for mental retardation reside in the cultural and familial environment, that the child's brain is without pathology, and that genetics are not influential.

Symptom patterns often are confusing and in many cases may change, leading to changes in diagnosis and assumptions about etiology. Chess (4) identifies a group of children who may manifest a specific type of dysfunction sometimes neuromuscular in nature, sometimes involving a specific sense organ. In other individuals, the symptoms may be more generalized, indicating diffuse damage, with resultant disorganization of functioning shown in increased irritability, decreased capacity for responding to stimuli, impaired impulse control, or decreased spontaneity. Some children within this group do not manifest a behavioral disorder; they may be relatively well-adjusted. Others may demonstrate varied symptoms indicative of a cerebral dysfunction: hypermobility, decreased or excessive attention span, distractibility or relative imperviousness to stimuli, hyper- or hypo-irritability, lability or monotony of mood, excessive dependency or inappropriate independence. Obsessive behavior may be observed in repeated questions, stereotyped gestures, or mechanically rhythmic body movements.

The difficulty of identifying an instance of primary mental deficiency derived from hereditary or constitutional defectiveness was stressed by Burgemeister (3). This difficulty has been lessened somewhat by more recent chromosomal finding that have in turn stimulated the increasing use of amniocentesis (2). Often observed is what might be called pseudo mental retardation, a functional or psychogenically determined condition. It can be differentiated from constitutional retardation accompanied by organic impairment only by extremely careful investigation. Organic impairment may be absent altogether. Many psychotic children act and function like mentally defective individuals; behavior problems are also frequently observed among mentally retarded children. Yet behavioral problems are not an inevitable concomitant of mental deficiency; they are most likely to appear when the environment demands more than the individual is capable of producing or giving.

Chess (4) cautions against diagnosing a child with mental retardation as an autistic child. The latter may resemble retarded or aphasic children in their failure to respond to the people who take care of them and in difficulty in learning to talk at the usual developmental time. An interesting observation about autism is offered by Rimland (18a) who finds a higher incidence of idiot savants (10 percent) among his autistic patients than among mental retardates (one in 2,000) or the general population (one in 3,000,000). There would appear to be a diagnostic problem here that is far from being resolved.

The frequent correlation of neurological damage with Childhood

Schizophrenia often leads to the rediagnosis of mental retardation as such children grow older, and the behavioral problems of adjustment abate (9). Retardation appears to be a more frequent concomitant of Process Schizophrenia than of the Reactive type. In both the child and the adult, Process Schizophrenia tends to result in greater intellectual deficit than in Reactive Schizophrenia, thus often confusing the judgment of variables in this area of research. Higgins (10) notes that retardates are judged to be Process Schizophrenics more often than to be Reactive Schizophrenics, and that Reactive Schizophrenics are more often called normal than are either organically damaged or mentally retarded individuals.

DIAGNOSTIC CONSIDERATIONS

If the individual child is to be understood and helped, the diagnosis must be based upon both etiology and relative levels of cognitive, sensory, and motor functioning. Chess (4) emphasizes the importance of a child's intellectual level in differential diagnosis. She contends that variability in levels of intellectual functioning at different times suggests a capacity to operate on a higher level and militates against the diagnosis of retardation. The schizophrenic child periodically will give some indication, however transient or partial, of intellectual functioning at or above the level expected of the child's age. Chess restrains any diagnostic leap with the reasonable caution that both retardation and schizophrenia may be present in the same child.

My observation is that brain-damaged children also often show variability in levels of functioning, comparable with that which Chess observes among schizophrenic children, and that these brain-damaged children may be incorrectly classified as mentally retarded. I have observed many young adults with Full Scale I.Q.'s as low as 50-55 who obtain prorated I.Q.'s of 135 in some subtests and zero prorated I.Q.'s in others. These young adults usually had been assigned to classes for mentally retarded in public school. The idiot savant, of course, uniquely exemplifies the wide range of skills possible in one individual, from an extraordinarily high level in one subtest to a generally low level in others (15).

Smith (21) finds that too often diagnosis of mental retardation is by default; the failure to establish brain damage is generally followed by the assumption that the brain is normal, allowing the further assumption of a genetic or cultural familial etiology. His study of 181 institutionalized mentally retarded adults suggests convincingly that their diagnostic classification was often inadequate simply because their examiners had not looked beyond I.Q. levels. Table 1 presents their original diagnostic classifications, the size of each diagnostic group, mean I.Q.'s and ages.

TABLE 1

Diagnostic Data for 181 Institutionalized Mentally
Retarded Adults in the Smith Study (21)

Diagnosis	N	Mean I.Q.	Mean Age
Cultural-familial	45	62.6	37.4
Congenital cerebral maldevelopment	56	62.5	38.4
MR with affective disorders	22	62.8	25.7
Unknown or other	24	71.6	39.6
Pre-, peri-, or early postnatal brain insults	34	60.6	36.0

The battery of tests administered provided four measures of cognitive functions and two of sensory and motor functions, the latter two generally considered independent of cognitive or intellectual level. The battery consisted of the Raven's Coloured Matrices (RCM), Peabody Picture Vocabulary Test (PPVT), Symbol Digit Modalities Test (SDMT), Memory for Unrelated Sentences (MUS), Double Simultaneous Stimulation (DSS), and the Purdue Pegboard (PP). Not one of the subjects obtained normal SDMT scores on either written or oral administration. PP scores were below normal in 98.9 percent. Additionally, 63.6 percent of the "MR with Affective Disorders," 58.3 percent of the "Unknown or Other," and 47.7 of the "Cultural-familial" group produced three or more errors on DSS.

Smith's study points to the error of a simplistic approach to the diagnosis of the mentally retarded, for example, to regard the cultural-familial group as composed of individuals with anatomically normal brains unfortunately limited to the lower end of the normal distribution curve of intelligence, a plight compounded by restriction of further intellectual development in their culturally deprived early environment.

Diagnostic evaluation must go beyond classification and establishment of etiology. It must provide a guide to active treatment. I.Q. testing, for example, should not be used merely for the purpose of segregating the mentally retarded in residences and institutions, but should suggest the basis for remediation and habilitation efforts. These efforts should use to the fullest the individual's stronger skills, while concentrating remedial work upon the weaker ones (12). Thus, adequate differential diagnosis requires the most careful scanning of as many types of cognitive, sensory and motor functions as can possibly be tested. Reliance upon a global I.Q. obscures the discriminating data that may identify areas of relatively intact functioning that have been progressing in spite of the child's damage in other areas. Unnecessary pessimism about outcome and reluctance to invest in therapeutic programs result when a child is labeled solely with a total I.Q. that falls in the Mentally Defective range. Differential analysis of functioning often creates more optimism, since this same child may have one or more functions that test within or above the Average range.

Do we do the patient justice? Are we correct when we label a child "mentally retarded" when one or more functions are observed to be at or near an Above Average level although *averaging* results in a much lower classification? The dangers in such labeling are that it discourages parents, teachers, and treatment professionals, creates pessimistic prognoses, and forestalls the very "in-put" of stimuli to the child's strong points and bulwarking of weak points that are known to make critical differences in ability to function. A statement of overall I.Q. should never be allowed to categorize a child. Meticulous diagnosis requires specific evaluations of each measurable function. Furthermore, the patient's social manner, his mode and rate of response, his employed vocabulary and use of metaphor must be recognized as *clinical data,* just as important as any fact of history or any test score in evaluating and planning for the individual.

The responsibility of the clinician in diagnosis and prescribing treatment is clearly stated by Durfee (7). He surveys literature reporting mental retardation as the diagnosis (rather, the misdiagnosis) when the real factors included such a wide range of situations as language problems, neuroses, autism, psychoses, Heller's disease, even a case of congenital deafness. Durfee cautions against professional "buck passing" and the tendency to accept past information and standing diagnoses rather than vigorously pursuing a current differential assessment.

Durfee's admonition also highlights the inadequacy of most diagnostic terms to make the needed statement about etiology. Identification of causative factors contributes a great deal to treatment planning where there is retarded mental function, while the term "mental retardation" alone contributes nothing.

This point may be illustrated with an example from the promising application of behavioral techniques—especially operant conditioning—in the education and training of the mentally retarded child (8). A considerable portion of this promise may reside in the use of parents as operant conditioners, thus moving to nip bad reinforcement schedulers in the bud, so to speak, and convert their force to the positive side. Behavioral investigations have established that the retarded child learns basic units—the simple conditioned reflex—as quickly as does the normal child. Hypotheses about the retarded child's difficulties with learning of a higher order include the possibility that attentional capacity is impaired, that he can make little or no use of mediating verbal responses, and that he has difficulty in forming higher level stimulus-response units. Obtaining the maximum from improved teaching procedures depends upon identifying and using the stronger, more intact functions in the child, hence upon identification and meticulous measurement of those functions.

Diagnosis must include also an assessment of the child's cultural and familial environment, of the extent to which these may be predicted to be constructive or destructive forces. In short, the parents and the family should be diagnosed as well as the child.

TREATMENT

Society, Crissey observes (6), is gingerly opening its doors to many among the mentally retarded. The gigantic sequestering institutions are slowly being replaced by community-based residences for small numbers of children, adolescents, and adults who attend school or work as well as live within a normal community instead of in isolation. Treatment interventions of all kinds are being helpful in facilitating this shift.

Parent counseling or psychotherapy is a significant aide in the constructive treatment of the child from the earliest days of identification of restricted functioning (16). Early engagement of parents' shock, depression, rage, ambivalence and rejection of the child can not only forestall brutalization, but also may contribute much to the child's ability to respond to special educational efforts. Parental input and participation, parental support and encouragement, have been observed by this writer to have the potential to move a child from the Mentally Defective to the Borderline Mentally Defective level, or from the latter to the Dull Normal level of mental functioning. Parental treatment may also be important in helping parents to minimize super-ego interdictions in their effort to control the child's behavior and to substitute positive reinforcement procedures instead, or to devise special educational approaches. Many parents need help in reducing a tendency to overprotect the child, a tendency that has a significant negative impact upon learning of all kinds, affecting as it does the sense of mastery. Parents often need help also in developing realistic understanding of their child's developing sexuality and their own fears about it.

Evaluation of the parents' ability and willingness to cope with these factors may influence the choice of a recommendation for care at home rather than residential training. Part of parental counseling may focus upon helping them help siblings shape constructive understanding of the child, especially to counteract distortions with realistic information.

Family therapy may be indicated where the siblings are old enough and also where the mentally retarded child is able to participate. Parents who fear for the impact on their normal children of having the mentally retarded sib at home may find their fears dissipated during the exploration and ventilation that family therapy permits. The therapist in couple counseling and family therapy must be acutely self-aware of personal attitudes and biases for or against the idea of family home care of the mentally retarded child. The therapist must exercise care not to influence unwilling, seriously masochistic, or otherwise ill-equipped parents and families to take on burdens they cannot cope with, or to impede loving and caring ones from deciding to keep the child at home when the therapist cannot empathize with that choice.

A useful overview of psychotherapeutic applications with the mentally retarded child is provided by Robinson and Robinson (19). Many retarded children have had little experience with play activities, and their use in therapy can be effective with adolescents and adults as well as children. Art therapy may be combined with play therapy, as in the use of music and dancing to encourage body mastery. In group therapy, play can promote more socialized behavior.

On a one-to-one basis, the therapist often must facilitate ventilation and catharsis and at the same time use the opportunity to set limits for the mentally retarded adolescent or adult, making clear that expression is welcome and acceptable in the therapeutic situation, but that in other life situations reality will require some limitation of expression. Reassurance is a frequently required therapeutic intervention, along with support. The therapist often finds it constructive to act as an advisor or advocate for the mentally retarded patient, intervening, explaining a situation to a teacher, a parent, or an employer where expecting the person to act on his own behalf is unreasonable. Frequently, goal-directed discussions of problems centering around important issues in life are useful. The therapist may suggest the area for discussion, suggest how to approach the discussion, and both initiate and move the discussion along with leading questions. An important feature to keep in mind when interpreting and reflecting with the mentally retarded patient is to use vivid concrete examples. An interpretation should be repeated in several different situations in order to reinforce the patient's comprehension. Role playing in psychodrama is an extremely useful technique, enabling retarded adolescents and adults to see themselves in relationship to other individuals and gradually to be able to predict reactions and responses.

Group therapy is also possible with the retarded adolescent and young adult. Many of the techniques discussed earlier are applicable to the group situation. Robinson and Robinson (19) especially value the group method because it minimizes the demand for abstract verbal comprehension by providing concrete, contemporary examples of human relationships which the patient can work on with other people. These can be defined and so controlled by the therapist that they are within the range of comprehension of the patients and hence are not overwhelming. Self-esteem is enhanced by the child's awareness through the group that other children have problems similar to his own. The skilled group therapist can, so to speak, titrate for the fearful child the amount of his participation in the group. Male and female co-therapist teams allow the development and exploration of transference feelings that otherwise might remain obscure.

All psychotherapeutic efforts with the mentally retarded must, to reiterate, minimize demands for abstract verbal comprehension and expression and focus on concrete skills for concrete problems of self-management and social relationships, especially those with peers. Another point worthy of reiteration is that the best psychotherapy for the brain damaged is the earliest possible development of those cognitive functions and skills that have been blocked by the cerebropathology. Special educational approaches to a child's specific disabilities based upon careful differential diagnosis, therefore, can be considered of primary psychotherapeutic value in bolstering a child's self-esteem and social adjustment. An illuminating illustration of the interaction of these forces is provided by the experiment reported by Krop and Smith (14). Their evidence indicates that mentally retarded children after training in drawing geometric figures obtained better Bender Gestalt scores and improved ratings in academic achievement and "socio-psychological" adjustment as rated by teachers.

PREVENTION

Prevention is an especially pertinent and compelling issue in both mental retardation and minimal brain dysfunction where the pathological impact of many controllable pre-, peri-, and early post-natal events and conditions are clearly established. This consideration brings the clinician face to face with the etiological force of poverty and with the preventive potential of political and social action to reduce its effects. While both mental retardation and minimal brain dysfunction strike all orders of society, statistics generally show them to be disorders of poverty and economic underprivilege. The incidence of brain disorders is positively related to the incidence of poverty (11). A study (17) shows that children of lower socioeconomic groups reveal a higher incidence of neurological signs. Anoxia and Rh incompatibility are not respecters of income level, of course. Children of middle-class parents undoubtedly are subject to brain injury before, during, and after birth. But the evidence mounts that the children of the poor are more frequent among the victims.

The National Children's Bureau of England reports (22) that by the age of seven, socially-disadvantaged children are behind middle-class peers in reading, school achievement, height, and mental development. The disadvantages are apparent at birth and increase with age. These conclusions are derived from a survey of 17,000 children born during 1958. In addition to being shorter, the poor children had more speech defects and poorer motor coordination. They were more likely to be hostile to teachers, and to be withdrawn and depressed. At age seven the reading gap is more than two years on the average. When this gap is projected into presumed I.Q. levels, the social nature of mental retardation is strongly suggested.

Economically deprived children need every personal resource they can muster to make their way out of their birth trap. Yet many economically deprived children are made especially helpless by the conditions of poverty: early malnutrition, poor prenatal and perinatal care, untreated or poorly treated febrile illnesses, and plenty of traumas to the head. All of the forces that injure the brain and impair its functioning are associated more frequently with life among the poor.

However, a study (23) finding that poverty is not primary was made in Westchester Country, just north of New York City. It suggests that being male and living in wealthier status are factors more frequently associated with brain damage. The area is not without poor people, but it heavily populated with the well-to-do. Another study (1) of children from all levels in a midwestern city reported that the *proportion* of minimally brain-damaged to normal children is the same across all socioeconomic levels.

Obviously, the statement that the children of the poor are more likely to be victims of brain dysfunction is contestable. Yet the face validity of the contention is convincing.

Psychologists and neurologists alone cannot alter the prevalence of the poverty that appears to underlie a substantial number of the tragic cases of mental retardation that we know to exist in our affluent society. That very helplessness may discourage many who would be moved to devote our professional lives to this single disorder. But we can continue to explore the relationship between deprivation and retardation and to assert its human costs while we work to allay them.

The established risk of being delivered of a mongoloid child (Down's Syndrome) for women over 40 has recently been drastically reduced by the development and widespread use of amniocentesis. The syndrome is linked to the appearance of an extra chromosome, making 47 rather than the normal 46 in the fetus. Geneticists have established that chromosome 21 undergoes spontaneous "trisomy" or tripling rather than the normal pairing (2). In amniocentesis, a needle is passed through the mother's abdominal wall and the wall of her uterus and through the amniotic sac. Amniotic fluid is withdrawn which contains sloughed-off fetal cells. These are cultured and examined for the presence of a forty-seventh chromosome. Where the extra chromosome is found, the mother has the choice of going ahead with the certainty of bearing a mongoloid child or terminating the pregnancy. Psychotherapy may be indicated to help the mother resolve any conflict that may exist within herself or between herself and her husband.

Educating women to the increased risk of bearing a mongoloid child when they become 40 is a significant preventive effort, along with discussion of the abortion option. Psychotherapists have an important role in these preventive efforts; many childless women over 35 enter psychotherapy with problems that are related to their childlessness. In arriving at their decision to have a child, which many of them do, awareness of the risk and the options available to them is strengthening should a crisis of decision arise.

The complex variables in the subject of mental retardation make any single hypothesis—whether it be genetic or cultural-familial causation—subject to both oversimplification and experimenter bias. Sarason and Doris (20) attempt to limit the risk of oversimplification by listing the areas of investigation necessary in mental retardation: psychology, biology, education, sociology, anthropology, and social history. Multivariate research design is required as a preliminary to unraveling the mysteries of this disorder. Equally important is the control of theoretical bias in all efforts to help the individual child; there is no single cause or type or effect of mental retardation. And there is no uniformly applicable intervention.

CASE ILLUSTRATIONS

1. *After placement in a class for mentally retarded children, a girl becomes "schizophrenic" and is hospitalized.*

When 13, T. became extremely upset following placement in a class for children of retarded mental development. She was hospitalized and described as confused, disorganized, withdrawn, delusional, and hallucinatory; the diagnosis offered was Childhood Schizophrenia. She had a difficult time in the hospital, was withdrawn and seemed unable to adjust to the ward routine, but finally improved and was discharged to her family's care. A second hospitalization occurred when she was 17. She had gone to Puerto Rico for a visit, stayed there for two months seeming to have a good time, but just before returning to the United States she became talkative, nervous, had suicidal ideas, and when she returned to the United States voluntarily re-entered the hospital. This time the diagnosis offered was Schizophrenia, Paranoid type. Thus, she came to a vocational agency at 18 with a multiple diagnosis—Mental Retardation and Schizophrenia. Her family was intact; she lived at home with her parents. Her father was employed.

Of her three brothers, the youngest was in a class for retarded children.

The agency psychiatrist commented: "The most striking thing about this young lady is her presentation. Judging from the history one would expect somebody who is quite difficult to communicate with. Quite to the contrary, she was very articulate and is able to carry on a very meaningful conversation despite the fact that she does have some difficulty with vocabulary. She was very clear about her feelings, her aspirations, the events that have gone on in her life, and certainly was able to tell me all those things that seemed rather important to her and important in terms of her life. She indicates that she has not been on medication for about three weeks, and apparently feels better without it. I could not elicit any delusional thinking, and although it has been stated that she has some difficulty with intellectual capacity I'm not able to make a determination about this. On this basis of what I have seen I would have great difficulties in making a diagnosis of Schizophrenia."

The patient was also seen by the agency psychologist, who reported:

"T. is an attractive, pleasant girl who looks sad, but is able to cut through it. In no way does she impress one as being psychotic. She has a speech defect of a moderate degree with a lisp and tendency toward mispronunciation that has nothing to do with an English limitation. Thus she will say "axe" for ask. Also she seems to have an anomia, which might be due to an English language limitation. When she said that she could not think of the word for powder puff in English but knew it in Spanish, I asked her to tell me what it was in Spanish; she pronounced the word as 'morta.' When I asked her to spell it, since it sounded so much like death, she spelled it 'morant.' As I tried to get her to be specific about this spelling her confusion mounted enormously.

"She is obviously of High Average intellectual endowment (she obtains a prorated I.Q. of 109 in Similarities and 106 in Comprehension), but has suffered severe deficits in several areas, particularly memory, attention, concentration, visual-motor, and peripheral-motor functions. On Information she obtains a prorated I.Q. of only 79, and it was clear here that the information available to her was attenuated by a memory loss. She spoke at this point of 'a big confusion in my life which makes everything confused for me.' Her difficulty in attention and concentration is evidenced by the low prorated I.Q. of 68 she obtains in Digit Symbol (finger dexterous work). Not only is she slow, but her figures are poorly performed; I believe this reflects difficulty with peripheral motor control. There is a perceptual-analytic difficulty also in the low prorated I.Q. of 68 she obtains in ability to assemble familiar objects. Here she showed spatial bewilderment, and even though she could recognize a part and associate it with a structure she could not properly locate it; with the Hand she said, 'I know this is a thumb, but I can't seem to get it in the right place.'

"The figure drawings show an intact body image to the extent that all of the major areas are properly represented, but there is a regressive quality, as well as a somewhat disorganized quality. Difficulties with reading and writing emerged, along with effort to deny these impairments and the great damage to her self-esteem as a result of them. Asked if she had any trouble writing, which I suspected from the beginning, she alleged that she did not. Asked to write a story, she wrote the following: 'A gilly in the class.' This led to her acknowledgement that she could not write, that she had great trouble reading also, that she had always had trouble reading and writing.

"Dual administration of the Bender Visual Motor Gestalt Test illustrates clearly the effect of memory attenuation upon her ability to function. The reproductions from memory are poorly organized; she loses the Gestalt, and one well-structured design in the shape of an arrowhead became a glob of dots when she attempted to recall it. On reproduction from direct copy there is much less tendency to lose Gestalt but there is a rotation and difficulty with peripheral motor control.

"The T.A.T. themes highlight a feeling of depression, of anger as a result of frustration, of the mother interfering with the pleasures and gratifications of the child. There is an in-turning of aggressivity against the self; this is much more denied than is sexuality, which is quite close to the surface and readily discussed by her; moral values around aggression are apparently of greater intensity than they are around sexuality. Her view of sexuality has long been hampered by fantasies of its sadomasochistic import, but she appears to be working through these quite well in recent years.

"Responses to projective queries indicate that she has felt deserted by her mother; her memories and dreams of childhood all have to do with separation from her mother and a feeling of being deserted and bereft.

"There are indications that in her heterosexual relationships, particularly to her current boyfriend, there has been a transference of major affective values from the mother. Her dream-life focuses around loss of him and the wish to have him treat her pretty much in a maternal way, in addition to being a sexual partner, which he is to her satisfaction. She has felt restricted and constricted much of her life by a number of forces: one is from her own perceived limitations induced by what may be cerebral damage; another is the prohibitions of her parents, who to this day are very much concerned about her and ride herd on her activities in restrictive fashion.

"It is well now to relate some of the test and interview findings developed from the suspicion of cerebral dysfunction. By way of review, at a relatively low range of the I.Q. scale there are 22 points difference between Performance, and Verbal I.Q., with Performance being lower than Verbal. The scale score for Comprehension is 9, for Object Assembly it is 5. This represents proportionately a considerable difference. As indicated before, attention-memory functions are also off at an average scale score of 6.

"T. had trouble academically from the very beginning and was placed in a CRMD class, most inappropriately, and with great damage to her self-esteem. This is one of the areas that caused her to feel depressed and damaged in self-esteem, and which has led to an explosive type of affect, since there are such strictures against aggressive acting out. It is also responsible for some of the suicidal ideation that she has had at times, but from which I think she is now very much alienated, so there would seem at this time to be no danger of suicidal acting out.

"She reports that she had a very high fever when she was about five years old and was in the hospital and placed in either cold water or cold packs. When she was about 10 she had her head bumped violently against the wall of an elevator by some man. When she was a child she caused herself to lose consciousness three times in one day by holding her breath and pressing against the carotid sinus. She experiences dizziness, double vision, choking sensations, tingling in the fingers. She also reports that she had experiences of things darkening and then suddenly lightening. She describes what may be altered states of consciousness, but which also may be intense fantasies built up around the wish for sexual gratification. She has had severe headaches, in which she felt that she was becoming an altered person; she also has experienced anger without having any reason for the anger. She becomes irritable sometimes, perhaps even explosive.

"This very attractive girl should be worked-up neurologically. There is a possibility of an ongoing psychomotor epilepsy. There appears to be definite cerebral damage impairing particularly memory, concentration, peripheral-motor activities, and perceptual-analytic functions. As I took her out to say good-bye, I noticed that she walked awkwardly. She told me that she trips, bumps into things, and walks in what she calls 'zig-zag.' "

2. *Neurological and psychological data disagree in a diagnosis of mental retardation.*

An 18-year-old girl, G., was referred to a vocational agency for training by a school for children with retarded mental development, from which she had been graduated. Her family was intact; her father was considerably older than her mother and not much involved with the daughter, but the mother was extremely so. G. listened to the radio, went to the movies, had a boy friend she saw occasionally, rode a bike, took piano lessons, played Scrabble, slept well, but was fearful of noises at night. When she was 15, a neurologist concluded from his examination: "There is no clinical evidence of convulsive disorder or focal brain lesion. The overall picture is one of mild moderate retardation, with some reactive anxiety."

She was examined by the agency psychologist who reported:

"G. is a very mature looking girl, lovely looking with long black hair and large brown eyes and a generous mouth. Her skin shows some neglect, typical of the impaired child. Her mouth exhibits a paralysis on the left side. She is left-handed, left-footed but right-eyed; this despite the fact that the left is her better eye. She is very co-operative and seemingly mature on a social basis. Her speech exhibits a slight stammer. Her affect is generally smiling and affable; one suspects immediately the primary defense of denial.

"The true status of her intellectual functioning is evident from the subtest scores obtained; they range from a high prorated I.Q. of 114 on Information to a low of 62 on the recognition of essential details. Ability to conceptualize is at the Average level. Comprehension is poor; I think we see here a difficulty in forming the associations required to move from the stimulus question to a response. Information is surprisingly wide and accurate: she knows the population of the United States, the number of Senators in the Senate, and can identify the Koran. Her difficulty in retaining several elements and manipulating them correctly appears on the Arithmetic subtest where she achieves a Mental Defective I.Q. of 67. Here she tended to add together the components in the question as the simplest process for her, rather than to execute the question itself which might require division or multiplication. An example of this is her response to this question: 'How many inches are there in 2½ feet? Her answer is '24½.' She completes the multiplication of 12 × 2 but then simply adds the ½. Another example is her response to the question: 'How many oranges can you buy for 36¢ if one orange costs 6¢?' Her answer is: '42.' Obviously she added the 36 and 6.

"There is an attention-memory deficit as well as a perceptual-analytic one. Digit Span is better than Digit Symbol, primarily because a physical-motor response of the hand is not involved in the Digit Span. Control of the pencil is relatively poor. She retains the general Gestalt of the figures, but her execution of them is a bit sloppy. Recognition of essential details is her poorest function, at a prorated I.Q. of 62; the assembly of familiar objects is not much better at a prorated I.Q. of 75.

"The Bender Visual Motor Gestalt Test shows a definite impairment of perceptual-analytic and psychomotor processes that is evidently on an organic basis.

"This girl cannot be considered mentally retarded on a genetic basis; there is clear evidence of innately Above Average or High Average verbal intellectual endowment. She may suffer from an anomia; frequently she gropes for the words she needs to explain herself, despite the fact that her vocabulary appears to be at the Average level. A good example of this came on the Picture Completion subtest when she wanted to say that the pole was missing from the flag; she said, instead, after struggling to find the word, 'the part where you have to hold it.' This could be related to her stuttering, or course. She appears to be cerebrally damaged, most specifically in a way involving attention-memory, perceptual-analytic, and psychomotor functions.

"The main thing to be said about her emotionally is her reliance upon denial. She obviously is affected by awareness of her limitations; her self-esteem is damaged, there is depression and anxiety. She handles all of this primarily by denial and by displacement. Thus, she will not recognize depression in herself but empathically feels unhappy about war conditions and the sufferings of other people. She has developed altruism to help her defend against her anger at her condition."

After several months in the workshop, G. became very anxious and hyperactive and was seen by the agency psychiatrist who questioned that ". . . this hyperactivity is the consequence of anxiety rather than the consequence of cerebral dysfunction. Motor activity secondary to cerebral dysfunction is similar to motor activity secondary to neurotic anxiety, or to anxiety precipitated by stressful situations, and I think we should be careful about distinguishing one from the other. The patient appears to be quite free of thought disorder or any other difficulty other than her incapacities and motor difficulty which are characteristic of cerebral dysfunction. She certainly has no psychotic process and seems to be a rather likeable girl."

3. *Two men, educated in classes for retarded children, produce contradictory psychodiagnostic data.*

Mr. W., a tall, pleasantly social man of 26, had been married for two years and had one child when seen for psychodiagnostic assessment as part of a vocational training program. He had been in classes for retarded children most of his time in school, leaving illegally at the age of 14.

He was found to be functioning at the Low Average level in perceptual-analytic tasks, achieving a prorated I.Q. of 94 in recognition of familiar details, and 88 in the assembly of familiar objects. In contrast, there was a marked deficit in attention-memory, with prorated I.Q. of 52 in Digit Span and 61 in Digit Symbol. Thinking processes were concrete, with difficulty in abstract conceptualization (prorated I.Q. of 64 in Similarities.) Data from the Bender were equivocal. Interviewing for neurological symptoms identified frequent sharp tingling in toes of right foot only, and rages without provocation. No event of etiological significance could be obtained. Depression and lowered self-esteem were apparently focused around a sense of desertion by his father in his childhood and embarrassment about his inability to read.

*   *   *

Mr. C. is married and has one child. He states with simplicity and conviction that he had been bright before he had meningitis and polio at the age of nine, and thereafter was in CRMD classes. He cannot read. His manner is courteous, attentive, thoughtful, and responsive. His employed vocabulary and use of metaphor suggest Average intellectual ability.

He achieved a prorated I.Q. of 81 in ability to conceptualize. Responses to Comprehension questions were marked by confusion and perplexity. Capacity for attention-memory was poor and worsened notably with complexity, as when required to recall digits backwards. In the perceptual-analytic area he did better when he could work without a guiding stimulus to follow (Object Assembly prorated I.Q. of 81) than when the visual field was complicated (Picture Completion prorated I.Q. of 55). The Bender showed a significant constructional confusion.

BIBLIOGRAPHY

1. *Alley, G. R., et al.:* Minimal cerebral dysfunction as it relates to social class. J. Learning Disabilities, 4:5, 1971.
2. *Benda, C. E.:* Down's Syndrome. Reported anon in Frontiers of Psychiat., 7:15, 1970.
3. *Burgemeister, B. B.:* Psychological Techniques in Neurological Diagnosis. New York: Hoeber Med. Div., Harper-Row, 1962.
4. *Chess, S.:* An Introduction to Child Psychiatry. New York: Grune and Stratton, 1969.
5. *Chess, S., et al.:* Disorders of Children with Congenital Rubella. New York: Bruner/Mazel, 1971.
6. *Crissey, M. S.:* Mental retardation: Past, present and future. Amer. Psychol.: August, 1975.
7. *Durfee, R. A.:* The misdiagnosis of mental retardation. J. Rehab., 35:1, 1969.
8. *Estes, W. E.:* Learning Theory and Mental Development. New York: Academic Press, 1970.
9. *Gittleman, N.* and *Birch, H. G.:* Childhood schizophrenia: Intellectual and neurological status, perinatal risk, prognosis and family pathology. Arch. Gen. Psychiat., 17, 1967.
10. *Higgins, J.:* Process-reactive schizophrenia. J. Nerv. Ment. Dis., 149-6, 1969.
11. *Hurley, R.:* Poverty and Mental Retardation. New York: Random, 1969.
12. *Karp, E.:* The why and wherefore of intelligence testing of the retarded. J. Clin. Child Psychol., 2:1, 1973.
13. *Kirkland, M.:* More psychiatrists focusing on mental retardation problems. Reported anon, Frontiers of Psychiat., February, 1972.
14. *Krop, H. D.* and *Smith, C. R.:* Effects of special education on Bender Gestalt performances of the mentally retarded. Amer. J. Ment. Defic., 73:5, 1969.
15. *LaFontaine, L.* and *Benjamin, G. E.:* Idiot savants: Another view., Ment. Retard., 9:6, 1971.
16. Mild Mental Retardation: A Growing Challenge to the Physician. New York: Group for the Advancement of Psychiatry, 1967.
17. *Pasamanick, B.:* Epidemiologic investigation of some perinatal factors in the production of neuropsychiatric disorder. *In* P. H. Hoch and J. Zubin (Eds.): Comparative Epidemiology of the Mental Disorders. New York: Grune and Stratton, 1961.
18. *Rensenberger, B.:* Key suggested to mental feats of idiot savants. New York Times, April 4, 1977.
18a. *Rimland, B.:* Infantile Autism. New York: Appleton-Century-Crofts, 1964.
19. *Robinson, H. B.* and *Robinson, N. M.:* The Mentally Retarded Child: A Psychological Approach. New York: McGraw-Hill, 1965.

20. *Sarason, S. B.* and *Doris, J.:* Psychological Problems in Mental Deficiency. New York: Harper and Row, 1969.
21. *Smith, A.:* Neuropsychological tests of 181 institutionalized mental retardates. Ann Arbor, Mich.: Neuropsychological Laboratory, Mimeo, 1977.
22. *Weintraub, B.:* British find poor children lag. New York Times, June 6, 1972.
23. *White, M. A.* and *Charry, J.* (Eds.): School Disorder, Intelligence and Social Class. New York: Teachers College Press, Columbia University, 1966.

CHAPTER 7

Depression

Psychotherapists more often see depression than any other complaint, except perhaps anxiety. Much is known about depression's causes and treatments. The almost tangible course of depression produced by the inward deflection of hostility and its lifting when interpreted and worked through is indeed a dramatic process, convincing evidence of the efficacy of psychotherapy. When one has treated many depressed persons, one almost automatically reviews the known psychological etiologies of depression and searches the history and present situation of the patient for inward deflection of hostility, loss of loved ones, a grief reaction, damage to self-esteem, or a major deception by an important person. Nonetheless, along with these, psychotherapists should look for other possible causes of depression, those with a physical basis.

Depression, for example, occurs episodically in senility, being characterized by rather shallow mood changes, in contrast to the deeper troughs of psychogenic depression.

Depression is in fact a frequent concomitant of neurological disorders; sometimes a neurological disorder goes unnoticed because the clinical observer is impressed by the depression and does not explore further.

Depression may be a predominant feature of epilepsy. Unlike psychogenic depression, the prodromal depression in epilepsy is sudden in onset and usually subsides with equal suddenness, although in rare cases it may last for several days. Suicide is rare in prodromal depression. Nicol (7) likens the rapid flow and ebb of seizure depression to a summer electrical storm, beginning with irritability and depression and clearing with a release of tension. However, it must be understood that depression may follow rather than precede a seizure (1).

Ictal depressions have also been investigated by Monroe (6); he too remarks their frequent sudden, seemingly inexplicable onset followed by equally precipitous and unexplainable remissions. They may last for only an hour or two or more days. They differ from psychotic depressive reactions in that they are accompanied by intense anxiety, usually of shorter duration than the depressions, but less motor retardation, less guilt, and generally fewer inferiority feelings. Monroe cites Yamada's observations that the ictal depression more frequently than psychogenic depression involves hypochondriasis, simple compulsive behavior (crying, laughing), disturbances of memory, hypermetamorphosis, and olfactory hallucinations. The latter are a frequent phenomenon of epilepsy. Episodes of explosive rage are frequent. On activation with Metrazol or Megamide the ictal depressions show paroxysmal abnormalities on EEG.

Depression appears in other neurological conditions as well. Nicol warns that in multiple sclerosis, euphoria is not the only mood change that occurs, that depression may be a feature of the earlier phases of this progressive disease, and if not comprehended as a possible link, the correct diagnosis may not even be suspected. Grief-like reactions occur as major symptoms in diffuse cerebral arteriosclerosis, paresis, tumors spreading across the corpus callosum, as well as multiple sclerosis. Intracranial pressure may result in apathy, accompanied by severe headaches, to be diagnosed as depression, when in fact a tumor, subdural hematoma, or other serious disease is the cause. Diseases of the neuromuscular system which leave a person weak, sometimes powerless, often result in depression, in reaction to the loss of control and mastery.

The depressive actions of certain drugs should be kept in mind by psychotherapists. According to Nicol these include Corticosteriods, Sulfonamides, Vitamin B12, Rauwolfia Alkaloids, Phenobarbital, and Chlorpromazine. Finally, Nicol states that there is sound evidence for associating some depressions with a deficiency of catecholamines in the brain (2, 7), and elation to a surplus of norepinephrine.

An interesting study has been made of the relationship of EEG findings to the affective psychoses by Assael and Winnik (1). Significantly higher incidence of abnormal EEGs was obtained from patients with affective psychoses in the depressive phase than from those with schizophrenia. Especially interesting is that the temporal lobe is a principal site for the "elaboration of affects in depressive psychoses."

Recently, a veritable flood of similar hypothetical speculations has followed upon the slowly accreting body of reliable data ascribable to differential functioning of the left and right cerebral hemispheres (see Chapter 15). Some of the hypotheses correlate affective disturbances specifically with disorders of the right hemisphere and schizophrenia with the left (see Chapters 3 and 5). The data, as reviewed by Parsons (8), are derived from differential hemispheric studies of gaze direction, electrical stimulation, electric convulsive shock, and amytal administration. To these may be added data from studies of EEG recordings (3, 4), some limited neuropsychological tests (9) and motoric laterality (5).

The hypotheses are interesting and invite continued study.

CASE ILLUSTRATION

1. *A man of 53, in psychoanalysis for a depression, is referred for psychodiagnostic evaluation of memory difficulties.*

The psychologist reported:

"O. complains of spotty memory, occasionally forgetting names and places. He is a compact, suntanned, healthy looking man, vigorous in manner, the successful head of a large business operation. He completed high school and perhaps a semester of college before entering business with his father. He was able to turn into a success a business that had been faltering. About three-and-a-half years ago he sold that business, took on another, equally difficult situation, which he has been moving towards more effective operation.

He quickly lets one know that his three children have developmental and emotional difficulties, that he feels in some ways that he has been a failure with them. He also intimates that his wife is an insecure woman, that she too has had emotional difficulties. O. is alert and responsive to the environment; he is interested in the objects in the office, he queries about them and offers comments from his own experience. He seems thoroughly related; there is no manifest sign of endogenous depression, though there are many evidences of a reactive depressive response as we talk about his memory deficits, his children's difficulties, and his own feeling of sexual disinterest in recent years.

"Emotionally there is considerable evidence of denial and repression. He is unable to supply any kind of dream history, neither recent, repetitive, nor childhood ones. This denial appears on the T.A.T. where he fails to observe the many sexual and aggressive features, despite the fact that he has a pressing sexual concern and is very con-

cerned about a general power stance and power specifically in relationship to people close to him. His sexual concern is evident in an
early memory—wetting his pants when he was about three and one-
half, implying a phallic concern at the time, possible voyeuristic excitement or fear of injury to himself. An incestuous theme is dimly suggested in one T.A.T. story where he fails to observe the pregnancy of
a woman but sees a man in 'control' of both an older woman and
younger woman.

"Object relations are disturbed, in the sense that he has a great
wish for closeness and feels its absence, with resulting susceptibility
to depression. He is proud of his interest in and altruism toward
people; he is concerned about their development and advancement.
One suspects that it is easier for him to express this concern and altruism when there is some degree of distance, so that he may find it
easier to maintain this attitude towards employees than with his own
family. His sexual interest is accompanied by a great deal of doubt.
Denial and disturbance in object relations are communicated in a story
in which a man is visiting someone whose parent is dying; the visitor
pretends to be depressed. One suspects that there has been an over-
idealization of his parents, more specifically his father, and that denial
of aggressivity and sexuality is tied in with this over-idealization, which
masks competitiveness and oedipal rivalry.

"The Figure Drawings reflect a rather disturbed body image. There
seems to be uncertainty in the sense of boundaries. There is some
indication of a struggle of power between male and female. There is
a marked concern about the well-being and integrity of his body.

"Perception of twins appears several times on the Rorschach, but
could not be explicated through association on his part; there is no
clue to the possible meaning for him except perhaps his wish for
some closeness, for an intense, intertwining closeness.*

"There is indication that a considerable charge of hostility has been
masked over the years, denied, converted into altruism and a sympa-
thetic concern for other people. There seems no particular danger of
this hostility erupting, so that its function in relationship to his present difficulties is difficult to perceive.

"The intelligence-test data indicate serious impairments in a number of areas. Verbal, Performance, and Full Scale I.Q.'s of only 109

---

* Dr. Rogers Wright suggests that this may reflect the patient's sensing of a
"neurologic splitting."

are patently incongruent with his business, social, and personal competence. His true level is indicated by a prorated I.Q. of 132 in Arithmetic, 126 in Digit Span, and 125 in Block Design. His prorated I.Q.'s for various subtests spread from this high of 132 to a low of 92—a range of 40 I.Q. points. In another view, scale scores are distributed from a high of 15 to a low of 7, again a large spread.

"Major deficits appear in the Verbal area. He achieves a prorated I.Q. of 102 in Information, 96 in Comprehension, and 102 in Vocabulary. These average to a scale score of 10 for the major verbal functions, contrasted with 13 for attention-memory functions. Evidence of impairment of perceptual-analytic functions is contained in the average scale score of 9 in these functions. He required twice the usual time to complete the Verbal Scale of the WAIS.

"The verbal difficulty essentially appears to be an aphasia, more specifically an anomia. Often he cannot find the word he needs, most specifically nouns and names. Thus, he cannot name four Presidents since 1900, but he can identify them when they are named and disagree when those before 1900 are named. He 'knows' the capitol of Italy, 'I have it on the tip of my tongue,' but he cannot find the exact word. He has some trouble recalling dates: Washington's Birthday is 'February 20th, possibly the 14th, no it is the 21st.' In Vocabulary definitions, 'tranquil' is defined as 'closing off something, not thinking of a problem.' On the Rorschach, in response to Card I, he says, 'I can't remember the name of this bird type; it stays up all night; it is not a bird, it is related to the rat. It flies around at night, and during the day it stays inside of a cave and it comes out at night.' For Card III, where he is trying to state his percept of twins, he says. 'People who were born at the same time, and have the same appearance, and they do the same thing at the same time; they are both warming their hands.' On the Picture Completion subtest of the intelligence scale, he seeks to identify Florida as the missing part of a map: 'The southeast part of the United States.' Wanting to identify 'stars' as missing from a flag, he says, 'There are not enough marks, meaning the states.' When he thought what he was assembling on one subtest was a buffalo, he spoke of it as 'Something that lived in the western part of the country. It is related to what we eat today. They were killed for their skins.' A 'stirrup' is 'Something you put your feet on when you ride a horse.' On the Heimburger-Reitan Quick Screening Test, he successfully drew a square, and named and spelled it. He drew a triangle, but could not name it, 'It is one-third of something.' He drew a cross but could not name it, 'It is for a church.'

"High-level ability with Arithmetic and recall of recent material—in Digit Span he is able to retain 8 digits forward and 6 in reverse—indicate no memory deficit when the stimulus is auditory. However, there is a memory deficit in the visuomotor area, so that on reproduction of the Bender Visual Motor Gestalt Test from memory, after a brief five second exposure, he tends to lose some degree of the Gestalt, a loss which does not appear when he copies the figures directly.

"Recognition of essential details is relatively poor at the prorated I.Q. of 99 in Picture Completion. His high-level performance in Block Design, where he achieves a prorated I.Q. of 125, is in sharp contrast with the prorated I.Q. of 92 he obtains in Object Assembly. The indication is that he is able to do effective work in the perceptual-analytic area when he has a visible stimulus around which to organize his motor response. But where the situation is more ambiguous and he must conceptualize the solution in his mind without such a guiding stimulus, as in Object Assembly, the deficit emerges.

"Observed too is a developing state of perplexity and confusion. This appeared to impair his Comprehension subtest performance; it was very evident on the Rorschach where he had difficulty visually organizing parts into a whole.

"While the necessary elements of an involutional depression are made available by his denial, there is no compelling evidence for such a state. There are features in his life which make for a depression, but most likely on a reactive basis. A man who values power and ability to command, he feels himself slipping and impaired in many areas, a form of impotence matched by the declining sexual interest. A recent mild heart attack further contributed to the depression.

"There is strong presumptive evidence for a cerebral dysfunction involving verbal expressive ability, a memory deficit for visual material, a perceptual-analytic deficit manifested as ambiguity of the stimulus increases. In addition he has marked difficulty in the verbal-conceptual area, evidenced by a prorated I.Q. of 96 in Similarities, a remarkably low score for a man of his manifest intellectual ability. His responses here were concrete. He can see no similarity between a fly and a tree, because, 'It grows from the earth; it doesn't have the living quality of a fly.'

"There is no conflict of lateral dominance: He is right-handed, right-eyed, and right-footed. He suffers no visual problems and reports no history of high fevers, head injuries, current dizziness, or tingling sensations in the extremities. He twice experienced unconsciousness; during the war, when he was in the Navy, he was unconscious briefly when someone applied pressure to the carotid sinus; there was a second similar event. Thirty years ago, he suffered severe migraine headaches. Twenty-five years ago, prior to the war, he recalls lying on a couch talking to himself. On rising, he found himself tremendously dizzy and unable to walk. This condition lasted two days, then gradually disappeared.

"The objective data obtained and the clinical impression combine to strongly suggest a neurological investigation in addition to psychotherapy for the emotional components."

Neurological Investigation

Neurological and EEG findings were normal or negative. Yet the patient's symptoms of memory loss and aphasia worsened. Despite the negative findings, the neurologist continued the patient under observation and repeated examinations, believing that his symptoms indicated brain pathology, albeit unidentifiable and defying localization.

BIBLIOGRAPHY

1. *Assael, M.* and *Winnik, H. Z.:* Electroencephalographic findings in affective psychoses. Dis. Nerv. Sys., 31:10, 1970.
2. *Dorfman, W.:* The recognition and management of depression. Psychosomatics, 11:5, 1970.
3. *Flor-Henry, P.:* Psychoses and temporal lobe epilepsy: A controlled investigation. Epilepsia, 10, 1969.
4. *Flor-Henry, P., et al.:* The neuropsychological correlates of the functional psychoses. Psychiat. Clin. Psychol., 3:34, 1975.
5. *Gur, R. E.:* Motor laterality imbalance in schizophrenia. Arch. Gen. Psychiat., 34, 1977.
6. *Monroe, R. R.:* Behavioral Disorders: A Psychodynamic and Neurophysiologic Analysis. Cambridge, Mass.: Harvard University Press, 1970.
7. *Nicol, C. F.:* Depression as viewed through neurological spectacles. Psychosomatics, 9, 1968.
8. *Parsons, O. A.:* The neuropsychology of depression. Mimeo, 1978.
9. *Taylor, M. A.:* Manic-depressive illness and schizophrenia: A partial validation of research diagnostic criteria utilizing neuropsychological testing. Comprehensive Psychiat., 16:1, 1975.

CHAPTER 8

Other Disorders with Equivocal Etiology

Six other disorders especially susceptible to confusion in diagnosis and thus to ineffective psychotherapeutic efforts are reviewed in this chapter. The psychotherapist is unlikely to encounter these disorders as often as he sees minimal cerebral dysfunction or epilepsy. But knowledge of them, awareness of their capacity to evoke or mimic behavior that resembles that found in functional disorders, underscores the need for caution in assigning diagnosis—and careful scrutiny of the possibilities.

A case in point is the tragically irrelevant diagnosis offered by a general practitioner, a pediatrician, psychiatrists and neurologists of a young girl, ultimately determined to be afflicted with dystonia musculorum deformans, as reported by the eminent neurosurgeon, I. S. Cooper (9).

The child began to limp when in the first grade. When X rays ruled out a suspected hip disease the general practitioner suggested that it was an emotional reaction to her first school experience, a position he maintained several months later after her leg twisted when she walked and she would fall. A hospital neurological work-up was within normal limits, and the child was referred to a pediatrician, who immediately passed her on to a psychiatrist who diagnosed a conversion hysteria, but prescribed no treatment. Again hospitalization for a neurological work-up; again negative findings, and again referral to a psychiatrist who advised psychiatric hospitalization. By this time the child was confined to bed, not to walk for about six years, her left arm and leg twisted and distorted by painful muscular contractions. The psychiatrists focused upon sexual incidents: bathing with her brother, having her pants pulled down by a neighborhood boy. Hospitalized for several months, she was put alone in a small room with a

235

closed, but unlocked door, and told that she could come out when she wanted to, when she was ready to walk out. The room was not cleaned. with the expectation that, revolted, she would want to leave it. During a subsequent hospitalization hypnosis was tried without benefit.

Finally, a transient neurologist, so-to-speak, recognized her disorder for what it was as he passed by during another hospitalization. And after six years of severe disability, grotesque deformity and unmitigated pain, the child was significantly helped by neurosurgery.

The disorders reviewed here all have the potential for a similar tragic comedy of diagnostic and therapeutic error.

NARCOLEPSY

This disorder of the sleep-wake cycle is often accompanied by vivid hynogogic hallucinations that may mislead the clinician to a psychiatric diagnosis. The disorder or sleep attack is manifested as a sudden and usually irresistible urge to sleep. Ordinary EEG procedures are usually unproductive, but continuous recordings in a sleep laboratory often show changes of diagnostic import. The psychotherapist is likely to read implications of schizophrenia into the hallucinatory manifestations, an error that can be avoided by taking a careful history that identifies the sleep disorder and its associated symptomatology. Shapiro and Spitz (23) illustrate the ease of misdiagnosis with the case of a woman originally diagnosed as suffering chronic undifferentiated schizophrenia on the basis of what were believed by the clinician to be psychotic hallucinations. She reported "Seeing people in my room," "Hearing voices from out of this world," and "Every night I see my mother and she's dead." After psychotropic medications failed, treatment with flurazepam produced remission, and psychotherapy then focused on the effects of having been diagnosed as mentally ill.

Narcolepsy is manifested in most instances by "sleep attacks," and is accompanied with varying frequency by catalepsy, hypnogogic hallucinations and sleep paralysis (23, 27).

Sleep attacks often emerge during periods when normal sleep patterns are disrupted, as during extended family disturbances, or irregular work schedules. The attacks are sudden and reversible; they may last from 15 seconds to one or two hours if the patient is lying down. While they occur most commonly when the patient is in a boring situation, they are also reported in exciting circumstances, as during coitus, even during a bombing approach. The attack can be delayed for minutes or hours. They are hazardous for automobile and other vehicle operators, and there is some evidence that sleepiness is responsible for more automobile accidents than is alcohol intoxication (27).

Catalepsy is a corollary symptom in about 70 percent of narcolepsy patients. It is a sudden weakening of localized or generalized muscle groups. When generalized the victim may slump to the floor, and may injure himself if on a ladder or near machinery. Characteristically, it is precipitated by surprise, laughter, anger or feelings of exultation, and lasts from a few seconds to a half-hour.

Hypnogogic fantasies occur in about 20 percent of narcolepsy patients. They may be both auditory and visual. As already indicated, they are largely responsible for the tendency to misdiagnose these patients as schizophrenic.

Attacks of *sleep paralysis,* usually of a flaccid nature, are reported in about 30 percent of these patients. They occur in transitional sleep-awake states, when the patient is either going to or waking from sleep. They last only a few seconds, the patient is usually conscious and can easily be aroused. Patients find these episodes frightening as they are usually accompanied by hallucinations of sounds or voices that are interpreted to mean the patient is in danger.

Obviously, hallucinations always necessitate careful diagnostic scrutiny. In addition to schizophrenia, the symptoms reported by narcolepsy patients should be differentiated from those of epilepsy, hypothyroidism, and hypoglycemia. The psychoanalytically-oriented psychotherapist must also scrutinize especially carefully any tendency to interpret sleep attacks and catalepsy as defensive and regressive processes initiated by ego-alien affects or impulses.

Medical treatment of narcolepsy has a relatively small armamentarium of drugs—amphetamines, monamine oxidase inhibitors, and tricyclic antidepressants—that may be used in combinations. Drug abuse and troublesome side effects are reported as problems. Abuse of the amphetamines particularly may produce hyperirritability or paranoia and other psychotic manifestations.

MULTIPLE SCLEROSIS

This disease of brain and spinal cord is marked by its slowly progressive course, and its periods of remission and acute exacerbation. Patches of the central nervous system demyelinate, producing a variety

of symptoms at different times in different patients that makes classification and common denominators difficult to establish.

Before the disease becomes recognizable the patient may experience
difficulty in walking and bladder control, dizziness, and emotional disturbances. Acute episodes usually are marked by visual disorders (partial blindness of one eye, double or dim vision, scotomas), weakness,
stiffness or fatigability of a limb, and, the most frequent symptom,
paresthesias in one or more limbs or on one side of the face. Aphasic
symptoms are rare. Neurological signs are many and varied. The patient may become euphoric, apathetic, or display poor judgment and
inattention. Mimicry of emotional disorders occurs and misdiagnoses
of hysteria, or even schizophrenia, are not rare.

The course and rate of progression of the disease are unpredictable.
Years may intervene between acute episodes, periods when the patient
functions effectively. Or the residues of acute episodes may leave the
patient dependent upon a wheelchair.

The cause of the disease is unknown. Among the hypotheses en-
tertained are: 1) infection by a slow acting virus, 2) an autoimmune
disorder, 3) toxic agents, 4) traumas, and 5) an abnormal blood clot-
ting mechanism.

Neuropsychological Correlates

The difficulty of making the necessary differentiation of multiple
sclerosis from other neuropathies and from psychiatric disorders is
noted by Goldstein and Shelly (10). Most neuropsychological studies
have not found evidence of cerebral damage. An exception is that by
Ross and Reitan (19), which has not been successfully replicated.
Others (7, 8, 14) have found little if any cerebral impairment.

Recent matched control studies by Goldstein and Shelly (10), and
Beatty and Gange (3) arrive at general consensus with earlier studies
by Reitan, et al. (18) and Matthews, et al. (14) in these findings on
neuropsychological testing:

1) the multiple-sclerosis patient shows significant motor dysfunctions;
2) mild cognitive deficits are detectable, especially as they involve
   motor tasks;
3) language, auditory perceptual skills and verbal intelligence
   appear unaffected.

Additionally, Beatty and Gange (3) report a high correlation between memory loss and motor dysfunction in multiple sclerosis that tends to disrupt the utilization of new verbal material.

Treatment

No medication of specific value has been discovered. Muscle training, passive movement, and massage of weakened limbs are advised. Fatigue is avoided, but the patient is encouraged to maintain activity as near normal as possible.

Psychotherapy should often be addressed to penetrating the denial that prevents the patient from dealing with the disease progress realistically. Support and encouragement facilitate accommodation to the residual limitations of acute episodes. Depression and rage are frequent reactions that benefit from ventilation and interpretations.

As some patients experience a loss of control of their own motor functions, the urge to control may be displaced and the effort to control family members may occur and set up intra-family stress. The patient may seek to dominate or control the actions of a spouse or children by manifesting inappropriate degree of concern about their behavior, or by complaining about their inattentiveness to the patient. When a good therapeutic alliance has been established, interpretation of such reactions may be candid and direct.

Psychotherapy with the multiple sclerosis patient is usually a long-term necessity, although some patients may require only short-term treatment from time to time.

DEVELOPMENTAL GERSTMANN'S SYNDROME

The history of this syndrome, whose very existence is seriously challenged, illustrates the uncertainties and dilemmas that characterize the diagnosis of many disorders, especially as in minimal brain dysfunction. During the 1920's Gerstmann identified a post-traumatic syndrome of unique specificity that embraced a quartet of symptoms: acalculia, agraphia, finger agnosia, and right/left disorientation. Constructional difficulties have been added to the syndrome by other observers. The correlation between these four was found not to be high, but when they occur it has been argued that the occurrence strongly suggests that the syndrome (25) was caused by damage in the left parietal area.

Other workers challenge the specificity of the syndrome, arguing that left parietal damage can exist without the full array of symptomatology being present, or that the syndrome is a component of an aphasis (5, 17). To counter this argument, cases of Gerstmann's without aphasia have been presented (17, 25), along with the contention that the high correlation between the syndrome and aphasia observed is probably due to simultaneous damage to the cortical areas underlying both.

To complicate the debate, the syndrome is observed in children rather rarely, and when found has often been associated with dyslexia. The etiology of the disorder in children has been added to the debate: is it developmental, constitutional or post-traumatic? In some children no event of etiological significance can be established; in others a traumatic or disease episode can be implicated. Furthermore, there are reports that dyslexia may or may not occur with the classical Gerstmann's symptomology; some children presenting the syndrome are superb readers, others are very much impaired.

Two cases are presented by Benson and Geschwind (4) that illustrate the diverse phenomena that may be associated with the syndrome to the confusion of the diagnostician.

A 12-year-old boy with a Verbal I.Q. of 131 and a Performance I.Q. of 101 had significant spelling, calculation and construction difficulties, finger agnosia, and right/left latency. Neurological signs were normal. Despite superb reading ability and intact speech and comprehension he encountered many difficulties in school. The authors concluded that he had a Developmental Gerstmann's Syndrome and recommended that the school allow him to take tests and present papers orally.

A 14-year-old girl presented low I.Q.'s (Verbal 79, Performance 75) that were depressed by poor levels in arithmetic and construction subtests. She also manifested poor finger identification ability; right/left difficulties, "grossly abnormal" writing, and some soft neurological signs. Speech and reading were good and she was passing all subjects except mathematics. Again a Developmental Gerstmann's Syndrome was diagnosed and certain undisclosed "corrective measures" were recommended to the school that enabled her education to proceed satisfactorily.

Very often agraphia is the most troubling aspect of the syndrome, causing severe learning problems. Where the child is bright and has good reading and speech ability educators may become confused, suspect malingering, and react to the child negatively. The emotional problems of the child with this syndrome can be severe, especially if there is failure to recognize the nature and cause of the agraphia and insistence that he develop normal writing ability. Allowing the child to report and be tested orally, or teaching him typing for these purposes, can avoid damage to the child's self-esteem and severe frustration to both child and teacher.

Case Illustrations

1. *Educational, social, and emotional difficulties in a bright 14-year-old boy diagnosed by a pediatric neurologist as having Developmental Gerstmann's Syndrome.*

L. was referred for assessment of current cognitive and emotional status. L. had been diagnosed two years before as having congenital Gerstmann's Syndrome, identified by the diagnostician as a specific cerebral deficit involving finger agnosia, agraphia, confusion of body laterality, and acalculia. In describing L.'s condition, Dr. X, neurologist, observed that the disorder results in considerable difficulty in being able to work independently, follow directions, and keep one's life ordered. Dr. X had made these recommendations to the excellent private boarding school from which L. was soon to be graduated:

1) An understanding of his difficulty by his teachers so they realize that his performance will not necessarily match up to their expectations.

2) Ability to take many of his tests and do much of his work verbally or through dictation rather than through the written form.

3) Help him to work on using typing to communicate.

4) Give him psychological support to help to reduce the negative behavioral influences, possibly on a continuous counseling basis.

5) To afford some special educational techniques in order to help him overcome some of his difficulties which can be arranged through Columbia University School of Education.

6) Possibly establishing a preceptor or big brother situation to help him with organization of his personal life and school assignments.

L.'s stay at the school has been a rather rough one for both L. and the school. Much of his behavior has seemed inexplicable to his teachers, with carelessness, eruptions of prohibited behavior, failure to work. The school felt unable to deliver some of the services suggested by Dr. X and disagreed with others, particularly in allowing him to use the typewriter instead of writing. L. has been receiving remedial teaching and psychotherapy.

L. is a fairly tall lad with a plump face, large eyes, soft mouth and nose. His manner is totally appropriate. He seems calm without any tension. His decorum was impeccable, relaxed and pleasant.

A psychological test report obtained two years ago attributed to L. a Verbal I.Q. of 127, Performance I.Q. of 109, and a Full Scale I.Q. of 121.

At this consultation, the following levels were obtained on the Wechsler Intelligence Scale for Children-R:

Information	15	(131)*	Picture Completion	12	(114)
Comprehension	12	(112)	Picture Arrangement	11	(106)
Arithmetic	17	(145)	Block Design	13	(121)
Similarities	16	(118)	Object Assembly	13	(121)
Vocabulary	16	(139)	Coding	10	(100)
Digit Span	13	(118)			

Verbal I.Q.   128
Performance I.Q.   112
Full Scale I.Q.   123

* Figures in parenthesis are prorated IQ's for each subtest.

The consultant's report follows: "Cognitively, there have been some significant changes since he was tested two years ago, although the Verbal, Performance, and Full Scale I.Q. remain relatively the same. Arithmetic ability has increased significantly from a scale score of 12 to one of 17. This is nearly 2 Standard Deviations of increment and represents a significant gain in this intellectual function. There has been an increase of 3 scale score points in Vocabulary from 13 to 16. This represents one Standard Deviation of improvement. He is operating at a Very Superior Level in both these areas at a prorated I.Q. of 145 and 139 respectively. Within the verbal area some other slight shifts upward in Comprehension and Digit Span are matched by some slight shifts downward in Information and verbal conceptualization.

"Within the Performance area there have been moderate improvements in spatial visualization functions, particularly in the ability to make constructions in conformity with external guiding stimuli and to assemble parts-to-wholes on the basis of his own mental idea of the parts-to-whole relationship. There has been a slight decrease in Picture Completion, the recognition of essential details, while perception of visually presented thematic material and digit substitution remain the same.

"The cognitive data reflect, therefore, a lad of Very Superior level intellectual endowment, who at the present time is functioning at that level in semantic comprehension, arithmetic reasoning, and information (which involves the storage and retrieval of old data) and at a Superior level in spatial visualization functions. There are ongoing deficits of moderate degree in verbal expressive ability and abstract verbal conceptualization, represented by prorated IQ's of 118 in Similarities and 112 in Comprehension. It is noteworthy that while these are areas of moderate deficit, that he functions in these in the Above Average range.

"Primary deficit appears to be in digit substitution, which requires symbol transformation and is intimately involved in reading and writing ability. Another area of significant deficit is in the comprehension of visually presented thematic material.

"L.'s handwriting and spelling are extremely poor. His Human Figure Drawing reflects a body image that is moderately distorted bilaterally. Right/left body parts identification is within normal limits, however. There is a possibility of a mixed lateral dominance involving the visual area particularly: He is right-sided in all hand and foot functions tested but mixed for the eye, using the right for close viewing and the left for distance viewing. The Hooper Visual Organization Test is within normal limits; this is a measure of ability to mentally manipulate visual elements without physical movements of the parts involved.

"Beneath L.'s appropriate, placid, friendly, social persona, there is evidence of conflict and intense affects. There is a well of sadness, a melancholia or depression which appears to overtake him from time to time. He makes a valliant effort to distinguish between these two, denies that he is subject to sadness, because that would, in his logic, necessarily be connected with a cause. Melancholia, however, which he acknowledges, cannot be assigned to any cause in L.'s system.

"The psychodynamic material also pick up a strong feeling of frustration: the reaction of a very bright lad observing a part of himself over which he seems to have no control, which he cannot bring up to his expectations or the expectations of others. L. appears to have a powerful drive to please his parents and authorities, and is subject to intense frustration because he often cannot do so.

"There is a well of aggression and anger here also, which appears to have a complicated origin. In part, it may be a familial quality that he shares, a result of the neurological deficit which produces hyperirritability and responsivity or an emotional reaction to his perceived deficits and the frustrations about them which make him angry because he feels impotent in relationship to them.

"L. also appears to anticipate injury, more on an emotional basis than on a physical one, although he translates it into physical terms. Thus his story for his Human Figure Drawing: "This man was very happy, until he was unfortunate. He was hit by a low flying rinoserous (sic!). But now he is happy again because he was accepted to M.I.T." This story not only reflects L.'s feelings about his difficulties but his ambition, his driving wish to achieve and succeed, to please himself and others. It also illustrates his use of humor to express anger at himself and others.

"L. experiences mounting tension, which derives from the several sources indicated here, and which often will lead to eruptions of behavior that may seem excessive. These appear to be safety-valve releases rather than defiance. Discipline preferably should not impose immobility, but allow him physical movement and discharge.

"L. attempts to handle his conflicts and feelings by denying that they exist. So he is likely to develop relative amnesia or forgetfulness for his involvement in many things. He is not prevaricating, but simply has repressed and forgotten. Another major defense is the use of jocularity to deny his concern about himself, his melancholic tendency, his sense of frustration and his anger, yet to express his anger. He attempts to develop controls; this has led to a moderate degree of obsessive compulsiveness in which he attempts to control by rigid procedures. While these are not manifest to any great extent, they reflect his involvement and concern about his situation. There is an element of negativism, of distrust, essentially, of authority's values and mores. This quality is often found in young people who feel that they have been deceived in some major way by their parents, and who express distrust in that way.

"L. has a very strong sense of identification with his father, and with his father's interests and activities. He intimates a yearning for his home, and perhaps some feeling of rejection. He may in part associate his learning difficulties with his being sent to a boarding school.

"There is evidence to suggest that when L. stops working he has become involved in sadness about his situation, has retreated within himself, is experiencing enormous frustration and negativism: One can expect this to occur and his functioning to be invaded from time to time by periods of intense affect that lead to outbursts of disruptive behavior, and also to defensive forgetting, leading to a failure to perform required tasks.

"L. needs the following elements to foster his continued development:

1) A challenging educational environment that will encourage the use of his intact, fine abilities.
2) Educational appreciation of his neurological deficits and the use of devices to circumvent them when possible.
3) Remedial training in his deficit areas.
4) Psychotherapy for his emotional problems.

"L. has the capacity for becoming an unusually fine adult, intelligent, sensitive, responsible, creative, humane. Educational planning may not be able to incorporate at one time all of the elements recommended, but they should be striven for."

GILLES DE LA TOURETTE'S DISEASE

This rare disease—only about 200 cases are reported in the literature (21)—is reviewed here because it epitomizes the ambiguity that surrounds the differential diagnosis of organic and functional factors and treatment in many disorders, not because the psychotherapist is likely to encounter this disease in his practice.

Three symptoms are said to characterize the syndrome: 1) *tics* that usually begin in small muscle groups of the face and gradually become generalized; 2) *coprolalia* or other involuntary explosive sounds (e.g., grunts, whistles); 3) *echolalia* or *echopraxia,* imitation of the vocalizations or gestures of another. The onset is in childhood or early adolescence. The child may appear hyperkinetic or show social problems, becoming aversive and manifesting behavior disturbing to others (e.g., sticking his tongue out, handling his genitals, stuttering, hissing, grinding his teeth). Concentration may be poor. The course of the disease is unpredictable. Often it is chronic, with alternating periods of remission and exacerbation; sometimes long-standing remissions occur

(1, 2). Originally described in 1825, the disease was formalized and given the name of Gilles de la Tourette, a French physician, in 1885.

Despite the rarity of the disorder, a lively debate continues about its etiology, particularly about whether there is a psychogenic contributant. Shapiro (21, 22) and Abuzzahah (1, 2) are adversaries in this debate, although the one does not appear in the bibliographies of the other.

Abuzzahah and Ehlen (1, 2) find it difficult to exclude either an organic or functional etiology in the disorder. Pathological evidence of brain tissue change is found in deceased Gilles de la Tourette patients; the disorder is known to follow brain injury and encephalitis; 50 percent of patients with the disorder have abnormal EEGs; and the disorder resembles hyperkinesis. They find the hypothesis for a psychological basis more speculative. The children are said to be compulsive and rigid, with limited and ineffective means for expressing the pent-up hostility they feel for their parents whom they wish to punish, except to release the hostile energy as tics and copralalia. Another psychological hypothesis proposes that these children have been exposed to an overwhelming emotional experience (a death, the primal scene) to which they do not know how to respond except with the tics and explosive vocalizations. In this hypothesis, the symptoms represent targetless overflows of affect and energy. In the preceding one, they are directed and purposeful. Finally, the absence of neurological signs in some patients is argued as supporting a psychological component.

Shapiro, et al. (21, 22) depreciate the significance of this argument, noting an erroneous tendency to label as psychogenic symptoms unaccompanied by "demonstrable organic pathology." They present a 16-year-long case history of a man with the disorder and analyze the judgment of his psychiatrist and psychologist to illustrate how symptoms may be convincingly but erroneously assigned a psychodynamic meaning. The psychologist likened the patient's tics and coprolalia to the actions of a paranoid schizophrenic who, after answering an examiner's questions, turns his head to speak in foul language to his imagined companion. The patient was treated by the psychiatrist for two years with psychotherapy and amobarbital and pentothal interviews. As these proved fruitless, he administered electroconvulsive and insulin-coma treatments, also without success. Finally, the patient was effectively treated with haloperidol, which has become the basic and preferred medication in this disorder (1, 2, 21, 22).

Shapiro *et al.* see the tics and other behavior as too poorly organized, and only partially affected by substituted *voluntary* behavior, to be labelled as compulsive. The view that the symptoms represent the action of defensive restraint, they argue, is disproved by the fact that when the patient is encouraged to express hostility, the symptoms increase: They decrease when the expression of hostility is avoided. They believe the patient observes this response in himself and learns to become a typical passive-aggressive personality. The disorder makes for emotional disturbance because the symptoms are bizarre, and because physicians iatrogenically increase psychopathology by prematurely diagnosing a psychological genesis; the patient fears he is crazy instead of having the reassurance of a neurological interpretation of his behavior.

Shapiro and his colleagues (21, 22, 26) cite the evidence supporting an organic etiology: 1) the 50 percent EEG abnormality among de la Tourette patients, and 2) the similarity of symptoms to those in established organic damage (they list about 25 organic disorders that need to be differentiated from de la Tourette); 3) the favorable response of EEG patterns to haloperidol; and 4) the high incidence of organic signs on psychological tests that suggest a CNS disorder of unknown localization. To these we may add pharmacological studies that demonstrate an exaggeration of tics in Gilles de la Tourette patients in response to norepinephrine in the brain (15). Shapiro *et al.* maintain that psychological conflicts are unrelated to the diagnosis and "irrelevant to the treatment" of the syndrome.

The evidence in Gilles de la Tourette is particularly difficult to sort out. Absence of organic evidence in some patients does not rule out the probability of a neurological disorder, as the review of epilepsy demonstrates, where therapeutic results are obtained with anticonvulsive drugs in patients whose EEGs are normal. The clinician testing a Gilles de la Tourette patient is wise to be alert to the interaction of both factors. While psychological factors cannot be assigned primary causative status, they must be considered as potentially powerful secondary forces. The bizarre symptoms and disturbing behavior in the child may easily evoke latent pathology or exaggerate it in the parents, thus creating stress within the family and a pattern of reactions that contributes to repressed hostility and patent rigidity. The impact upon both self-image and body-image is obviously enormous, and promotes aversiveness.

Psychotherapy alone has not been successful. Abuzzahah and Ehlen

(2) report this failure, along with unproductive outcome with hypnotherapy, milieu therapy, and behavior modification. The major tranquilizers, especially haloperidol, have proved most effective and are established as the primary treatment for both young children and older patients in whom the syndrome has been long present. Stimulants and antidepressants have not been effective. Azuzzahab and Ehlen advise the simultaneous use of medication and psychotherapy, the latter often involving the parents. Treatment should begin as soon as possible to avoid entrenchment of symptoms and to minimize the development and influence of secondary gains.

THE 14-AND-6-PER-SECOND POSITIVE SPIKE PATTERN ON EEG

The *14-and-6-per-second positive-spike pattern* (PSP) is one equivocal neurobehavioral condition in which the diagnosis depends upon firm establishment of the neurological criterion, while some doubt remains about the behavioral correlates. These behaviors are often similar to those that psychotherapists encounter among emotionally disturbed patients. Awareness of the possibility of this positive-spike pattern (PSP) on the electroencephalogram as a source of such behaviors increases diagnostic caution and may modify treatment approaches.

Six symptom pictures are correlated by Greenberg (12) with the positive spike pattern: 1) autonomic dysfunctions involving headaches, nausea, vomiting, and episodic abdominal pains; 2) seizure disorders; 3) behavior disorders; 4) isolated acts of intense rage and violence; 5) nonepileptiform medical or neurological disorders; 6) personality traits of affective blunting and superficial emotion with ruminations about hostile impulses and the feeling that something is wrong with one's body.

The PSP is a specific wave pattern which Greenberg defines as fairly constant wave forms in which the spikes are positively deflected, unlike the usual abnormal findings in epilepsy in which the spikes are negatively deflected. The positive spikes appear usually in conditions of drowsiness or light sleep, through the leads on either side of the head from the posterior temporal and occipital areas. The contralateral ear or linked ears serve as the reference electrode. Greenberg states that positive spike patterns are ordinarily accompanied by other abnormalities of recordings; slow wave activity from the right posterior section is also found in about 25 percent of the EEG recordings that demonstrate positive-spike activity. In a study of 14 patients with *14-and-6* in his private practice, Greenberg (11) found that only six produced EEG records uncomplicated by posterior slowing or seizure phenomena.

Monroe (16) finds the autonomic symptoms associated with the 14-and-6 pattern suggestive of epileptoid phenomena: they appear abruptly, are transitory in nature, and disappear precipitously. The behaviors associated with the episodes, while impulsive and explosive, are usually skilled, coordinated, and well-planned, hence differing from usual psychomotor phenomena associated with epileptic seizures. The episodic, autonomic symptoms respond well to anti-convulsant drugs, favoring a therapeutic diagnosis of an epileptic disorder. The behavioral manifestations respond less well to the anti-convulsant drugs and somewhat better to psychotropic medications.

Seldom occurring in infancy, the pattern presents a gradual increase in incidence with age up to a certain point, reaching a peak among those at about the age of 14 or 15, with frequencies between 20 to 30 percent among unselected school children. Thereafter, there is a gradual decline until the age period 20 to 24, where frequencies of 9 percent have been recorded. Between the ages 25 to 30 the incidence is 1 percent. An incidence of 0.5 percent is observed in the general population between the ages of 30 to 40. The pattern has not been reported among subjects over 50 years of age.

Various areas of the brain have been implicated in the localization of the 14-and-6 pattern. The limbic system has been more frequently mentioned than other areas. Initially, according to Greenberg, the investigators Gibbs and Gibbs believed that the positive spiking pattern reflected an epilepsy of the thalamic and hypothalamic regions. Etiology appears to lie in head injuries, encephalitis, and birth injury; a possible genetic factor is suggested by the high familial concordance which has been demonstrated.

The occurrence of behavior disorders in association with the 14-and-6 positive spike pattern is reviewed by Boelhouwer, *et al.* (6). They state that the incidence is about 20 percent when the behavior disorders tallied are limited to hyperactivity, temper tantrums, impulsive behavior, fire setting, antisocial behavior that is skillfully directed and executed, assaultiveness, against oneself or others. When *any* form of disturbed behavior is present and counted in the history, the percentage increases to 60 percent. Patients with 14-and-6 spiking were more frequently diagnosed by psychiatrists as having organic brain syndromes, significant medical social pictures involving enuresis, encopresis, temper tantrums, and other complaints than were controls.

A significant feature of the etiological and developmental picture appears to be the nature of family relationships and the occurrence of serious organic illness. Greenberg (13) compared hospitalized patients with right occipital-lobe damage (aged 16-30) with those with 14-and-6 positive spiking and those with negative or normal electroencephalographic readings. Most significant was the higher incidence of protracted illnesses in childhood among the patients with positive spike patterns. These patients also were significantly underemotional and demonstrated higher incidence of blunted affect than did the right-occipital brain-damaged group.

In another study Greenberg (12) associated the blunted, underemotional affect component accompanying 14-and-6 per second positive spiking with a disrupted family milieu. When the family milieu was less disturbed, the 14-and-6 patient tended to be more aggressive in his behavioral disturbance; less aggressivity and less clinging dependency are associated with the more disrupted family milieu. Boelhouwer *et al.* (6) also explored the relationship of environmental factors as an interacting force with the 14-and-6 positive spiking. They studied two groups of adolescent and young adult patients who manifested behavior disorders. One group also demonstrated positive spiking, the other was without this EEG characteristic. Special attention was paid to the detection of soft neurological signs; no differences were found between the groups in this respect. Enuresis and convulsions occurred more frequently in the positive spike group, but not with statistical significance. Only toxemia during pregnancy was significantly present in the mothers of the positive-spike group patients. Poor physical health appeared to characterize the positive-spike group, as did overprotectiveness by the mother. Seemingly contrary to Greenberg's findings, acts of aggressiveness and assaultiveness were more frequent in the positive-spike group. However, they do not separate those with intact and disrupted family environment, as did Greenberg.

A relatively high incidence of 14-and-6-per-second positive-spike patterns in young schizophrenics is reported by Shagass (20), who believes that the clinical picture in schizophrenic disorders is significantly affected when the 14-and-6 pattern and the mechanisms which presumably underlie it are present.

Treatment

Patients with the 14-and-6 positive-spike pattern respond favorably to certain drugs. Boelhouwer cites a better response of the 14-and-6 positive-spike group to a combination of Thiordazine and Diphenyl-hydantoin than to either drug alone.

Smith *et al.* (24) cite significant improvement in Verbal I.Q. among 14-and-6 patients with the use of Ethosuximide, an anticonvulsant medication. Performance I.Q. change was not significant. As might be expected, the Full Scale I.Q. change was significant but at a lesser level than the Verbal I.Q. Psychomotor and personality tests did not change. The study is interesting in that it was made upon patients who had already been receiving the medication; the experiment continued some on the drug, while others were placed on a placebo, a double-blind series. All but one of the 10 subjects receiving the drug showed an increase in Verbal I.Q.

Greenberg, having identified the family milieu as interacting with the neurological phenomenon, stresses the importance of family therapy in the treatment of 14-and-6 patients to work through the feelings of guilt and the cross-charges of blame between parents and child, parent and parent, child and siblings.

He further notes that these patients often experience affective aloofness, a sense of isolation from others, and of not caring about them, which when ego-alien perplexes the patient, who is nonetheless unable to do anything about the feeling of interpersonal distance. The aloofness may be complicated by the experience of protracted childhood illness that heightened dependency upon parents and in turn upon their surrogates. Affective re-education may become the central task of therapy. The aloofness may be defined for the patient and his family as a function of the cerebral dysfunction, and they may be told that the difficulty often ameliorates with maturation and appropriate training in how to recognize and respond to the needs of others and of himself.

Involvement of the family in therapy is frequently imperative in such situations, to identify for them the source of the patient's difficulties, to enroll them in the re-education program, and to prepare them for understanding and accepting the deficits that remain after therapy and re-education. Moreover, amelioration of the patient's difficulties, which may have given the family a scapegoat or conversely may have bound them in a mutual effort to bear the family burden, may lead to emergence of other underlying family pathology, for which they will need help.

Case Illustrations

An unusual opportunity to study the 14-and-6 pattern was provided Zitrin *et al.* (28) when they discovered the pattern in three members of a family. Their primary patient, a 17-year-old white male, and his father and sister, all produced EEG records with 14-and-6 positive spiking. The pattern appeared in the boy's tracings both awake and asleep, but only during sleep recordings for the father and sister. The pattern did not appear in the mother's tracing during either type of recording. The EEG of the maternal grandmother was normal, and there was no history of mental or neurological disease in her family. The father's parents were not available for study. Behavioral disturbances were identified most strongly in the family members with the 14-and-6 pattern, less so in the mother with a normal EEG.

The boy had been admitted to a psychiatric hospital with complaints of difficulty in functioning in school and in concentration, pressure feelings in his head, constipation, and enuresis, which began three months before admission. Precipitationg circumstances were believed to be the increasing difficulty of his high-school courses, increasing pressure from his parents to do well, and moving away from the neighborhood in which he had grown up and where he had lived near his maternal grandparents.

The labor of his birth lasted four days and delivery required forceps. While his father was in the service, the boy for the first two years of life could not fall asleep unless his mother slept with him. When the father returned, the boy was allowed to cry for four or five hours until he fell asleep alone. He had trouble learning to suck, was a poor eater until four, did not speak until he was nearly three, when he was discovered to be partially deaf because of obstructing adenoid tissue, which was removed. His hearing and speech improved although he continued to manifest a speech difficulty.

He was rather isolated, preferred being alone to being with peers. Although he never liked school, he did well until the third year of high school, when his grades deteriorated. While he appeared to crave affection from his parents, he did not confide in them. No destructive behavior was reported.

On admission he was shy, laughed inappropriately, talked to himself, "showed looseness of associations, blocking, inadequate and inappropriate affect, impaired judgment and insight, and often appeared to be autistic."

Psychological testing did not produce evidence of organicity. On a short form Wechsler-Bellevue test he obtained an overall I.Q. of 100, and prorated I.Q.s of 119 in Picture Arrangement (his best function), 104 in Similarities, and 91 in Comprehension. His figure drawings were like those of younger and psychotic children.

In the hospital he stored rocks and a knife in his room. He set a fire in the waste basket in his room. There was no assaultive behavior towards others. The hospital diagnosis was Hebephrenic Reaction in a pre-existing Schizoid Personality.

The father, 39, had been the illegitimate child of a promiscuous woman who abandoned him when he was three years old. He grew up thereafter in a foster home. His foster mother remained interested in him so that when he had trouble in a boarding school when he was about ten he returned to live with her and remained there through high school, where he did well. He continues to be fond of his foster mother and remains in touch with her. He joined the Merchant Marine when he was 18 and married his wife, who was pregnant, when he was 21. He gave up the heavy drinking that had been his custom while in the service. He is easily moved to rage, screams, breaks dishes and furniture and sometimes beats the children. He deprecates his wife, makes all important decisions, and is generally aggressive. He has worked rather steadily as a truck driver. He refused to cooperate with psychological testing.

The mother, 35, is shy, fragile, easily moved to tears. She is the oldest of four children. In early childhood she often held her breath until she fainted. Her shyness increased at age 13 after a period of tomboyishness. She disliked her mother's domination and moved away from her neighborhood three months before their son entered the hospital.

On the short-form Wechsler-Bellevue test, she achieved an overall I.Q. of 119, 128 in Similarities, and 95 in Picture Arrangement. She showed a conflict between dependency upon her mother and hostility for her. Reality testing was considered adequate.

The sister, 14, was born in an easy labor of three hours. She ate well, walked at 14 months, and talked at 18 months. Like her mother she, too, for a while held her breath until fainting. She was outgoing and played well with other children. She liked school and did above-average work. She disliked her brother, argued with her father, and complained that her mother was not available to her. Her I.Q. on the short-form Wechsler was 124, with prorated I.Q.s of 136 in both Similarities and Comprehension. No evidence of organicity was found. Projective techniques suggested anxiety, depression from in-turned rage, some feelings of depersonalization, oscillating reality testing, and confused sexual identification. Her figure drawings were typical for her age. About one year after her brother came home from the hospital, she ran away from home, was found and brought back to enter psychiatric treatment. There had been no earlier history of behavior disturbance.

Zitrin and her colleagues find the correlation between EEG pattern of the 14-and-6 with behavioral disturbance to be far from convincing but at least suggestive and worth of exploration. Their major point would appear to be their observation that the clinically critical periods of individuals with 14-and-6 emerge only in relationship to stressful familial and environmental factors. Such precipitants, of course, are not unique to individuals who show the 14-and-6 positive-spike pattern.

PHYSIOLOGICAL DISTURBANCES OF CORTICAL FUNCTIONING

Cortical functioning may be disturbed by a variety of physiological malfunctions, with concomitant alterations of mood and behavior. Those that result in cerebral anoxia are of special interest since this condition may result in extremely strange behavior that is hard to diagnose. Among the processes that cause cerebral anoxia are heart disease with reduced cardiac output, severe asthma, a hyperactive carotid sinus which may induce fainting episodes, breath-holding spells, hyperventilation which alters the oxygen-carbon dioxide balance in the blood and leads to dizziness, and hypoglycemia.

For nearly half a century severe hypoglycemia—hyperinsulinism producing lowered blood sugar—has been associated with cerebral dysfunction. Yet the disorder remains difficult to separate from its emotional and psychological concomitants. If prolonged, hypoglycemia results in anoxia of nerve tissue because nerve cells become affected in a phylogenetically regressive order, apparently related to differences in metabolic rate. Thus the cells of the cortex are first affected, the older brain and the brain stem are last affected.

The condition may arise from any of a host of causes: insulin overdosage in diabetic patients, disturbances of the nervous system, endocrine disorders, tumors of the pancreas or pituitary, liver disease, alcoholism, lesions of the hypothalamus and brain stem, intestinal surgery, and protracted diarrhea.

The symptoms emerge rapidly with the decline of blood sugar, and may resemble either psychiatric or neurological disorders; confusion, tremor, anxiety, irritability, hunger, nausea, dullness, apathy, agitation, restlessness, poor judgment, disorientation, impaired perception, altered states of consciousness, coma, and seizure phenomena. The hypoglycemic effect upon the brain is diffuse, not localized, so that alteration of all brain-behavior functions is possible. The EEG picture corresponds with the clinical findings, showing alterations early in the attack, with diffuse, non-localized disturbances.

The suddenness of onset, the effect upon higher functions, the intense anxiety and irritability, often mislead the clinician to diagnose a functional disorder, especially an anxiety or conversion reaction. Obviously, a pre-existing neurosis or psychosis may become aggravated by the emergence of hypoglycemia. In all cases the diagnosis is facilitated if the patient's emotional functioning prior to the suspected hypoglycemia can be established.

The diagnosis of hypoglycemia ultimately depends upon laboratory analysis of the blood-sugar level over a five-hour period. Careful attention to the association of eating patterns with behavioral reactions is important in taking the history. Prompt relief of seemingly neurotic or neurological symptoms upon the ingestion of sweets is strongly suggestive of hypoglycemia and may warrant laboratory studies of the patient's blood.

The neurological and psychiatric aspects of this biochemical disorder have been presented briefly by Zivin (29), who cites two cases that merit recapitulation.

A 22-year-old man manifested bizarre automatic behavior that suggested temporal-lobe epilepsy. In the army, he would come to consciousness in the mess hall, clad only in underwear, having taken his outer clothes off while experiencing a blackout. Neurological and EEG studies were made, but not blood-sugar analyses. After his discharge from the army, his mother observed one morning before breakfast that he seemed detached and was behaving automatically. Attributing his state to hunger, she gave him a sweet beverage. His behavior quickly altered, he became aware of his surroundings, and was astounded to learn how he had behaved during his lapse. Hospitalization followed.

EEG readings showed generalized cerebral involvement without seizure discharges, a pattern considered compatible with hypoglycemia. High levels of insulin were found consistently in the blood; sugar levels were consistently low. A tumor of the islet cells of the pancreas was suspected and confirmed upon surgery. Blood-sugar levels returned to normal and remained there following removal of the tumor. The patient returned to school and is said not to have manifested either significant emotional problems or automatic behavior. This patient's case is noteworthy because his behavior so resembled psychomotor epilepsy that biochemical possibilities were at first overlooked. His psychological history of adoption and early problems in learning and behavior further delayed the biochemical exploration.

Zivin's second case is a 40-year-old man, clearly a long established neurotic usually reacting poorly to stress, who began to experience anxiety, detachment, muscle spasms, and tightening of the throat without having been exposed to stress situations. Inquiry established that these newer symptoms most frequently emerged in mid-morning or late afternoon, or during both these inter-meal times. Blood-sugar examinations clearly associated his exaggerated symptoms with lowered glucose levels. A high protein diet and sedatives alleviated these episodes and decreased their frequency but did not eliminate them; ingestion of sugar quickly mitigates those that now occur. The significant feature here is the exaggeration of already established neurotic patterns by a hypoglycemic condition.

BIBLIOGRAPHY

1. *Abuzzahah, Sr., F. S.* and *Ehlen, K. J.*: The clinical picture and management of Gilles de la Tourette's syndrome. Child Psychiat. Human Devel., 2:1, 1971.
2. *Abuzzahah, Sr., F. S.* and *Ehlen, K. J.*: Tourette's Syndrome: A Guide For Parents. University of Minnesota, Undated.
3. *Beatty, P. A.* and *Gange, J. J.*: Neuropsychological aspects of multiple sclerosis. J. Nerv. Ment. Dis., 164:1, 1977.
4. *Benson, D. F.* and *Geschwind, N.*: Developmental Gerstmann syndrome. Neurology, 20:3, 1970.
5. *Benton, A. L.*: The fiction of the "Gerstmann's syndrome." J. Neurol. Neurosurg. Psychiat., 24, 1961.
6. *Boelhouwer, C., et al.*: Positive spiking: a double-blind control study on its significance in behavior disorders, both diagnostically and therapeutically. Amer. J. Psychiat., 125:4, 1968.
7. *Brown, S.* and *Davis, T. K.*: Mental manifestations and the emotional and psychological factors in multiple sclerosis. Assoc. Res. Nerv. Ment. Dis., 2, 1971.
8. *Canter, A. H.*: MMPI profiles in multiple sclerosis. J. Consult. Psychol., 15, 1951.

9. *Cooper, I. S.:* The Victim Is Always The Same. New York: Harper and Row, 1973.

10. *Goldstein, G.* and *Shelly, C. H.:* Neuropsychological diagnosis of multiple sclerosis in a neuropsychiatric setting. J. Nerv. Ment. Dis., 158:4, 1974.

11. *Greenberg, I. M.:* Cerebral dysfunction in general psychiatric office practice patients. Xerox, 1970.

12. *Greenberg, I. M.:* Clinical correlates of fourteen and six cycles per second positive. EEG spiking and family pathology. J. Abnormal Psychol., 76:3, 1970.

13. *Greenberg, I. M.:* Development and clinical correlates of disrythmia. Arch. Gen. Psychiat., 21, 1968.

14. *Matthews, C. G., et al.:* Neuropsychological patterns in multiple sclerosis. Dis. Nerv. Syst., 31, 1970.

15. *Meyerhoff, J. L.* and *Snyder, S. H.:* Gilles de la Tourette's disease and minimal brain dysfunction. Amphetamine isomers reveal catecholamine correlates in an affected patient. Psychopharmacologia, 29:3, 1973.

16. *Monroe, R. R.:* Episodic Behavioral Disorders. Cambridge, Mass.: Harvard University Press, 1970.

17. *Poeck, K.* and *Orgass, B.:* Gerstmann's syndrome and aphasia. Cortex, 2, 1966.

18. *Reitan, R. M., et al.:* Cognitive, psychomotor and motor correlates of multiple sclerosis. J. Nerv. Ment. Dis., 153, 1971.

19. *Ross, A. T.* and *Reitan, R. M.:* Intellectual and affective functions in multiple sclerosis. Arch. Neurol. Psychiat., 73, 1955.

20. *Shagass, C.:* Neurophysiological studies. *In* L. Bellak and L. Loeb (Eds.): The Schizophrenic Syndrome. New York: Grune and Stratton, 1969.

21. *Shapiro, A. K.* and *Shapiro, E.:* Clinical dangers of psychological theorizing: The Gilles de la Tourette syndrome. Psychiat. Quart., 45:2, 1971.

22. *Shapiro, A. K., et al.:* Tourette's syndrome: Summary of data on 34 patients. Pre-publication copy. Mimeo, Undated.

23. *Shapiro, B.* and *Spitz, H.:* Problems in the differential diagnosis of narcolepsy versus schizophrenia. Amer. J. Psychiat., 133:11, 1976.

24. *Smith, W. L., et al.:* Psychometric study of children with learning problems and 14-6 positive spike EEG patterns, treated with Ethosuximide (Zarontin) and placebo. Arch. Dis. Childhood, 43:231, 1968.

25. *Strub, R.* and *Geschwind, N.:* Gerstmann syndrome without aphasia. Cortex, 10:4, 1974.

26. *Wayne, H. L., et al.:* Gilles de la Tourette's syndrome: electroencephalographic investigation and clinical correlation. Clinical EEG, 3, 1972.

27. *Zarcone, V.:* Narcolepsy. N. E. J. Med., 288:22, 1973.

28. *Zitrin, G., et al.:* 14 and 6 CPS positive spike in a family. Arch. Gen. Psychiat., 9, 1963.

29. *Zivin, I.:* The neurological and psychiatric aspects of hypoglycemia. Dis. Nerv. Syst., 3:19, 1970.

II

APPLICATIONS FOR THE
PSYCHOTHERAPIST

"A principle of exploitation operates in effective neuropsychodiagnosis—the exploitation of the merits of any procedure that clarifies the relationship between brain function and behavior. Each therapeutic discipline offers something to the others here." This passage from the introduction to this book is repeated here as the starting point for the following guidelines for application by the psychotherapist.

Many influences must be sought to identify brain pathology and recognize its effects upon behavior, a complex and difficult matter. Only with openness, flexibility, willingness to recognize and use the products from all methods can the limitations of any single hermetic system be overcome.

Attitudes and biases, of course, influence much of our professional behavior, even our scientific behavior. One attitude must be explored here: the psychotherapist's tendency toward pessimism about neurological impairments. A serious impediment to the development of neuropsychodiagnostic acumen has been the general dread of immutability in neurological disorders, the notion that all such disorders doom the patient to an unchangeable lifelong limitation, while psychogenic disorders are often regarded consciously or unconsciously as relatively subject to improvement. The psychotherapist particularly is optimistic about prognosis in psychogenic disorders. Training and experience instill the expectation that most psychological problems are modifiable: a conflict can be resolved, a regression reversed, a failure to progress overcome by appropriate stimulation and support.

In sharp contrast, neurological difficulties arouse pessimism. Somatically based, etched into or cut out of human tissue, they are viewed as

259

irreversible. A scar is permanent, and there is as yet no transplanting of brain tissue. A lesion can be excised only along with some surrounding brain tissue, further damaging the patient. The psychotherapist may be reluctant to risk his therapeutic optimism by discovering that the behavior or learning problem he sees and hopes to ameliorate is neurologically determined. We know that in purely psychogenic disorders a therapeutic alliance based upon the mutual expectation that the patient will get better is most likely to produce exactly that result. Some therapists thus reason that manifest behavioral disturbance is the only treatable aspect of a maladjustment, and that knowledge of etiology neither helps treatment nor guides it.

Psychotherapists will be motivated to acquire knowledge of the neurological elements in diagnosis only as we can foresee a beneficial application of that knowledge. While such applications are not now abundant, even those few now possible make significant differences for the individual patient in whose situation the neurological elements figure. A real danger is that defense of one's optimistic outlook may limit consideration that the possibilities include a neurological element, and result in a professional and scientific act of denial. In fact, its result can be the opposite of its intention, if certain optimistic realities available when a cerebral function is accurately diagnosed are missed by the therapist. That early discovery of proliferating lesions can be lifesaving is obvious. Less well-recognized but real are the optimistic possibilities for treatment of the obscure, non-lethal minimal cerebral dysfunction once discovered.

If depersonalization, severe depression, anxiety, or a learning impairment is found to have some neurological basis, the patient's psychotherapy can be based upon realistic goals, not obfuscated by the hopeful misapprehension that the causation is purely psychogenic. Patient and therapist are rescued from protracted and futile battering against what appears to be an inflexible pathology. Such rigidity often prevails exactly because the intervention is wrong for the physical facts. The patient departs with self-esteem badly damaged and feeling that he is beyond help or, if he has a stronger ego, believing that psychotherapy is a fraud. The therapist, if candid, confronts his failure and searches for an insight he may have failed to achieve or an interpretation he neglected to offer. Or he can always catalogue the patient as resistant.

Accurate diagnosis can forestall many such futile forays and minimize aimless groping in others. A seizure disorder that simulates schizophrenia, with altered states of consciousness and panic-level anxiety but without convulsions, can be controlled and relief of symptoms achieved by proper medication. Under very careful controls similar assistance can be provided to some school-age children who show hyperkinesis and concentration difficulties. When neurologically-based symptoms are recognized and properly treated, the truly psychological aspects of the patient's problems become discernible and available for psychotherapy. Many cases of hyperkinesis, for example, do *not* require medication if properly diagnosed and treated with individual learning techniques and psychotherapy. With such programs, many children may be taught to tolerate and adjust to their hyperactivity.

When a neurologically-based cause of a learning disability is differentiated from among possible alternatives, teaching strategies can be developed to mobilize the child's more intact functions, and instruct him in tactics to circumvent or surmount his disabilities.

When amelioration of an impairment is genuinely impossible, as in untreatable neurological situations, the diagnosis becomes a reality requiring adjustment. That task replaces the anxiety and torment of uncertainty. Self-reproach for not getting better can be reduced or removed. Psychotherapy directed to the task of engaging the harsh reality is in fact more promising than the pursuit of a psychodynamic that is nonexistent or greatly overweighed by the neurological component.

CHAPTER 9

Diagnosis and Causality

Some psychotherapists are opposed to preliminary diagnosis; others mildly and rather vaguely consider it a good idea; still others actively urge it as a precaution to assure that insight-uncovering therapy be eschewed for a patient potentially psychotic. In general, diagnosis is neither prominent nor valued in psychotherapy. But if the therapist is to give any weight to the neurogenetic element in behavior, he must be prepared to make a careful diagnostic scrutiny and to use all his findings in charting the course of therapy.

Psychodiagnosis as a specialty of psychologists, despite its early development, has not grown as has psychotherapy. Psychodiagnosis has not kept pace in the development of information; it does not enjoy the same respected place in the curriculum; it does not elicit the same enthusiastic response of students or the sense of urgency both patients and therapists give to the treatment process. Why has this aspect of psychology been allowed to decline?

DIAGNOSIS OF DIAGNOSIS

The limitation of mere nosology has been a major deterrent. Nosology, however refined, does not illuminate etiology, or guide the selection of treatment methods, or estimate prognosis. Still less does a label, however accurate, comprehend the individual human drama each person brings into treatment. Consider only a few aspects of the complex process we call schizophrenia. Psychogenic schizophrenia may arise as a failure of progression, or as a result of regression. Thus some schizophrenic individuals with the latter patterns respond well to analysis, a therapy held by many to be indicated only for persons with a diagnosis of neurosis. Give something a name and the search for its meaning becomes less compelling. Or worse, give something a name

263

and categorical meanings rather than individual meanings come to mind. These lull the therapist, mitigate his anxiety, dull his inquisitive drive to find the particular in the individual.

Another obstacle has been the attitude of some psychotherapists that they can proceed helpfully in treatment without a formulated plan of intervention for the patient, that revelations will occur as treatment slowly proceeds. These therapists are not concerned with the development of an adequate psychodiagnosis, since they do not believe it necessary. Some even hold that action by the therapist is undemocratic and deprives the help-seeker of his autonomy and individuality. But the patient desires relief from emotional stress; he may seek to change his life style, to overcome blocks to behavior that deprive him of gratification and achievement, to master acute anxiety, to halt and reverse the invasion and impairment by primary processes of the functions of his ego, to restore his emotional state to some former equilibrium. He seeks help. An adequate response to his reasonable wish to be benefited by his interchange with us requires that we be equipped to help him. I believe that this equipment includes an attitude of purpose, of intention. Only if no purposeful action is expected from the therapist, need he not prepare himself for action. Only if he is expected merely to react, reflect, interact, is he free of the responsibility to decide that his response to the helpseeker is the most probably helpful of all those available.

Psychodiagnosis has suffered also from a sense of timelessness with which some therapists approach their therapeutic reponsibility. Consider the lassitude that may be read in this advice, "If we settle back to work with a patient in a long-term program it does not matter so much how vague the focus may be; eventually we will be able to score" (7). Though it was not the writer's intention, the young therapist may conclude that since psychotherapy is governed by chance, he may consort with the patient until, fortuitously, he is able to help him. His only influence to cast probability in favor of the patient will be to offer his services for as long as necessary—forever if need be, until the patient tires of him, or in perhaps too many instances, he of the patient. To oppose this drifting is not to argue that some individuals do not benefit from being in therapy all of their lives, either with one therapist, or moving occasionally from one to another therapist. But it is to say that such a sense of timelessness makes the need for assessment and decision seem less compelling, to the detriment of many patients.

One encounters, too, the argument that psychodiagnosis requires taking a case-history. Since this step, the argument continues, fosters use of analytic-inferential-deductive processes, it is dehumanizing, and "contact" with the patient is lost. This argument is made against the case-history methodology itself, rather than against a dehumanizing manner of obtaining a history. In truth, the way the method is applied determines whether or not it will be dehumanizing. Human contact is made by a person pursuing a goal; methods will reflect his intention and his style. The case-history method in the hands of an examiner is himself; he will not become an empty chanter of questions unless he is empty. Perhaps this disparagement of the analytic-inferential-deductive process is the most serious obstacle to using diagnosis to contribute to treatment. The argument implies that one cannot think and be empathic at the same time. Yet this combination of activities is the basic demand upon the therapist—a requirement difficult but possible. Empathy is essential, as are impulse control and the use of highly developed secondary-thought processes. The therapist tending to the hysterical will probably spontaneously stress the affect component; in the more obsessional, the cognitive will be more prominent. But the therapist need not fall on either side. Passionate allegiance to either affect or cognition alone is not of help to patients. The therapist must be humane but knowledgeable as well. Heritage, background, life, and personal insight provide his affective qualities; his training often consists largely of expanding his knowledge, ideally with personal therapy; his development as a therapist is the ongoing synthesis of all the ways he experiences his own existence.

Two powerful psychoanalytic biases impede the development of psychodiagnosis. One holds that the data available at the beginning of treatment are insufficient for a valid diagnosis, that diagnosis must await the virtual completion of treatment, when all the needed data become conscious, hence available. Many analysts reject this bias in practice, but the literature, where views are open to the scrutiny of colleagues and elders, is murky. Efforts to determine if a patient is "analyzable" are encouraged, clearly an effort at diagnosis, but not one that leads to a forthright recognition that a meaningful diagnostic procedure is needed. Perhaps such development will be fostered by a study of failures. When, at the end of a protracted psychoanalytic procedure, a patient is judged to be unanalyzable, judgments of alternative procedures might be made from the vast amount of data then at last accessible to the analyst, and an effort made to relate hints or indications available early in the treatment to the finding that the patient cannot benefit.

The keystone of this psychoanalytic bias against diagnosis is confusion about the source of the data available to the psychoanalytic procedure. Human behavior even during free association is seldom if ever purely unconscious, but at most derivative from unconscious sources, and in many respects strong clues are as readily available at the beginning as at the end of an analytic procedure. Diagnosis is a hypothesis. A hypothesis is a device to guide an experiment; it does not follow its completion, except as it may lead to another experiment. The consequence of this particularly persistent analytic bias is clear: since psychodiagnosis preliminary to treatment is regarded as impossible, the effort receives little attention. Like an unfavored child, its development suffers from neglect.

The second bias against diagnosis among psychoanalysts arises paradoxically from one of the most powerful spurs to diagnosis—determinism. Freud's perception that psychic phenomena heretofore inexplicable were determined was so potent that psychotherapy was strongly influenced for decades along deterministic lines. The concept is a magnificant one for its power to stimulate inquiry: the phenomenon under observation is not accidental; it has a cause: what is it? But the concept becomes stultifying, and precludes inquiry rather than stimulates it, if one is convinced that etiology is always limited to psychogenic conflict or psychic trauma. Then attention is not directed to alternative or contributing determinants, social or physical. That the suffering mind is always presented in a body has been overlooked in the dazzling light of the newer revelations of psychological causes.

Diagnosis suffers also because diagnosticians have not used fully the increasingly available information about the effects of culture upon human behavior, nor those of genetics, physiology, and neurology. We are usually aware that the normal behavior of an individual from a comparatively simple rural or semi-urban culture may appear aberrant to a city-reared therapist, and that judgments must be made within the context of social difference. But we make only token acknowledgment of the complexity of interaction when a person of one culture tries to comprehend a person from another quite different. Moreover, the diagnostician operating within his own culture is not much better off. In some respects we are virtually retarded in the attitudes we bring to the understanding of the contribution of our own culture to behavior. As a single example, the role of expectation in shaping human behavior and in creating contentment or conflict has only recently begun to get attention. And what do we really know, what can we validly say, about the behavior of youth alienated from society? Do we really grasp any of the elements in dropping-out? Active nihilism? Racism? Sexual exploitation?

The impact of genetics is even more obscure, obfuscated as it is by partisan loyalty in the nature-nurture controversy. There is promise in the work on chromosomal variants and criminal behavior. Perhaps the investigation of schizophrenia through the study of twins would have greater usefulness if it became concerned more with behavior and less with nosology.

The purpose of this book is to stress that physiological and neurological processes often produce behaviors that correspond with those that arise psychogenically and can be confused with them. It would be overly generous to say that therapists are "somewhat aware" of the possibility that disturbances of calculation, perception, language, attention, retention, and execution revealed in psychological testing may be caused by lesions of the brain. In the teaching of psychological testing attention is paid to the presence of lower psychomotor scores as the index of brain damage. But this is a narrow view indeed. In his review of clinical manifestations of these behaviors, the psychodiagnostician seldom considers alternatives other than the psychogenic. The teaching of psychodiagnosis simply has not kept pace with the information generated by neuropsychology about the behavioral manifestations of cerebral lesions or of epilepsy, for example. Nor has it followed the hypotheses forthcoming from work in electroencephalography. Faints, fits, falls, depersonalization, bad trips, hallucinations, depressions are some of the behaviors that require differential diagnosis; any of them may be determined neurologically or physiologically, some culturally, as well as psychogenically. Few if any behaviors do not warrant consideration of alternatives and scrupulous consideration of all possible factors that affect the diagnosis and in turn the prognosis and treatment of a troublesome human condition.

To repeat, diagnosis and therapy are artificially separated in practice and diagnosis is not emphasized. Further, psychodiagnosis has been largely apart from the mainstream of contemporary developments in related sciences. The psychodiagnostician, of course, cannot blame himself if data from those fields available to him are few. He cannot use what is not there. But he is responsible for asking questions and for making known what he needs. He is even more responsible for using such information as is available. It is here that psychodiagnosis has tended to fail itself.

Perhaps zeal for diagnosis is dulled by the comforting notion that one's own particular treatment (psychoanalysis, behavior therapy, tranquilizing drugs, marathon encounters, whatever) is after all the most efficacious for the largest number of people. Differential assessment and selective application of a treatment approach, therefore, are not a persuasive necessity. If "my therapy is the only true therapy," then my analysis, operant conditioning, psychotropic medication, or intensive group experiences, or whatever, is the answer. Disinterest in diagnosis is a logical consequence of such belief. Yet psychoanalysis is not the only therapeutic application of psychoanalytic theory, nor is the use of hierarchical approaches to a dreaded situation solely the property of behavioral theory. Different theories of personality often lead to the use of very similar techniques. A single personality theory will allow the use of many therapeutic approaches. Psychoanalytic comprehension of defensive structure in the personality, for example, may lead either to an uncovering approach, or to efforts to restrain and repress. Diagnosis, properly emphasized, can strengthen therapy, whatever its theoretical base may be.

So the first order of business for the psychotherapist who wishes to apply concepts of neuropsychodiagnosis is to value diagnosis as a function in his practice. An attitude of skeptical inquiry concerning the cause and sometimes the causes of any symptom will lead him to consider as possible any and all etiologies, until each is evaluated and discarded or elevated to the status of "probable."

THE PSYCHODIAGNOSTIC FORMULATION

Because a set of facts on probable etiology, treatment intervention, and prognosis have so much more value in psychotherapy than mere nosology, I have suggested elsewhere (6) that a "psychodiagnostic formulation" is preferable to a diagnostic label. This formulation results from the therapist's answers to a series of implied questions. These are seldom if ever posed directly, but rather guide the therapist through an inquiry that permits formulation in his own mind of a reasonable statement of cause. He can then select interventions based upon that statement. These questions provide the structure for a neuropsychodiagnostic inquiry as well as a purely psychodiagnostic one.

1) *What is the presenting complaint?* The complaint is the manifest

reason the individual seeks treatment. It is the discomfort or the source of such discomfort that motivates patients to give up time and money and to allow the invasion of their privacy necessary to provide relief. The therapist is first concerned with whether the complaint presented is the real trouble, or a mask or a derivative expression of the real problem.

2) *What is the precipitating cause of the complaint?* Behavioral and psychological disturbances often are illuminated when one learns details of the circumstances in which the patient became aware of the complaint. Such inquiry may elicit facts concerning the nature of the stimulus which precipitates the disturbance; these in turn tell something about the impulses with which the patient is uncomfortable or is struggling, and can become evocative of a history of preceding related events. If precipitating events make no psychodynamic sense in relationship to the complaint, their absence may suggest that an etiology other than the psychogenic is involved.

3) *What are the antecedent analogues of the present situation?* The search for antecedents to the present situation traces data that will strengthen or weaken a tentative hypothesis postulated on the basis of the presenting complaint and the precipitating circumstances.

Identification of a situation similar to the present one at an earlier stage in development will confirm a hypothesis about psychodynamics, reassure the therapist about his first view of the causes of the individual's disturbance, and heighten his confidence in the therapeutic ventures he is likely to undertake. Even when the present situation does not duplicate preceding events, either precisely or in part, these earlier incidents may provide information that rounds out understanding of the forces inherent in an emotional disturbance. Failure to find related past events may suggest that the disturbance is indeed of recent origin —an important fact for treatment and one usually increasing the probability of a favorable prognosis.

4) *What are the meanings of the symptoms?* Symptoms are generally understood as indications of something other than themselves, and can be considered at three levels of meaning: (a) their universal meaning as the product of conflict, trauma, or deprivation; (b) their generic meaning established through clinical experience and psychoanalytic investigation, e.g., in depression, the dynamics frequently causal are inward deflection of rage, loss of love, damage to self-esteem, or deception, and (c) the specific individual variations of general symptom

dynamics, e.g., express prohibitions against anger in the patient's family.

When the psychotherapist is able to understand the patient's symptoms on all these levels, his confidence in a purely psychogenic etiology is vastly reinforced. When such understanding is weak or lacking, he must consider further exploration through interviewing or psychological testing. Or, again, he must entertain possible causes other than the psychogenic.

5) *What is the state of the ego system?* Some function of the ego is involved in every emotional disturbance or behavioral disorder (3). Knowledge of the various ego functions, the manifestations of their disturbances, and ability to evaluate both the strength and weakness of each function permit the therapist to focus upon needed changes and to select interventions (1) predictably effective with specific ego weaknesses. Eleven functions have been systematically studied and described by Bellak and Hurvich (2): reality testing, sense of reality, judgment, regulation and control of drives, object relations, thought processes, adaptive regression, defensive functioning, stimulus barrier, autonomous functioning, and synthetic functioning.

Identification of a weakened function is not in itself sufficient warrant to undertake the strengthening of that function by any specific intervention, even though the intervention may have been clinically tried and found effective in seemingly similar conditions. Different causal pathologies, neurological as well as psychological, may produce a similar ego deficit. Conflict over rage or sexuality, for example, may result in aversiveness in object relations, but so also may fear of lapses in a person suffering *petit mal.* Aversiveness in object relations in an aphasia victim can be based in fear of communication difficulty. The final ego expression may be similar, but the effective therapeutic intervention would be different for each patient. Etiology, therefore, is a crucial variable in the use of ego-function description and evaluation as a guide to treatment.

6) *What shifts are necessary to restore homeostasis?* If the cause is psychic conflict, presumably resolution will reduce symptomatology; if traumatization, the gradual discharge of affect and the restoration of competence. If the cause is the physical one of prodromal anxiety in a paroxysmal disorder the control of seizures will be necessary. This question seeks to pinpoint the alteration—emotional or familial, or physiological or neurological—necessary if the patient is to experience relief from his complaint. The formulation follows the lead provided

by Freud's structural hypothesis of ego, id, and superego, which illuminated the imbalance between these structural components of the personality induced by neurosis, and suggested how balance might variously be restored, in one person by strengthening of ego through either increasing or weakening a defense, in another by mitigating or diverting an impulse, and in still another by increasing or decreasing the superego.

7) *What interventions are most likely to produce the shift needed to restore homeostasis?* Here the selection of an intervention must not be limited by the training or theoretical bias of the therapist, but rather by the reasoned conclusion that one selected from among the total array of possible interventions probably has more capacity to shift the balance in this specific individual suffering from an observed and comprehended disequilibrium. A major consideration in this question is should there be any intervention at all, an important caveat for which I am grateful to Dr. Herbert Fensterheim. Experience may warn that any intervention may make a bad situation worse, or that the patient's ego strengths or real-life resources are inadequate for coping with the strains that therapy, however supportive, must inevitably evoke. The therapist is well advised to try explicitly to state for himself the extent to which he should intervene.

8) *What therapeutic allies are available?* Allies to the therapeutic process reside within and without the patient. The inner allies are the patient's motivation, the strength of ego functions that may be called upon to bolster weaker ones, the capacity and desire for pleasure and for work. Allies external to the patient include people who may be able to relate to him in supporting or abetting his therapeutic progress. A patient with defective judgment may be induced to accept the counsel of a friend who has a more rational approach to matters than the patient has been able to exercise. The availability of friends and family as safeguards in suicidal danger needs no stressing here.

9) *What shall be the general procedure of this therapy?* The effort to order priorities within therapy is based upon consideration of the importance of the various goals to be achieved and their effects upon the quality of the patient's life and his future. It includes consideration also of the reasonableness of expectations, since one goal may be easily reachable, while others may require long periods of training or the slow uncovering of dynamics.

When a neurological problem is seen as possible, the first priority may be a neurological examination to focus the diagnosis, as when a proliferating lesion is suspected. Or it may be a medical consultation and a period of anti-convulsant medication when subictal states are creating anxiety. Or the first step may be a series of family conferences, as when altered attitudes toward a child with minimal brain dysfunction are needed to relieve parental pressure upon the child.

10) *What is the prognosis?* This question compels the therapist to review all of the foregoing questions and their answers. Some evidence (5) indicates that clarity of comprehension by the therapist of the dynamics of a psychogenic disorder increases the favorable nature of the prognosis. Other studies (4) suggest that expectation of patient improvement by both therapist and patient is a powerful spur to beneficial change. The role of motivation, of capacity for insight, of strength of ego are all to be considered here. In neurological problems, the prognosis may hinge upon the established efficacy of an anti-convulsant or hyperkinetic drug, or the length of interval from injury, or upon factors in the physical realm, such as the mass of a lesion. Even when these are immutably pessimistic, the responsible therapist must know them, and serves the patient best when he does.

When the therapist wishes to add the neuropsychodiagnostic area to his inquiry, as I advocate, these ten questions must be further pursued with more detailed questions, focused on the neurological experience of the patient. These are the subject of the next chapter.

BIBLIOGRAPHY

1. *Bellak, L.* and *Small, L.:* Emergency Psychotherapy and Brief Psychotherapy, Second Edition. New York, Grune and Stratton, 1978.
2. *Bellak, L.* and *Hurvich, M.:* A systematic study of ego functions. J. Nerv. Ment. Dis., 148:6, 1969.
3. *Bellak, L.:* The psychoanalytic concept of the ego and schizophrenia. *In:* L. Bellak and P. K. Benedict (Eds.): Schizophrenia: A Review of the Syndrome. New York: Logos Press, 1958.
4. *Frank, J. D.:* The role of hope in psychotherapy. Int. J. Psychiat., 5, 1968.
5. *Malan, D. H.:* A Study of Brief Psychotherapy. London: Tavistock Publications, 1963.
6. *Small, L.:* The Briefer Psychotherapies, Revised Edition. New York: Brunner/Mazel, 1979.
7. *Wolberg, L. R.:* Technic of short-term psychotherapy. *In* L. R. Wolberg (Ed.): Short-Term Psychotherapy, New York: Grune and Stratton, 1965.

CHAPTER 10

Details of the Neuropsychodiagnostic Interview

The frequency of equivocal neurological conditions in psychotherapeutic practice combines with the capacity of neurological and psychological disorders to mimic each other into a reasonable requirement that each applicant for psychotherapy be assessed for the operation of neurological factors. The therapist must be willing therefore to shift his approach from the less-structured psychodiagnostic interview to the highly-structured neurodiagnostic inquiry. Psychodiagnostic interviewing involves fewer specific questions, and tends to rely upon associative thinking, a process which, if not free in the traditional psychoanalytic sense, is influenced by the patient's concern with his difficulties and his wish to be helped. The neuropsychodiagnostic inquiry is specifically structured by the requirement to survey as much as possible of the brain-behavior relationship.

Content for such an inquiry is discussed here: the queries suggested may be added to the psychodiagnostic inquiry as the therapist finds them appropriate to the patient, to his own style, and to the specific situation. Generally, the less-structured psychodiagnostic inquiry should precede the neurodiagnostic questions, so that the more freely associational responses are not stilled by the specific questions necessary later.

THE HISTORY AND ETIOLOGICAL POSSIBILITIES

The history is focused upon identifying any insult to the body or any developmental abnormality that may have etiological and diagnostic significance. Six major areas of neurological import are usually pursued.

273

1) The birth process: Any information the patient may have about his prenatal and birth events is sought. Does he know anything about these? Did his parents speak of these? Was his mother bed-confined because of bleeding? Was his birth difficult? Protracted? Was he premature? Did he require incubation? Did his mother have rubella? Was she ill in any other way? Was she emotionally disturbed? The victim of an accident? Was there Rh incompatibility? Was there false labor? How long was labor? Was he post-term, hence larger and subject to more pressure? Were instruments used? Medications given? Is there any knowledge of his condition immediately following birth? Was he phlegmatic? Were there any problems about breathing, suckling, or swallowing normally? Were there convulsions? Any deformation of the head? Was caesarian section performed? This area is usually most ambiguous, buried in unavailable records, unrecorded information, layers of forgetfulness, and distortions of memory. Nonetheless, it should be pursued. If the patient is a child, the parents should be interviewed and the pediatrician asked for information.

2) Developmental history: Psychotherapists usually are accustomed and trained to make inquiries about the emergence and maturation of developmental landmarks such as feeding habits, toilet habits, posture control, emergence of ability to sit, stand, walk, speak, dress. To these should be added specific inquiries about any sensory or motor problems, and any early learning difficulties.

3) High fevers: Their cause, symptoms, duration, treatment, and sequelae are queried. It is well to pursue a history of any reaction to inoculations of various kinds, since a severe reaction may be equivalent to a serious disease episode. Was the patient convulsive or delirious during any febrile experience?

4) Accidents involving injuries to the head: Were they accompanied by unconsciousness? Vomiting? Bleeding from the ears? If unconscious, how long? Was the patient hospitalized? How long? Was the patient examined by a physician. Were any special procedures undertaken? EEG? Skull X-rays? CAT scan? Neurological examination? Can reports of these be obtained? Among psychiatric populations, a history of electro-convulsive therapy may be an important etiological factor related to residual memory and cognitive defects, among others.

5) Anesthesias: Did the patient undergo surgery? How many times? For what? Duration of anesthesia in each case? Type of anesthesias used? Sequelae, if any? Heart surgery, on the increase as techniques are refined, continues to result in a rather high incidence of post-opera-

tive neurological complications. Hemiplegia, agnosias, blackouts, and giddiness have been reported (3).

6) Poisoning: Foods? Chemicals or gases other than anesthesias? Drugs? Paints? Sprays? Over-doses? Concern is growing about the possible adverse effects of medications used in infancy and childhood.

SPECIFIC NEUROPSYCHODIAGNOSTIC QUERIES

The therapist observes the patient's motor behavior from the moment of greeting in the waiting room, during the walk to the consulting room and throughout the interview. Gait, posture, rate, and character of movement are observed. Visible skin is scrutinized for scars, which are investigated in the inquiry. These sometimes lead to accounts of faints, assaults, or injuries of etiological consequence.

Any speech disturbance such as slurring, slowness of reaction, articulation difficulties, perseveration, or grammatical failures is noted. Special care must be given to evaluating speech and the thought processes inherent in it. Too often there is a tendency to ascribe motor difficulties to neurological causes only and thought disturbances to psychogenic ones only. Vague answers, unresponsiveness to requests for elaboration, and seeming lack of insight may be denial in the psychogenic sense, but they also may reflect an aphasia. Illogical statements may derive from a schizophrenic inappropriateness or looseness of associations, but they also may be the product of organic impairment.

The major sensory experiences, motor expressions not usually observable in the office directly, developmental progressions, and integrative capacities are explored through queries such as the following:

1) Does the patient have any knowledge about his motor development? That is, does he know when he began standing, walking, running, balancing?

2) Does he consider himself more clumsy than most people? Does he drop things? Bump into things? Stumble or fall often?

3) Was the patient ever hyperactive, or sluggish, slow moving, inactive?

4) Does the patient recall any difficulties in learning? To read? To write? Do arithmetic? Do not be put off from these queries by the fact that the patient may be a college graduate or a Ph.D. A learning disability may still be present. In this connection, a hearing difficulty may impair acquisition of language. Comprehension and expression both may be affected so as to suggest an aphasia or a thought disorder.

5) Has he experienced blurred vision or double vision, even when his eyes have been corrected, if necessary? Do moving lights disturb him (flickering TV, strobes, automobile lights at night)? Do moving lights make him tense, edgy, uneasy?

6) Has he experienced phosphenes—hallucinations of light flashes darting by the side of the eyes in the dark, or seeming to explode?

7) Has he experienced dizziness, especially dizziness not caused by drugs, heat, hunger, fever, hyperventilation, or asphyxia? Has he fainted under such circumstances? Has he had to hold on to keep from falling down because the environment tilted suddenly?

8) Has he heard ringing sounds, high-pitched sound, or an unintelligible rapid voice? Laterality, if present, should be determined.

9) Does he experience tingling sensations in the fingertips or toes? These are sometimes experienced as electric-like buzzings, as if the person has received a shock. They may be described as itching, with need to scratch the member. Do these members become numb without cause? These sensations must be differentiated from the commonplace feeling after a limb has "gone to sleep" and is recovering. If these sensations have been experienced, inquiry should be made concerning laterality: both sides or one?

10) Does he become angry without apparent cause?

11) Has he experienced blackouts? These are episodes in which a person, talking with or listening to someone, suddenly is unable to hear even when his name is called, or hears the other person but is unable to respond. These states must be differentiated from preoccupation from which the person can be aroused to respond to a call.

12) Has he experienced altered states of consciousness? These may be reported as feelings of depersonalization. Or the person, fully awake, suddenly begins to dream. He is aware that he is both awake and dreaming. The experience is often frightening; the patient may fear insanity or that he is the victim of mysterious and dangerous forces. These states need to be differentiated from daydreaming which can be ended at will or in response to a summons.

13) Has he experienced an aura-like state in which he has felt strange? Or feared that some nameless, shapeless, unfocused danger may befall him? In such states the patient may be fearful of leaving the home or may require companionship for security. Obviously, these states must be differentiated from both phobias and free-floating anxiety states, a process of differential diagnosis not always easy.

14) Automatic behavior is investigated. Has the patient been doing

things he was unaware he was doing? Or started out with one destination in mind and found himself at another, without memory that he had decided to alter his course? Or without memory of how he got to the place where he suddenly finds himself?

15) Favored medications are investigated. Sometimes a clue to a psychomotor epilepsy is found when a patient relates a fondness for some of the older anti-convulsive drugs (such as the amphetamines and the barbituates). Patients may report that such drugs give them a sense of calmness and security, of evenness and composure that they lack without them.

16) Disturbances of body image are explored. Has the patient had the impression of alterations in the size of hands, feet, or head?

17) Has he experienced distortions in the apparent shape, and size, or distance of objects?

18) Has he experienced impairment of movement, gesturing, walking?

19) Have there been disturbances of speech, reading, calculation, musical skill?

20) Has he experienced difficulty with memory? If so, is it general? Of events? Material just read? Does it involve words? Inability to say or write the right word?

21) Has there been any sudden alteration of audition? Increased sensitivity to sound? Music seeming to change into noise? Has there been any fluctuation in the comprehension of speech?

22) Is there increased sensitivity to taste? To smell? A favorite odor becoming unpleasant, then pleasing again?

23) Has the patient experienced any disturbance of spatial orientation? Taking wrong turns? Putting his arm into the wrong sleeve?

24) Has he experienced any impairment of reading? Recognizing numbers, letters, musical notations? Has the visual field become constricted or limited in any way?

25) Has the patient experienced writing difficulties in forming letters or words or numbers?

26) Has there been any change of efficiency in writing and reading? Is writing less fluid? Reading less rapid?

27) Has there been difficulty in arithmetical processes? Does the patient recognize numbers when written or spoken? Can he do mental calculations?

The manner in which the patient affirms or denies the experiences asked about these questions is an important clinical datum, influencing the diagnostician's evaluation of the likelihood that the symptom is indeed present. I have been impressed by the unequivocal affirmative response of some patients, coupled with the convincing clarity of their description when asked to give an example or illustration of the experience being queried. Some responses are hesitatingly negative, as if somthing vaguely familiar has been touched upon, but not quite brought into sharp cognitive focus. Other responses are hesitating affirmative, and suggest that the patient may not have understood, or may be suggestible. In all cases, the request for examples and descriptions is routine to guard against suggesting what is not present.

DETERMINATION OF "HANDEDNESS" AND LATERAL DOMINANCE

"Handedness" is an extremely important clinical datum of potential significance for both diagnosis and research, as discussed in Chapter 15. Most people are right-handed, and so, as with speech, their "handedness" is controlled by the left hemisphere of the brain. However, there is a considerable degree of partial left-handedness and ambidexterity, so that in left-handed and partially left-handed people, the right hemisphere may assume more control over speech functions than is usual.

"Handedness" may have diagnostic and localizing significance. If a right-handed person demonstrates a right hand weaker than his left in the absence of muscular disease, a left-side of brain difficulty may be suspected. Or if the left hand is significantly weaker than is expected in a right-handed person, a right-hemisphere involvement may be suggested. The patient, therefore, is questioned carefully as to "handedness." Obviously, the use of the hand in writing helps determine this function. Additionally, the patient may be asked to go through the motions of driving a nail, opening a door, shaking hands, throwing a ball, using a fork.

The dominance of the legs is explored by having the patient go through the motions of kneeling, kicking an imaginary ball, stepping on an imaginary bug to establish which limb is used.

A first step in determining eye dominance is to establish relative visual acuity of the two eyes. Does the patient have a good eye and a bad eye? If the patient needs glasses, they should be worn during this part of the examination. Two conditions of viewing should be checked:

close and far. For the former the patient is asked to put a hole in a 3 x 5 card to one eye, close the other eye, and peer at an object on the table before him. For far-viewing dominance the patient is instructed to stand at one wall or corner of a room while the examiner stands at an opposite wall or corner as far apart as the room permits. The patient extends one arm pointing the index finger of that arm at the examiner and sighting along it with one eye closed. The dominance of the eyes may be explored also by having the patient look through a paper tube as if it were a telescope. Luria (2) suggests a useful eye-dominance test: to have the patient, with both eyes open, line-up a pencil held vertically in his hand with a vertical line on the opposite wall. While maintaining this alignment, the patient's right eye is covered (or is closed); then the left eye is covered with the right eye remaining open. Should the pencil appear to move to the right when the right eye is covered, and not move when the left eye is covered, the right eye is dominant. The opposite result, movement of pencil to the left when the left eye is covered with little or no movement to the right when the right eye is covered, demonstrates dominance of the left eye.

Determination of ear dominance requires dichotic listening instrumentation and is generally not convenient for the psychotherapist to explore.

"Handedness," "sidedness," or dominance are not always clear-cut. Lateral dominance may vary from hand to eye to foot in the same person, or within the organ tested. In the latter case a person may be ambidextrous, or show a mixed dominance for the eye or the foot, or for two or all of the organs tested. This kind of finding confounds the determination of any lateralized dysfunction so that the psychotherapist should be wary in interpreting the observations made.

PROJECTIVE QUERIES

The foregoing neuropsychodiagnostic queries obviously do not include all brain-behavior relationships. They do cover the major sensory modalities, paroxysmal phenomena, motor abnormalities, language problems, and learning difficulties. Moreover, they often elicit, by way of association, accounts of significant behavior not specifically covered by the queries here suggested.

Another type of query—the projective question—has similar power to evoke associations that sometimes lead to a neurological clue, as well as supply the psychodynamic material to which they are addressed. Thus a patient, asked for the worst thing that ever happened in his life, may recount loss of a loved person, a serious automobile accident, or a subictal state. Ten such subjects for questions are suggested here. Obviously the inventive clinician can readily add to them.

I am grateful to Dr. Bernard Landis for his ideas in this area of inquiry. He suggests that literary individuals may be asked for their favorite literary hero and heroine, for example. A politically-oriented individual may be invited to fantasy that he has just become president of the United States and asked to identify three major decisions he would make at once in that office. Dr. Molly Harrower developed the Most Pleasant-Most Unpleasant Concepts questions as a drawing test. A related approach in France (1) asks children to draw the Land of Fear and the Land of Joy. Any of these may be posed as questions for oral response rather than drawing.

The points I explore are these:

1) The earliest memory of an event or experience in the patient's life, the age at which it occurred, and the feeling associatd with the experience.

2) A dream history that includes any dream during childhood that is recalled, recurrent dreams, and one or two recent dreams.

3) What does the patient consider to be his best quality, trait or characteristic? His worst?

4) What does the patient consider to be the best thing he has done in his life? The worst?

5) What does the patient consider to be the best thing that ever happened to him? The worst thing?

6) If the patient could relive his life what would he change? What would he keep the same?

7) What is the most pleasant thing the patient can imagine or think of? The most unpleasant?

8) If the patient had three wishes that magically could come true what would he wish for?

9) What favorite joke does the patient have?

10) What has been the worst, the most serious problem in the patient's life?

Interviewing data, of course, are most subjective and their interpretations relative to the diagnostician's experience. Among the gross subjective evaluations the diagnostician makes is whether or not the patient is psychotic or mentally retarded. This evaluation must in large measure be based upon the patient's social manner in relating to the diagnostician, his comprehension of questions, his responsiveness, his spontaneous vocabulary and mode of expression, his perception of relationships, and his insight into the goal inherent in the questions being asked of him. *These clinical impressions may be crucially important to the diagnostic outcome and must be weighed heavily.* Given the strong clinical impression that the patient is *not* schizophrenic, his rambling verbosity and illogical statements may emerge more clearly as manifestations of an aphasia and seem less likely to be loose associations and contaminations.

In a related fashion, the impression of social competence in a person said to be mentally retarded, or with a Full Scale I.Q. of 65, can lead to the discovery of Above Average, even Superior level, capability in specific functions alongside of severe impairment in other functions, and in turn to a diagnosis of brain damage.

Aside from occasionally obtaining those irrefutable facts that almost beyond doubt identify a brain lesion, the diagnostician is constantly asking himself, "Is there anything about *the way* this person walks, moves, speaks, feels (haptically), sees, hears, reads, writes, thinks, feels (emotionally), approaches problems, solves problems, shifts from one set to another—is there *anything* about this person that arouses suspicion of organicity?"

When organicity is suggested clinically, the diagnostician seeks objective data. Psychological testing is a major source of such data, reducing subjectivity, though not eliminating it, by permitting the application of standardized tasks in standardized fashion.

BIBLIOGRAPHY

1. *Boucharlat, J., et al.:* Le test du pays de la peur et du pays de la joie. Annales Medico-Psychologiques, 2:4, 1970.
2. *Luria, A. R.:* Higher Cortical Functions in Man. New York: Basic Books, 1966.
3. *Morgan, D. H.:* Neuro-psychiatric problems of cardiac surgery, J. Psychosom. Res., 15, 1971.

CHAPTER 11

Psychological Testing

The value of psychodiagnostic test instruments depends on the skill and sensitivity of the clinician who administers them. The data he derives from the tests may mean nothing to him in the face of a theoretical bias, or because of his inexperience. Yet in the same data an obscure relationship between items, or some innocuous sounding patient responses could arouse an "aha!" response in the experienced clinician open to all possibilities. The astute clinician notes matters of personal style, of preference for working with one task but not with others or approaching the test examination in an *order* different from the usual. This chapter assumes no magic for psychological tests, but stresses that they are extensions of the clinician. Matarazzo (36) wisely cautions that when a person's life history contradicts psychological-test results, the examiner should hesitate to diagnose on the basis of the tests alone. Of intelligence level specifically, Matarazzo observes that the life history generally is the more reliable.

The most widely used psychodiagnostic test battery is based upon a broad survey of intellectual function (usually one of the Wechsler scales) and an emotional exploration with projective techniques (usually the Rorschach, the Thematic Apperception Test, and the Human Figure Drawings). Individual psychodiagnosticians may vary from this model by adding other instruments (the Bender Visual Motor Gestalt Test, House-Tree-Person Test, for examples) or by substituting for projective techniques the quantitative analysis of the Minnesota Multiphasic Personality Inventory.

The basic battery with some additions indicated below has proved in my practice to be a practical, efficient, and reasonable *preliminary* step in both neuropsychodiagnosis and psychodiagnosis. After handedness and cerebral dominance have been established as part of the Interview, I consider these following essential to the total diagnostic scrutiny and a necessary prelude to the treatment process:

1) The Wechsler Scales (WAIS or WISC);
2) The Bender Visual Motor Gestalt Test; or the Benton Visual Retention Test;
3) Tests of lateral hemispheric functioning;
4) Projective techniques: Rorschach, Thematic Apperception Test, Human Figure Drawings.

To these the clinician may add additional tests when data from the basic battery suggest a cerebral dysfunction, in order to probe for corroborative evidence.

The psychotherapist unfamiliar with neuropsychological testing and the rationale that underlies it might at this point read the section on Psychological Techniques in Chapter 17. He should keep in mind that no single test score, ratio, pattern, or derivation alone can be counted on to diagnose brain damage. The assumption that organic brain damage is a single, unitary entity that may vary in "degree but not in nature" is without foundation (36), a fact that cannot be overstressed. The brain perceives, processes, and responds in many different ways. The modalities of so-called input and output are relatively few, and relatively manifest to the examiner. But the internal processing methods that intervene between input and output are much more numerous, obscure, and inferential. The psychological-test battery seeks to assess these many modalities, but in fact only begins to address some among them. The psychotherapist who uses the basic psychological battery is not attempting to substitute it for the wider, deeper survey of the neuropsychological test battery, but rather to identify any possible modality dysfunction (s) that would require referral for neuropsychological and/or neurological consultation.

THE WECHSLER SCALES

These long-established scales—the original Wechsler-Bellevue (WB), the Wechsler Adult Intelligence Scale (WAIS), and Wechsler Intelligence Scale for Children (WISC)—are potent diagnostic instruments. Their power, which derives from the diversity of functions examined in the subtests, had been obscured somewhat by the search for single test indicators of brain damage. Also the "Hold-Don't Hold" dichotomy of the Wechsler Scales does not reflect the variety of deficits possible when certain areas of the brain are damaged. Wechsler himself reported that some subtests of the early Wechsler-Bellevue Scale were more sensitive than others to deterioration and brain damage, and that some functions measured by the Scale held up while others were more likely to be impaired (57, 58). Evidence that this Hold-Don't Hold or Deterioration Scale is not diagnostically effective has been rather consistent (8).

Another impediment to recognition of the diagnostic value of the Wechsler Scales has been the tendency to suspect brain damage only when Performance-Scale scores are significantly lower than Verbal-Scale scores—a tendency that ignores the possible impact of left-hemisphere damage upon verbal functions which is a well documented cerebral hemispheric phenomenon. However, even when neuropsychological research took hemispheric functional differences into account, and produced data that related Verbal I.Q. deficits to left-hemisphere damage and Performance I.Q. deficits to right-hemispheric damage, the conclusions were challenged by other researches. Matarazzo (36) in his monumental fifth edition of *Wechsler's Measurement and Appraisal of Adult Intelligence* reviews eight studies between 1958 and 1971 that would indicate that patients with left-hemisphere damage do less well on Verbal subtests than on Performance subtests, and that patients with right-hemisphere lesions do the reverse. Patients with bilateral damage tended to perform more like right-hemisphere damaged patients, that is, do better on Verbal than Performance subtests. These conclusions were challenged by others, notably Smith (52, 53) who reported that his own study of large numbers of patients with lateralized lesions and the studies of others could not confirm the differential lateral sensitivity claimed for the Verbal and Performance I.Q.'s. Examination of the nature of the individual subtests in both Verbal and Performance Scales, which is attempted below, makes clear that the one is in fact not purely verbal nor the other purely performance. Aggregate I.Q. scores may obscure marked deficits in specific subtest functions. Diagnosis appears better served when subtest scores and performances are considered individually, instead of relying upon comparisons of the Verbal I.Q. with Performance I.Q. (15).

Still another misapprehension about Wechsler signs has resulted from a tendency to assume schizophrenia when a patient succeeds with difficult items of a subtest after failing easier ones. This assumption has a corollary that the brain-damaged patient reaches the limit of his capability on a subtest and thereafter consistently fails. Both these assumptions rest upon another and questionable assumption: that there is a perfect relationship between the gradient of difficulty established by item analysis for a subtest and the capacity of the brain to do problems of increasing difficulty. But failure at lower levels coupled with success at higher levels need not mean schizophrenia. Rather it may mean that the "more difficult" problem contained words or concepts, or required processes that remained intact within the individual's brain or for which he was able to establish alternate routes, while the representation within his brain of the elements of an "inherently easier" problem were impaired, destroyed, or interfered with by the particular damage he had suffered.

A fourth deterrent is resistance to using the Wechsler in a combined clinical-statistical fashion, that is, to comprehending the individual brain-behavior characteristics required by each subtest in addition to the scale score it produces. Matarazzo's survey (36) reported only research efforts on the diagnostic sensitivity of the Verbal-Performance I.Q.'s. No data were available to illuminate the neurodiagnostic import of intra-individual subtest scatter, which is, as detailed below, where the clues appear. Luria (33) does the Wechsler scales an injustice and overlooks their clinical potency, I believe, when he regards them as psychometric instruments rather than a clinical method. Had he approached their use with his superb clinical acumen, they might have risen in his esteem; certainly he could have made valued contributions to their application as clinical instruments.

Fundamentally, it is the ability to illuminate a brain function and the behavior relative to that function that makes any test valuable to the neuropsychodiagnostic process. When the test in addition permits clinical observation as well as quantification, its value is vastly enhanced.

As early as 1954, Klebanoff et al. (30), observed that while the overall scores of the Wechsler were relatively insensitive to brain damage, the subtests had significant discriminatory power. This has later been confirmed. Reitan (45) in 1965 cited his own experiments and those of Reed et al. (44) to demonstrate that Wechsler's-Scale variables consistently showed more differences between brain-damaged and normal groups than did measures of concept formation, alertness, and motor functions. The explanation rests in the varied effects of different brain lesions and the capability of the subtests to assess some of the possible effects on the functions.

The Wechsler scales tap many functions. Language skills, receptive and expressive, are required to understand and respond to questions and to follow instructions. Computational ability is tested. Capacity for attention and recall, both long- and short-term, is assayed. Construction praxis is evaluated. Concept formation is required. Graphomotor skills are reviewable. Thought processes are exercised. Sequencing is required.

Most of the functions enumerated are testable on a relative continuum of difficulty established by the item analysis used in their construction. The scoring and scaling procedures permit one function to be compared quantitatively with all others, an essential in neuropsychodiagnosis. The diagnostician, knowing for each subtest the stimulus modality employed, the nature of the response required, and the intervening function of integration involved, is able to use their results clinically. The six subtests that constitute the *Verbal Scale* all employ an auditory stimulus and require an oral-verbal expressive response. Each subtest taps a different function or, more precisely, a set of functions: the cerebral process taking place between stimulus and response.

Information taps relatively old memory; it requires recall of names, dates, and geographical, literary, anatomical, and other information. Both the storage and retrieval of this old data are tested.

Comprehension requires the exercise of judgment, reasoning, and abstract thinking, and assesses awareness of social amenity.

Arithmetic requires mental calculation.

Similarities requires concept formation and associative and abstract thinking.

Digit Span measures recent memory and capacity to attend and concentrate.

Vocabulary evaluates comprehension and expression of word meaning.

All five subtests of the *Performance Scale* depend upon a visual stimulus. The response requirements and the output are varied, as are the functions tested.

Digit Symbol evaluates simple matching accuracy and speed and requires a manual-motor response that can be evaluated for control and placement. Involved are capacities for learning, attention, memory, and sequencing; all of these are mental functions.

Picture Completion requires recognition of essential details in a parts-to-whole relationship, and judgment. The response required here is an oral-verbal expressive one, unlike the other Performance subtests.

Block Design is a constructional task involving spatial relations and figure-ground separation, requiring a motor response.

Picture Arrangement requires thematic perception and construction, with a motor response.

Object Assembly is also a constructional task, involving spatial relations ability and a motor response. Three of the four items of the WAIS and two of the WISC Object Assembly subtests involve representations of the human body and hence may tap the body-image function.

Analysis of the scales by Witkin, *et al.* (59) has identified three major factors:

1) *Verbal,* consisting of Information, Comprehension, and Vocabulary.

2) *Attention,* consisting of Arithmetic, Digit Span, and Digit Symbol.

3) Perceptual-Analytic, consisting of Picture Completion, Block Design, and Object Assembly.

These correspond with the three major factors in the Wechsler scales, apart from the "*g*" factor, discussed by Wechsler (57):

1) *Verbal comprehension,* consisting of Vocabulary, Information, Comprehension, and Similarities.

2) *Non-verbal or performance,* consisting of Picture Completion, Picture Arrangement, Block Design, and Object Assembly.

3) *Memory,* consisting of Digit Span, Digit Symbol, and according to the age of the subject, Arithmetic and Information.

Wechsler also presents a personal communication from F. B. Davis reporting on the differences in scale scores between pairs of WAIS subtests, differences significant at the 15 percent level. The average difference is three scale-score units; the range is from two to four points. Differences in excess of three scale points alert the diagnostician to a pathological process. This factor-analytic approach may be used clinically by averaging the scale scores for the subtests making up each of Witkin's factors and comparing the factors on the basis of such average scale scores.

I have found this method somewhat limited in sophistication. First, it does not consider the overall I.Q. level of the patient being examined. A difference between Verbal and Perceptual-Analytic factors of three scale points has far more pathological significance when the patient's Full Scale I.Q. is 100, and even more so when the I.Q. is lower, than it does if the Full Scale I.Q. is 140.

The averaging of subtests into a factor-average scale score may also tend to conceal an extreme deviation in a specific function. For example, for a given patient the average scale score for the Verbal factor may be 12, while for the Attention factor and the Perceptual-Analytic factor it may also be 12. Thus, no difference appears. But examination of the contribution of each subtest to the average factor score may tell quite another story. In the Perceptual-Analytic factor, both Picture Completion and Block Design may be 14, while Object Assembly is eight. Within the factor, therefore, one function is six scale units below the others, twice the average for all differences reported by Davis to Wechsler, and strongly suggestive of pathology.

Considerable clinical insight can be derived from careful consideration of the differences in modality and process required by each subtest and the manner in which the patient deals with each task. Block Design and Object Assembly are both constructional tasks, both involve a visual stimulus and a motor response. But in Object Assembly the patient must form a mental conceptualization of the whole from the parts, without an external representation of the whole, as is the case in the Block Design subtest where a drawing of the required whole is the visual stimulus. In some patients, the increased ambiguity of the Object Assembly items may reveal a deficit in ideation that would not be identified by the somewhat more structured and guided Block Design. Another patient whose difficulty is separating or interpreting figure-ground relationships may do considerably better on the Object Assembly, with less figure-ground interference or conflict between stimulus card and puzzle parts, than on the Block Design, where he must integrate his construction with an external model. In some patients this situation may appear rather dramatically, with a very poor Block Design in contrast to a much better Object Assembly. The drama may appear in Object Assembly; the Hand, the most ambiguous item, will be done quickly, earning top speed credits, while the other three items will be done far more slowly, albeit accurately. A related phenomenon in the use of the Bender Visual Motor Gestalt Test is reported by Koppitz (32), who observed that some brain-damaged children find the sight of the stimulus card confusing; these children prefer to look at the card, put it out of sight, and draw the designs from memory.

Whatever else the Similarities and Comprehension subtests measure, they both call upon verbal expressive ability. It is in this latter function that they differ markedly. Most items of Similarities can be answered with a single word response (furniture, directions, food, metals, etc.). In contrast, most Comprehension items require a more extended response that involves propositional thinking, the interrelating of at least two ideas into a conclusion. Very often, various dysphasic disorders are apparent in differences between these subtests. Low-level Comprehension accompanied by high-level Similarities suggests a verbal expressive defect of propositional thinking as indicated. The reverse situation (high Comprehension, low Similarities) indicates a deficit of verbal concept formation. When both are low, a major aphasic disorder is suspected; usually this is accompanied by low Vocabulary, so that the entire Verbal factor produces an average scale score supporting the presumption of dysfunction. The Picture Completion subtest may uncover sufficient difficulty in word-finding ability to suggest an anomia that can be present with or without a deficit in propositional expression or abstract conceptualization. We should recognize too that capacity for abstraction (à la Goldstein) is tested by some items of Comprehension as well as by Similarities. Indeed, these items, those that ask for meanings of metaphors, appear to require a higher level of abstraction than the capacity for single quality associations required in Similarities.

Clinically, it is useful also to scrutinize the point in each subtest which presents a marked increase in complexity or requires a shift in approach. On Block Design, the increase in number of blocks to nine with item 7 is in itself an imposition of more difficulty, presenting a more heavily populated test environment and a more complicated visual field. In addition, there is the further complexity of the need to shift from a 2 x 2 square to a 3 x 3 square. Then the actual complexity of the design itself is to be considered. Item 7 of the Block Design appears far less difficult than item 8, so that with some patients the examiner may not observe marked difficulty with the other requirements until the design difficulty is increased. Digit Span can be understood as presenting a linear increase in difficulty based simply upon the increase in number of digits the subject must remember, until recall in reverse order is required and the patient's capacity for attention and recall becomes vastily more burdened. It well may be that for Picture Arrangement and Object Assembly, as well as Block Design, the mere increase in number of units (pictures or parts) is enough added difficulty to overtax the capacity of a brain-injured person, although, of course, this factor cannot be divorced from the inherent difficulty of the item itself. In any case, brain-injured persons are observed to "fall apart" under pressure, and increase of difficulty of any kind may constitute that pressure for them, and should be recognized clinically.

Wechsler himself has had a somewhat limiting effect upon the use of his scales in neuropsychodiagnosis. He tended to limit his assessment of the scales' values mainly by statistical standards, and not to credit sufficiently the clinical applications in individual patients. So he finds the most general impairments in cases of organic brain disease are in visual-motor functions, ability to shift, memory, and in synthetic ability. He concludes that these patients do consistently better on Verbal Scale tasks than on the Performance Scale and that brain damage of whatever origin will produce a typical test syndrome, *if* the damage is sufficiently extensive, a significant proviso.

His conclusion probably is a valid one: massive brain damage will produce a loss in general intelligence. However, it does not account for findings which differentially implicate the left and right cerebral hemispheres: in adults some lower verbal subtest scores generally are associated with left-hemisphere damage in a right-handed person, while some lower performance subtest scores in a right-handed person are associated with right-hemisphere damage.

Beyond this, Reitan (46) investigated the hypothesis that brain damage may be diagnosed in the presence of little or no difference between Verbal and Performance Scale scores when one of the sensitive subtests (Similarities or Block Design) is markedly low. The significance of the absence of a difference between Verbal and Performance scales in such a situation, Reitan hypothesizes, is indication of a static rather than a proliferating lesion.

The sensitivity of subtests of the Verbal Scale to left-hemisphere lesions and of the Performance Scale to right-side damage has led to a great deal of research (31, 38, 39). Localization of functions in the cerebrum is discussed in Chapters 14 and 15. Parsons and Vega (38) reaffirmed factor-analytic findings that Vocabulary and Block Design subtests have the highest loading respectively on the Verbal and Perceptual Organizational factors, and that these factors are respectively associated with the left-hemisphere and right-hemisphere function. Similar results associate deficits on the Similarities subtest with left-hemisphere damage and Object Assembly deficit with right-hemisphere damage. Significantly lower means on Picture Arrangement are associated with right-hemisphere lesions by McFie and Thompson (35). McFie (34) reports consistent findings of dysfunction in Digit Span, Similarities, and Arithmetic in left-hemisphere disorders, while Picture Arrangement, Block Design, and Object Assembly are linked to right-hemisphere damage. The reader will note that these lateralizing signs refer to specific subtest scores rather than Verbal and Performance I.Q.'s.

This reported ability of some Wechsler subtests to lateralize brain damage in adults is solid argument against reliance upon any single test pattern as indication of organicity. However, equal sensitivity was not found for the Wechsler Intelligence Scale for Children (WISC) in a study of subjects with a mean age close to ten years (43). (Presumably, lateralization of function has been completed and then damaged in the adult patient, while it may still be developing in the child. Nonetheless, the same attention to differences between subtest functions on the WISC as is practiced with WAIS appears a good clinical procedure.)

The Wechsler scales permit the introduction of two procedures often productive of clues to brain damage: *testing the limits and the application of stress.* These procedures are possible without altering the standardized scoring, as they are instituted after the usual administration and scoring as an additional step.

A deficit in the attentional factor can be checked by readministering the Digit Symbol subtest, for example, with the request that the patient attempt to go faster on the second trial than he had done on the first. Ability to increase speed without loss of accuracy of location and form would suggest that the poorer first effort was not due to an organic factor but to an emotional or motivational one. Loss of speed and/or decreased accuracy may be strongly suggestive of the fatigability associated with organic conditions, after consideration is given to muscle weakness, depression, or regressiveness.

Stress can be added to the Block Design by readministering the subtest with the request that the patient now construct the designs block by block in a plane rotated 90° from the orientation of the design, in the approach of Satz (50).

Limits may be tested in a number of ways. On the Digit Span, should the patient fail to retain, say, six digits forward on two trials, a third set of six digits may be offered. Failure on the third trial confirms the limit of capability; success does not alter the scoring as a failure but brings it into question as a true limit. The requirement to recite the digit series backwards adds stress to the situation, and unusually large differences between the forward and backward series should not be assigned automatically to anxiety. Limits may be tested also by extending the time on the most difficult item failed by the patient on Arithmetic, Block Design, Picture Arrangement, and Object Assembly. Another technique is to tell the patient who has reached the allowable limit on Information, Comprehension, Similarities, Arithmetic, Picture Completion, Block Design, Picture Arrangement, or Object Assembly that there is another solution or arrangement for the last item or two he has taken and failed. He is asked to attempt a solution different from the one he had offered. Or a patient may be told that his construction of a Block Design or Object Assembly item constains an error. Can he find and correct it? This procedure may help distinguish between a true dysfunction and carelessness.

Another form of limit-testing is to request an explanation from the subject of any of his solutions or responses that appear unusual or perhaps bizarre. In Arithmetic, one may ask "How did you get that answer?" Or the patient may be asked to rethink his original answer without being told it is incorrect. In Vocabulary, Similarities, and Comprehension, one may ask "Tell me more about what you mean." On Picture Arrangement, one may ask the subject "Tell me the story as you see it," and with unusual arrangements on Object Assembly, one may ask "Tell me about this construction. Explain it to me."

I have found it helpful to estimate the capability of a patient to respond to additional clues beyond those provided by standardized directions of administration. The technique is analogous to the use of backgrounds of varying degrees of interference in assessing visual recognition. On Block Design, the examiner may construct part of the solution of the items the patient has failed, and then have the patient attempt to complete the design. The examiner begins with a small portion of the design and constructs larger portion if the patient is unsuccessful with the help provided by the first partial construction. Similar procedures can be followed with Picture Arrangement and

Object Assembly. Questions may be asked about Picture Completion items to direct the patient's attention to a consideration necessary for correct response. For example, if for the crab (item 15) the patient says "Some legs are missing," the examiner may ask after the entire test is finished, "How many legs are missing here?" while again showing the picture of the crab. Information about ability to respond to additional clues can be helpful to teachers of the patient, especially in remedial efforts, and to work supervisors in establishing how much of a field must be present for the patient to be able to carry the task on to completion.

A diagnostic problem difficult to clarify wtih the Wechsler scales has been the differentiation between organic brain-damage conditions and schizophrenia. Wechsler reports, without citing sources, that Performance functions are more adversely affected than Verbal functions in most mental disorders (with the exception of acting-out individuals), as well as in organic brain disease. One resolution of this difficulty may be implied in the effort by Birch and Walker (9) to differentiate brain-damaged and schizophrenic children in their ability to identify the Block Design item they had been unable to construct. This effort is based upon earlier work by Birch in association with Bortner, which demonstrated that both brain-damaged adults and brain-damaged children correctly identified the design they had failed to construct properly, while schizophrenic patients were less able to do so. DeWolfe (17, 18) found that schizophrenics do less well on Comprehension and better on Digit Span than do brain-damaged patients. Watson (56) seeking to replicate these findings confirmed them in one hospital population but not in another.

A related effort at differential diagnosis utilizing the Similarities subtest with children advocates an error-analysis approach, actually a clinical orientation to test data. Hall and La Driere (23) found that emotionally disturbed children more often offered an expansive error or a conceptually inadequate response, whereas the responses of brain-damaged children were characterized by restrictive errors, such as "don't know," or no response.

Success in lateralizing brain damage with some Wechsler subtests has spurred efforts to use them in localizing sites and identifying types of lesions. Such capacity of the subtests to localize must be considered hypothetical at this time; indeed such precision is not required of the psychotherapist who is seeking to rule out or rule in the possibility of brain damage and the need for specialized consultation.

A graphic demonstration of the value of Wechsler scales in neuro-psychodiagnosis is the inclusion of nine WAIS measures in the "key" approach to diagnosis developed by Russell, et al. (49). In addition to the Verbal, Performance, and Full Scale I.Q.'s, they use the Digit Symbol, Digit Span, Vocabulary, Similarities, Block Design, and Object Assembly subtest scores.

THE BENDER VISUAL MOTOR GESTALT TEST AND THE BENTON VISUAL RETENTION TEST

The Bender Visual Motor Gestalt Test is, as Koppitz (32) cogently observes, a complex visual-motor task that involves at least four identifiable stages: 1) perceiving the stimulus; 2) understanding what is seen; 3) translating the perception into a planned motor act; and 4) the motor act itself. In it, the patient is asked to copy designs of relatively simple nature.

Impairment in the functions tested, therefore, may be either receptive or expressive. Koppitz finds that most often, but not always, impairments of both processes are involved.

Long-established indications of organicity from the Bender are: rotations of the designs from the axis in which they are presented; distortions in reproduction; collisions in which designs are run together; disproportion between components of the design; use of circles, loops, or lines for dots; use of angles or straight lines for dots; use of angles or straight lines for curves; and perseverations.

A clinically rich developmental approach to the Bender has been evolved by Koppitz. All the distortions observed on the Bender occur in the productions of all children at some point in their development. Age norms are essential, therefore, since a distortion if age-appropriate is not significant; if, however, it persists beyond the age of expected additional capability, it bears diagnostic import.

Incidence of rotation increases with lower I.Q., so that this factor must be considered in evaluating a patient's drawings.

Several scoring systems are available for an effort to objectify interpretation. Among these are the Pascal-Suttell (40) scoring system, the Koppitz system (32), the Hutt-Briskin system (27), and the Hain method (22). The Pascal-Suttell system differentiates two types of rotation: type I is the usual rotation of 45 degrees or more; type II includes special instances of rotation on designs 4, 5, 6, and 7, and rotation of more than 45 degrees of design A and part of design 3.

Freed (20) uses this differentiation to show that non-psychotic neurological patients produced significantly more type II rotations than did psychotic and neurotic patients.

Some clinicians have found it useful to incorporate a memory component into the administration of the Bender by asking the patient, after the usual administration procedure, to draw as many of the designs as he can recall. The procedure is difficult to evaluate because of the intelligence factor, the varying complexity of the designs, and the decreasing time interval from exposure of the first design to the last.

My preferred procedure has been to introduce a memory component *before* the usual administration, using only designs A, 3, and 4. Each is exposed for a five-second interval, removed, and the patient is asked to reproduce it from memory. The usual style of administration then follows, using all of the designs. Comparison can be made of each design reproduced from memory and on direct copy; the variables of intelligence, design complexity, and time interval are eliminated.

Additional stress can be introduced by using Canter's Background Interference Procedure (13). The Bender is first administered in the usual way except that each design is drawn separately on its own sheet of blank paper. Other test material (WAIS, Rorschach) is then administered to facilitate extinction of memory of the designs. Then the patient is requested to draw the designs again, each upon its own sheet of paper which now contains a background of intersecting curved lines placed at random.

From her work with children, Koppitz (32) has identified clues in Bender drawings to the presence of brain damage. These are quite applicable to adults. Brain damage, if it impairs the complex receptive-expressive visual motor function assessed by the Bender, results in regression in that function. Her suggested clues are:

1) Excessive time.

2) Tracing designs with the finger.

3) Placing finger on the part of the design being drawn.

4) Preferring to draw from memory because sight of the card is found to be confusing.

5) Rotating the card and the paper to draw and then returning the paper to the correct position after the drawing is done.

6) Uncertainty about the number of dots and circles, despite several checkings of them.

7) Hasty drawings are made first, then erased and corrected with much effort.

8) Expression of dissatisfaction with drawings and efforts to correct them.

Some of these are similar to Piotrowski's (41) clues to brain damage on the Rorschach. Both the Rorschach and the Bender are visual-perceptive tasks, although the Bender requires a graphomotor response, and the Rorschach an oral-verbal expressive one; increased time, tracing, and anchoring with the finger have been observed to be spontaneous aids to an impaired visual-perceptive process.

Research evidence in support of the ability of the Bender and of Canter's variation, the Background Interference Procedure, to identify brain damage has been equivocal. Brain-damaged patients were significantly differentiated from psychiatric groups by scorings of their Bender reproductions, but not by their time scores, in a study by Rosecrans and Schaffer (47). Brain-damaged patients in a group did more poorly than a non-brain-damaged group when scored with the Koppitz Developmental score, Parsons, et al. (37) found. The Hutt-Briskin scoring system is reported by Johnson, et al. (28) to be relatively effective in identifying brain damage only with patients of Borderline or Dull Normal I.Q.'s. Mosher in reviewing Hutt's book (26) comments that the Bender is correlative only in the most obvious cases of brain damage. And Tymchuk (54) finds the Bender less effective in individual cases than in differentially diagnosing groups of brain-damaged persons from the non-brain-damaged. He suggests exploration of a scoring system that would combine evaluation of both errors and time.

Canter hypothesizes that his Background Interference Procedure (BIP) applied to the Bender can distinguish between brain damage and schizophrenia because of the mild arousal conditions the BIP presents (12). Kenny (29) found the BIP discriminated brain-damaged children from both emotionally disturbed and control groups better than did the standard Bender. Adams, Kenny and Canter (2), however, note that the BIP is much less sensitive to brain damage in children than in adults. Adams (4) found the ability of the BIP to contribute to the diagnosis of brain damage in mentally retarded children uncertain and that it did not discriminate hyperkinetic boys from controls (17). And Adams (3) in another study observed little difference between the Bender and the BIP with a group of heterogenously brain-damaged adults and a non-brain-damaged adult group of psychiatric patients, although the brain-damaged group made more errors on the Bender and deteriorated more on the BIP.

Smith (51) reminds us that the Bender Visual Motor Gestalt Test was not designed to explore possible brain damage but rather disturbances of psychological, emotional origin. He recommends instead the use of the Benton Visual Retention Test (7). The scoring system is well illustrated and easy to follow. Normative standards are provided for evaluating children and adults according to both "number correct" and "error" scores that take age, sex and intelligence levels into account. Three equivalent forms of the test are provided. Recall or memory is incorporated in the administrative design; in addition to direct copy of one of the forms, the patient is asked to reproduce the designs from memory five, ten and/or 15 seconds after exposure. Additionally, Smith observes that the designs incorporate right and left peripheral figures that are sensitive to homonymous hemianopsia and to unilateral spatial inattention. Two administrations of the test (one from recall, the second from direct copy) take only about ten minutes.

TESTS OF LATERAL HEMISPHERIC FUNCTIONING

These tests are the only additional procedures to be added to the standard psychological assessment battery. Their value is that the patient provides his own norm for comparison; he is not being compared with groups of other patients but with himself—one side of his body against the other, one type of function against another.

The Heimburger-Reitan Method

An easily administered test for lateralizing brain damage was developed by Heimburger and Reitan (24). They utilize four of 36 tests of aphasia that comprise the original Halstead-Wepman Aphasia Screening Test. Their choice of tests exploited the well-established dominance of the left hemisphere for language functions and of the right hemisphere for spatial and constructional tasks.

The subject is separately shown a line drawing of a square, of a triangle, and of a Greek cross. He is asked to copy each of the drawings without lifting his pencil from the paper, then to name each figure, and finally to spell the name of each.

Then the examiner says an unexpected sentence, "He shouted the warning." The subject is asked to repeat this sentence, to explain it, and finally to write it.

The tasks are simple, and none has been practiced by most patients. Language skills, naming, spelling and explaining are required. The first three tests also assess constructional praxis. The authors acknowledge that the test is not entirely ideal, but report that it still does a good job of separating patients with left-hemisphere damage from those with right-side lesions. The four simple tests are useful in checking upon hypotheses concerning language or spatial dysfunctions derived from administration and scoring of the Wechsler scales. These tests are utilized in the neuropsychological "key" method developed by Russell, et al. (49). They use a five-point rating scale for scoring the drawings of the Greek cross. Drawings illustrating each point on their scale are presented as guides, and the clinician just beginning to use the method will find these especially helpful.

Motor Tests

Simple and quickly administered motor tests assessing lateralization are the Purdue Peg Board, finger-tapping speed, and strength of grip. Strength of grip, of course, is measured by a dynamometer; three trials are run and an average obtained for each hand.

Instrumentation for testing speed of finger tapping can be constructed relatively cheaply; electronic circuity is used, so that strength is not being tested. The finger completes the circuit, the electrical impulse activates a counter. Three trials of 10 seconds each are administered for each hand and an average figure derived for each hand. Halstead utilized the finger-tapping speed test in his battery by measuring the dominant hand only. Reitan advocates its application to both hands, finding that damage to the left hemisphere, for example, will affect not only verbal skills but speed and strength of the contralateral hand.

The simple beauty of these methods is that each patient provides his own control. Suspicion of a lesion is created when the dominant hand is slower than the other hand or when the non-dominant hand is significantly slower than the dominant hand. In my experience, the non-dominant hand usually averages ten fewer contacts than the dominant hand in a ten second period on the finger-tapping speed test in an undamaged individual. Research is needed to establish norms and grades of significant difference.

Increasingly, I have come to rely on the Purdue Pegboard (14, 42, 55). Each hand is tested separately starting with the preferred hand, and then both in use simultaneously. The three procedures are then repeated and the results for each are averaged. The entire administration takes only about 10 minutes. Scoring is simple and norms are available (14).

PROJECTIVE TECHNIQUES

Projective techniques are not found in the batteries employed by most contemporary neuropsychologists, although originally Halstead showed the Rorschach blots on a screen and used multiple-choice questions about them in search of perceptual deficits, and Reitan has some early publications on the Rorschach. Despite the development of rating scales for Human Drawings and the early proliferation of systems of organic signs in the results of Rorschach, neither of these instruments has been used widely in identifying or lateralizing brain damage.

However, many pathological phenomena appearing with administration of the Human Figure Drawings and the Roschach may arise from neurological rather than psychological causes. Differentiation of organicity from psychogenesis from the projective tests alone is not possible, but when coupled with data from the WAIS and tests of lateralization, the value of projective data even on the neurological side increases.

At their most objective level, the Human Figure Drawings and the Rorschach involve specific processes: the Figure Drawings require grapho-motor representation of a mental concept of the human body; the Rorschach is a visual-perceptual stimulus requiring intermediate processes of recognition, integration, and naming, and an oral-verbal expressive response. Where lesions affect these functions or parts of them, administration of the techniques may reveal the dysfunctions.

On the Human Figure Drawings, distortions comparable to those appearing on the Bender or the Greek cross may appear, and difficulty in handling the pencil and controlling the drawn line may be observed; bilateral asymmetry may be prominent. On the Rorschach, pronounced difficulty in arriving at a perception satisfactory to the patient may be indicative of a dysfunction. This difficulty is identical with Piotrowski's Impotence sign, in which the patient is aware that his response is inadequate but is unable to improve it.

When certain pathologies appear, awareness of the possibility of more than one explanation leads the diagnostician to careful review of the data from the WAIS, the lateralization tests, the history and the special interviewing. On the Figure Drawings, robot-like drawings may reflect neurological disturbances in body image *or* rigidity of thinking and feeling. Over-emphasis upon detail may reflect the uncertainty of an organically-impaired individual *or* the careful control of the obsessive. Fragmentation of the body parts may arise from neurological difficulty in coalescence *or* the ego disruption of schizophrenia. A body outline rendered in short, separate, overlapping lines may be the expression of the schizophrenic feeling of vulnerability and failure of individuation through separation *or* the organically impaired patient's inability to sustain production of a line of more than a very short length.

Burgemeister (11) reviewed the various systems of Rorschach organic signs—Piotrowski (41), Hughes (25), Ross and Ross (48), Dorken and Kral (19), and Baker (5)—and found that their diagnostic valence could be weighted in any number of causal directions. From her own research and clinical experience, Burgemeister identified the Rorschach indices of greatest value in suggesting organicity as follows:

1) Piotrowski's *repetition of responses,* when it occurred in a person of upper-level intelligence.

2) Piotrowski's *perplexity* sign.

3) Piotrowski's *impotence* sign.

4) Piotrowski's *automatic phrasing.*

5) *Perseveration of content,* with inability to vary content when asked to do so. (Note: this is a limit-testing technique.)

6) *"Pickiness,"* or assigning major prominence to small details.

7) Indications of feeling of threat to integrity of the self in the content of responses.

8) Impairment of organizational ability.

9) Personalization of responses, suggesting impairment in abstract thinking.

10) Prominence given to a color in a response with passive content.

11) Catastrophic reaction of anxiety, or inability to muster a response.

Burgemeister emphasizes that the value of the Rorschach in neuropsychodiagnosis is dependent upon its integration with other test data. The uncertainty of Rorschach findings for neuropsychodiagnosis is apparent in the use of the technique in assessing the personality of epileptics. Mixtures of organic and neurotic features prevailed in the populations studied by Delay, *et al.* (16). Pathology was manifest in the *experience type* obtained. The epileptics tended to be either of a constricted type with relatively good social adjustmnt, or an extratensive type with poor social adjustment. Thus, the root pathology is not differentiated by the Rorschach; it could arise from the organic disease or from the individual's response to his disorder.

Baker (5) believes that the use of the Rorschach in neurodiagnostic efforts has stressed the intellectual aspects of the subject's approach to the blots rather than his emotional response. The Rorschach's value, she suggests, is in revealing a person's emotional reaction to the change in his ability to cope that he undergoes as a result of brain damage.

The clinician must consider both dimensions—the intellectual and the emotional—in assessing brain damage. Skill in this combined approach comes only with experience.

The single most important quality for the psychotherapist to develop in relationship to emotional disturbances is caution and skepticism concerning any single explanation or etiology. This necessity is stressed by the predicament in Rorschach diagnosis, a predicament shared by all psychodiagnosis: many similar symptoms are to be found among brain-damaged, physically ill, and functionally disturbed individuals.

Baker obviously had this predicament in mind as she reviewed some of the difficulties in differential diagnosis using the Rorschach:

1) The many hysterical symptoms associated with emotional response to brain damage are similar to those observed in psychosomatically and somatically ill persons.

2) The patient with *both* a functional psychosis and mild brain damage may defy differential diagnosis.

3) Perhaps the most difficult differential diagnostic problem is that presented by the person of low intelligence, poor education, and immature hysterical personality.

The value of projective techniques in neuropsychodiagnosis is related to their ability to detect dysfunction in the *nature of the process involved in the task they impose,* and in the individual's response to the alteration in adaptive ability produced by brain lesion. Birch and Diller (10a, 11) hypothesize that anatomical damage to the brain produces either subtractive or additive alterations in behavior. A lost sensory capability is illustrative of a subtractive alteration. Or, additively, a lesion may produce psychological disturbance unrelated to the amount of tissue destroyed. In this schema of brain-behavior relationships, amount of tissue loss does not necessarily correlate with degree of psychological disruption.

To test their hypothesis, Birch and Diller performed a unique experiment in which ten hemiplegic patients were divided into two groups of five each: those who exhibited Piotrowski's signs of organicity on the Rorschach and those who did not. From this dichotomy they were able to predict features of the examination postulated to be consequences of neurophysiological disturbances identified as "additive," such as labileness, disorientation, convulsions. In a reverse experiment, a second group of ten hemiplegics were divided into groups of five each on the basis of whether they exhibited "additive" or "subtractive" features. From this dichotomy it was possible to predict the presence of Piotrowski's signs; correlation of +.77 was obtained between the number of additive features and Piotrowski's signs.

The authors conclude that features associated with organicity on the Rorschach are a reflection of neurophysiological rather than neuroanatomical disturbance. They found that the most helpful of Piotrowski's signs are not unique to the Rorschach but appear also with other types of behavior. Low percentage of Popular responses and low percentage of Good Form were useful in distinguishing between their two groups of patients. Lower Response Total and paucity of Human Movement responses were not so helpful, because they also reflect depression and their appearance therefore may be caused by the individual's reaction to his illness rather than being primarily a result of neurodisintegration. The most effective Rorschach indicators were those shared with other clinical groups: Impotence and Perplexity. Perseveration was not so valuable, appearing in 90 percent of the organic patients and 50 percent of the non-organic patients. Scores and signs from the Rorschach test can be associated with brain damage, but the absence of organic signs does not mean that the individual does not have brain damage. Birch and Diller conclude that the Rorschach is not sensitive to brain damage *per se* but rather to the emotional-behavioral consequences of brain damage.

Two years later Birch and Belmont (10) turned from traditional scoring methods of the Rorschach to consider the kind of demands the Rorschach task imposes upon an individual. They identified three stages or levels of function inherent in the Rorschach task:

1) *The visual-verbal task.* The subject looks at a complex stimulus and gives an oral-verbal expressive report of his perception. Visual sensory input is related to the symbolic process; the figure-ground shading, shape, and color are organized within the person's ideational capability and content. The end result of a complicated process, the patient's response is a single Gestalt. Scoring for this task is "Well-Defined" or "Poorly-Defined."

2) *The perceptual-analytic task.* This is the response to the inquiry, in which the subject is asked to identify the components of the stimulus that entered into his response. This analysis requires an active review of possible blot qualities and characteristics, but may evoke new responses to the original percept. Scoring here is "Well-Analyzed" or "Poorly-Analyzed."

3) *The verbal-visual task.* This task requires the patient's response to the testing of limits. A percept not reported by the subject is suggested to him, to see if he can alter his original perception in accordance with the verbal suggestion. The subject's ability to offer a conception in accord with the verbal suggestion is scored "Accepted" or "Rejected."

The authors compared the protocols of 18 left-hemiplegic patients in the seventh decade of life with 16 orthopedic patients of the same age, but not neurologically damaged. The protocols were scored in Klopfer's manner, then rescored for the three task levels described above. The major difference observed was in the perceptual-analytic task: the brain-damaged group had greater difficulty analyzing perception into component and contributing parts. No differences of significance were observed in the visual-verbal or verbal-visual tasks. Traditional scoring found some of the brain-damaged group less productive, while others were similar to the non-damaged group in response total. Clarity of percept was inversely related to productivity: patients with low productivity offered higher proportions of clear-cut percepts at the visual-verbal level than did high productivity patients. Low productivity was also associated with better performance at the perceptual-analytic and verbal-visual tasks.

Belmont and Birch (6) speculate that the low-productivity group may have achieved a relatively constricted area of adequate functioning—similar to patients described by Goldstein who functioned well as long as the environment was limited, constant, and clearly defined—by limiting sensory input or their responses to it. The higher-productivity group, unable to develop such protective insulation, continued to react to a wide array of stimuli with inadequate responses. These findings are reminiscent of the observations by Delay, *et al.* (16) of bipolar Rorschach "experience" types among epileptics, with constriction more frequently associated with better social adjustment than was the case among the "expansive" type.

An extensive analysis of Rorschach organic signs is available in the Handbook by Goldfried, *et al.* (21) for the psychotherapist who may wish to pursue matters of validity and reliability in detail.

Generally, the Thematic Apperception Test (TAT) is not useful in neuropsychological diagnosis. Occasionally, perhaps rarely, a *severe* anomia, visual-perceptual difficulty or oral-verbal expressive disorder is apparent. But these, because severe, are likely to be more objectively evaluated by the Wechsler tests.

BIBLIOGRAPHY

1. *Adams, J., et al.:* The relationship between the Canter Background Interference Procedure and the hyperkinetic behavior syndrome. J. Learn. Dis., 7:2, 1974.
2. *Adams, J., et al.:* The efficacy of the Canter Background Interference Procedure in identifying children with cerebral dysfunctions. J. Consult. Clin. Psychol., 40:3, 1973.
3. *Adams, J.:* Comparison of task-central and task-peripheral forms of the Canter BIP in diagnosing brain damage in adults. Percept. Motor Skills, 33:3, 1971.
4. *Adams, J.:* Canter Background Interference Procedure applied to the diagnosis of brain damage in mentally retarded children. Amer. J. Ment. Deficiency, 75:1, 1970.
5. *Baker, G.:* Diagnosis of organic brain damage in the adult. *In* B. Klopfer (Ed.): Developments in the Rorschach Technique, II. Yonkers, N. Y.: World Book, 1952.
6. *Belmont, I.* and *Birch, H. G.:* "Productivity" and mode of function in the Rorschach responses of brain-damaged patients. J. Nerv. Ment. Dis., 134, 1962.
7. *Benton, A. L.:* Benton Visual Retention Test. New York: Psychological Corporation, 1955.
8. *Bersoff, D. N.:* The Revised Deterioration Formula for the Wechsler Adult Intelligence Scale: A test of validity. J. Clin. Psychol., 26:1, 1970.
9. *Birch, H. G.* and *Walker, H. A.:* Perceptual and perceptual-motor dissociation: Studies in schizophrenic and brain damaged psychotic children. Arch. Gen. Psychiat., 14, 1966.
10. *Birch, H. G.* and *Belmont, I.:* Functional levels of disturbance manifested by brain-damaged (hemiplegic) patients as revealed in Rorschach responses. J. Nerv. Ment. Dis., 132, 1961.
10a. *Birch, H. G.* and *Diller, L.:* Rorschach signs of "organicity": Physiological basis for perceptual disturbances. J. Proj. Tech., 23, 1959.
11. *Burgemeister, B. B.:* Psychological Techniques in Neurological Diagnosis. New York: Hoeber Med. Div., Harper & Row, 1962.
12. *Canter, A.:* A comparison of the background interference procedure effect in

schizophrenic, non-schizophrenic and organic patients. J. Clin. Psychol., 27:4, 1971.

13. *Canter, A.:* A background interference procedure to increase sensitivity of the Bender Gestalt Test to organic brain disorder. J. Consult. Psychol., 30, 1966.

14. *Costa, L. D., et al.:* Purdue Pegboard as a predictor of the presence and laterality of cerebral lesions. J. Consult. Psychol., 27, 1963.

15. *Davis, W. E., et al.:* Categorization of patients with personality disorders and acute brain trauma through WAIS subtest variations. J. Clin. Psychol., 27:3, 1971.

16. *Delay, J., et al.:* Rorschach and the Epileptic Personality. New York: Logos Press, 1958.

17. *DeWolfe, A. S.:* Differentiation of schizophrenic and brain damage with the WAIS. J. Clin. Psychol., 27:2, 1971.

18. *DeWolfe, A. S., et al.:* Intellectual deficit in chronic schizophrenia and brain damage. J. Consult. Clin. Psychol., 36:2, 1971.

19. *Dorken, H.* and *Kral, V. A.:* The psychological differentiation of organic brain lesions and their localization by means of the Rorschach test. Amer. J. Psychiat., 108, 1952.

20. *Freed, E. X.:* Actuarial data on Bender-Gestalt Test rotations by psychiatric patients. J. Clin. Psychol., 25:3, 1969.

21. *Goldfried, M. R., et al.:* Rorschach Handbook of Clinical and Research Applications. Englewood Cliffs, N. J.: Prentice-Hall, 1971.

22. *Hain, J. D.:* The Bender Gestalt Test: A scoring method for identifying brain damage. J. Consult. Psychol., 28:1, 1964.

23. *Hall, L. P.* and *La Driere, LaV.:* Patterns of performance on WISC Similarities in emotionally disturbed and brain-damaged children. J. Consult. Clin. Psychol., 33:3, 1969.

24. *Heimburger, R. F.* and *Reitan, R. M.:* Easily administered written test for lateralizing brain lesions. J. Neurosurg., 18, 1961.

25. *Hughes, R. M.:* A factor analysis of Rorschach diagnostic signs. J. Gen. Psychol., 43, 1950.

26. *Hutt, M. L.* (Ed.): The Hutt Adaptation of the Bender-Gestalt Test. 2nd ed. New York: Grune and Stratton, 1969.

27. *Hutt, M. L.* and *Briskin, G.:* The Clinical Use of the Revised Bender-Gestalt Test. New York: Grune and Stratton, 1960.

28. *Johnson, J. E., et al.:* The relationship between intelligence, brain damage, and Hutt-Briskin errors on the Bender-Gestalt. J. Clin. Psychol., 27:1, 1971.

29. *Kenny, T. J.:* Background interference procedure: A means of assessing neurologic dysfunction in school-age children. J. Consult. Clin. Psychol., 37:1, 1971.

30. *Klebanoff, S. G., et al.:* Psychological consequences of brain lesions and ablations. Psychol. Bull., 51:1, 1954.

31. *Koestline, W. C.* and *Dent, C. D.:* Verbal mediation in the WAIS Digit Symbol subtest. Psychological Reports, 25:2, 1969.

32. *Koppitz, E. M.:* The Bender Gestalt Test for Younger Children. New York: Grune and Stratton, 1963.

33. *Luria, A. R.:* Higher Cortical Functions in Man. New York: Basic Books, 1966.

34. *McFie, J.:* Assessment of Organic Intellectual Impairment. London: Academic Books, 1975.

35. *McFie, J.* and *Thompson, J. A.:* Picture arrangement: A measure of frontal lobe function. Brit. J. Psychiat., 121:564, 1972.

36. *Matarazzo, J. D.:* Wechsler's Measurement and Appraisal of Adult Intelligence. Fifth Edition. Baltimore: Williams and Wilkins, 1972.

37. *Parsons, L. B., et al.:* Validity of Koppitz's Developmental Score as a measure of organicity. Percept. Motor Skills, 33:3, 1971.
38. *Parsons, O. A.* and *Vega, A.:* Different psychological effects of lateralized brain damage. J. Consult. Clin. Psychol., 33:5, 1969.
39. *Parsons, O. A., et al.:* Agitation, anxiety, brain-damage and perceptual-motor deficit. J. Clin. Psych., 1963.
40. *Pascal, G. R.* and *Suttell, B. J.:* The Bender Gestalt Test. New York: Grune and Stratton, 1951.
41. *Piotrowski, Z.:* The Rorschach ink-blot method in organic disturbance of the central nervous system. J. Nerv. Ment. Dis., 86, 1937.
42. *Rapin, I., et al.:* Evaluation of the Purdue Pegboard as a screening test of brain damage. Develop. Med. Child Neurol., 8, 1966.
43. *Reed, J. C.* and *Reitan, R. M.:* Verbal and performance differences among brain injured children with lateralized motor deficits. Percept. Motor Skills, 29, 1969.
44. *Reed, J. C., et al.:* The influence of cerebral lesions on the psychological test performance of older children. J. Consult. Psychol., 29, 1965.
45. *Reitan, R. M.:* Psychological effects of cerebral lesions in children of early school age., Mimeo, 1970.
46. *Reitan, R. M.* and *Heineman, C. E.:* Interaction of neurological deficits and emotional disturbance in children with learning disorders: Methods for differential assessment. Indiana University Medical Center and Fort Wayne Child Guidance Clinic. Mimeo, undated.
47. *Rosecrans, C. J.* and *Schaffer, H. B.:* Bender-Gestalt time and score differences between matched groups of hospitalized psychiatric and brain-damaged patients. J. Clin. Psychol., 25:4, 1969.
48. *Ross, W. D.* and *Ross, S.:* Some Rorschach ratings of clinical value. Rorschach Res. Ex., 8, 1944.
49. *Russell, E. W., et al.:* Assessment of Brain Damage. New York: Wiley-Interscience, 1970.
50. *Satz, P.:* A block rotation task: The application of multivariate and decision theory analysis for the prediction of organic brain disorder. Psychol. Monog., 80:21, 1966.
51. *Smith, A.:* Neuropsychological testing in neurological disorders. *In* W. J. Friedlander (Ed): Advances in Neurology. New York: Raven Press, 1975.
52. *Smith, A.:* Certain hypothesized hemispheric differences in language and visual functions in human adults. Cortex, 2, 1966.
53. *Smith A.:* Verbal and nonverbal test performance of patients with "acute" lateralized brain lesions (tumors). J. Nerv. Ment. Dis., 141, 1965.
54. *Tymchuk, A. J.:* Comparison of Bender error and time scores for groups of epileptic, retarded, and behavior-problem children. Percept. Motor Skills, 38:1, 1974.
55. *Vega, Jr., A.:* Use of Purdue Pegboard and Finger Tapping performance as a rapid screening test for brain damage. J. Clin. Psychol., 25:3, 1969.
56. *Watson, C. G.:* Cross-validation of a WAIS sign developed to separate brain-damaged from schizophrenic patients. J. Clin. Psychol., 28:1, 1972.
57. *Wechsler, D.:* The Measurement and Appraisal of Adult Intelligence. Baltimore: Williams and Wilkins, 1958.
58. *Wechsler, D.:* The Measurement of Adult Intelligence. Baltimore: Williams and Wilkins, 1944.
59. *Witkin, H. A., et al.:* Psychological Differentiation. New York: John Wiley, 1950.

CHAPTER 12

The Neurological Consultation

From the variety of diagnostic procedures suggested here, evidence may accumulate to suggest to the psychotherapist that some of his patient's behavior and suffering may be neurologically determined. To summarize, grounds for suspecting a neurological implication are indicated when:

1) The history includes events or conditions of etiological significance, such as birth injuries or difficulties, traumas, febrile episodes, prolonged anesthesias, poisonings, certain diseases, or persistent learning difficulties, school problems, or behavior disorders.

2) The patient complains of paroxysmal phenomena or the therapist detects them, involving any sensory modality, or such factors as balance, altered states of consciousness, memory losses, or automatic behavior.

3) The psychological-test data reveal a variation among brain functions that exceeds the usual expectation for variation on the Wechsler scales, or pronounced organic indications on the Bender, the lateralization tests, or the projective techniques.

4) Disturbing emotional states (such as anxiety, depersonalization, *déjà vu* experiences, depression, hypochondriasis) cannot be clearly connected in psychodynamic terms to etiology, precipitating circumstances, or meaning to the patient.

5) A sudden emotional change has occurred which cannot be ascribed to specific precipitating circumstances, and the change is accompanied by disturbances of sleep, ravenous hunger and/or thirst, metabolic disorders, or changes in sexual appetite.

6) The patient complains of a gradual alteration in vision, hearing,

307

touch, motor control, balance, or skills such as typing or playing of musical instruments, or the therapist uncovers such changes.

Suspicion becomes probability and increases as the data from one source is bulwarked by confirming data from another source.

If the clinical review is convincing enough, the therapist faces the question: What to do next? Proceed with psychotherapy and keep the symptoms under observation? Refer the patient to a neurologist for examination?

An intermediate step is available here in which we can discharge our ethical responsibility not to make judgments beyond our training, while safeguarding the well-being of the patient and avoiding unnecessary alarm to him. This step requires that the psychotherapist develop profession liaison with a neurologist. The neurologist must be knowledgeable about and respect cognitive and behavioral manifestations, able and willing to evaluate data from the history, clinical observation, and psychological tests communicated to him by the psychotherapist, and willing to arrive at an estimate of the probability that neurological and related instrumental examinations are justifiable. The cooperating neurologist should be known to practice persistent care in exploring for symptomatology in the face of a patient's anxiety or depression, language difficulties, limited intelligence, and perhaps seemingly psychotic behavior.

Within such a professional liaison, telephone consultations can serve to guide the psychotherapist. When the probability justifies neurological exploration, the therapist must present the patient with the possibility that some of his symptoms may have a neurological base, and that the success of psychotherapy may depend upon appropriate medical treatment for a neurological condition if it is found to exist.

If the neurologist suspects, from the data given to him by the therapist, that an expanding lesion is present, and the patient's life is at stake, the therapist must make every effort to persuade the patient to cooperate with the neurological exploration. How far the therapist goes in making the danger to life explicit will depend upon the probabilities delineated for him by the neurologist. He may in case of eminent danger to life make a flat-footed statement of such danger, coupled with the offer to continue therapy centered around the critical matter of the patient's rejection of a possibly lifesaving recommendation or his denial of a life-endangering possibility

If the neurologist suspects a static lesion of long standing, a neurological examination may be of value in that it may set realistic expectations for the psychotherapy. Or prescribable medication may be expected to ameliorate the symptoms somewhat. Such good fortune might be obtainable for patients with the paradoxical reaction to amphetamines in minimal brain dysfunction, or for patients with psychomotor epilepsy who can be relieved with one of the several available anti-convulsants.

This telephonic neurological consultation, therefore, should be part of the practicing equipment of the psychotherapist, just as is regular consultation with other professional specialists.

An important factor in the use of neurologic consultation is the therapist's willingness to face his own, often unconscious, reaction to the very idea of a neurological lesion. (Dr. Rogers Wright has prodded me into this reflection.) While we cannot minimize the potentialities for pain, loss of function, and death as possible concomitants of a brain lesion, nor the dread of these, we cannot hide from them if they exist. Nor should we ignore the vast reassurance and relief that can be given a patient when mysterious symptoms are elucidated. The facts must be sought.

CHAPTER 13

Implications for Treatment

Two major principles to guide the treatment of the brain-damaged person were discussed in earlier chapters on specific conditions. (Chapter 2 *Minimal Brain Dysfunction;* Chapter 3 *Epilepsy;* Chapter 4 *Aphasia and Dysphasia;* Chapter 5 *Schizophrenia;* Chapter 6 *Mental Retardation;* Chapter 8 *Other Disorders with Equivocal Etiology.*)

1) The patient should not be categorized automatically into a general group with all other brain-damaged individuals; his limitation in functions and his emotional problems in relationship to his limitations must be individually assessed. Children with damaged brains may suffer from any type of psychiatric condition (16). Not all, for example, become disorganized; some, in a defensive reaction, become compulsively orderly to a degree that may approach the pathological, in a desperate effort to maintain control over their world and themselves (5). The life task of individuation and separation from the parents, as another example, is more difficult for the brain-damaged child and adolescent, but its impact often varies according to the stage of the psychosexual development and the quality of the supporting family and culture.

The brain-damaged person is handicapped. When his brain damage is severe and manifest, he is clearly subject to the same internal and external stresses that other physically handicapped persons experience. But in the cases of minimal, equivocal conditions of cerebral dysfunction, the handicap may not be grossly manifest. The victim may perceive his limitations rather specifically, or vaguely sense that something is wrong with him, that there are tasks that he cannot master. To the outsider—parents, teachers, friends—he may seem inept, stubborn, unmotivated, negativistic. Shelsky (17) has shown that a visible impairment is not necessarily more injurious to self-concept than one that it

310

is not manifest. Anxiety, depression, self-doubt, withdrawal, and lowered self-esteem are the lot of both the manifestly and the minimally brain-injured person, although not always in the same way or degree.

2) Treatment of the brain-damaged individual requires multiple efforts which may draw upon remedial instruction, special training, environmental manipulation and structuring, medication under expert guidance, psychotherapy, counseling, social casework with the patient and his family, or behavioral modification. Indispensable to the therapist is a roster of special services and training available in the community. Among the possibilities, the therapist must be able to assign priorities in a treatment program. Where self-esteem is badly damaged by cognitive failure, remediation or "ortho-education" may take precedence over psychotherapy, or initially only supportive interventions may be indicated (15). An overly-tense or hyperactive patient may best be first helped to develop skill in relaxation through basic meditation procedures (21), hypnosis (20), operant conditioning (6, 8, 11) or biofeedback procedures (4, 14). An adult victim of recent brain damage, weighted with a negative self-concept not readily expressed in words, may respond initially to an art therapy approach (9). Or the parents rather than the patient may be selected as the first focus for intervention when a child whose behavior they find hard to manage is evoking destructive responses from them (19).

A schema applicable to the treatment of the brain-damaged person is suggested in the work of Kraines (13) with neurosis. He postulates that the cortex interacts with the hypothalamus in what he calls the "emotional circuit" to produce neurotic reactions. In this schema, the cortex, which has no emotional tone itself, analyzes a stimulus conceptually, activates a response pattern in the hypothalamus, from which impulses activate the subcortical nuclei, endocrines, viscera, and musculature. These impulses then return through the recticular system and the thalamus to be integrated in the limbic system. Kraines reasons that the ideal therapeutic program for neurosis would have two thrusts: 1) improving cortical conceptualization of stress situations through psychotherapy; 2) reducing hyperactivity in the emotional circuit by physiological means (drugs) and conditioning procedures (reciprocal inhibition, operant conditioning, and hypnosis).

Whatever one's view of his thesis that neurosis is more than a psychic reaction, it can be reversed or changed in emphasis to conceptualize the brain-damaged individual, whose damage also almost always involves a psychic reaction. Kraines' two elements of treatment retain validity with the brain-damaged person. To these must be added a third and fourth treatment effort often required for the brain-damaged individual: alteration and control of his environment, and special instruction.

The traditionally trained psychotherapist—whatever his orientation —may well overlook one or more of the additional treatment efforts the brain-damaged patient will need. The psychoanalytically-oriented therapist is likely to pursue modification of cortical conceptualization through resolution of an assumed, but not necessarily extent, conflict. The behavioral therapist and the drug-prescribing therapist are seeking a neurophysiological quieting. The rehabilitation worker and the remedial teacher strive for the acquisition of a new or substitute skill. The family therapist will attempt to obtain improved communication and understanding within the family. The neurologically-impaired individual will probably need all of these efforts in his behalf simultaneously if he is to be saved from a confrontation with catastrophe.

Brain damage does not preclude the advisability of insight-oriented psychotherapy. It does, however, mandate departures from the customary psychodynamic conceptualization of symptoms and behavior, conflict as a cause, insight as a cure. The treatment of the brain-damaged has thus benefited from the work of Goldstein (10), who sensitively mapped the narrow, fragile separation between failure and catastrophe for the brain-damaged individual. Usually, the impairment of cerebral functions contributes to difficulty in discharging tension by impairing capacity for successful adaptation, depending upon the nature of the functions and/or the degree to which they are impaired. Some impaired persons will be unable to tolerate shifts because of the tension inherent in the shifting process. Some cannot sustain a close relationship, which they may very much need, if bearing tension is necessary to sustain the relationship. Failures in these and other adaptations interfere with self-realization; they endanger the very existence of the individual, and forbode catastrophe for him.

The brain-damaged person, Goldstein observes, spontaneously develops protective mechanisms to forestall anxiety and the catastrophic fear: he may deny his incapacity; he may withdraw from activities and interpersonal contacts in order to avoid failures; he may become compulsively involved with the activities which he finds he can master, where his competence is unquestioned, and where he avoids confrontation with failure. These *protective* mechanisms, Goldstein argues, must be carefully understood as different from *defensive* mechanisms in the psychodynamic sense. Compulsive behavior, for example, in both the brain-damaged and neurotic person may originate as defense against anxiety. In the former, it is born of inability to function or as a way to keep from feeling overwhelmed by a shifting external environment. In the latter it arises from conflict. Goldstein reasons that treatment, therefore, of the brain-damaged individual should focus upon prevention of catastrophe. The therapeutic task is to help the organism make a new adjustment to life through both physical and psychological means, despite abnormal functioning.

In this effort, every and any type of intervention that can reasonably be understood to help a given individual avoid a specific failure has a respected role: medications to reduce hyperactivity, to mitigate anxiety arising from failure or contributing to failure, to restore metabolic equilibrium in brain cells; remedial instruction to increase the power of intact functions, to strengthen weak ones with repetition or to develop new pathways; a special program in a rehabilitation-workshop to develop new employable skills for those that had been lost, or to develop them where they have not before existed; environmental manipulation and structuring to withdraw the patient from activities where he must fail, to place him in those where he can succeed, to modify others to the extent necessary for him to succeed with them, to control the demands placed upon him by family, covertly or overtly; psychotherapy to provide unchallenging understanding, and to strengthen the reality testing he needs to cooperate with necessary medical and instructional programs, to select areas of success and avoid those of failure, to improve impulse control, repair damage to self-esteem, and improve object relations.

There are within the psychoanalytic literature at least two familiar rubrics that may serve the psychodynamically oriented therapist well, with which he may be comfortable:

1) Kardiner's (12) conceptualization of the traumatic neurosis as a failure of adaptive capacity, and his prescription for the development of new and the restoration of old "action syndromes," that is, competence in specific adaptive functions.

2) Bellak's (2, 3) ego-function assessment as a guide to psychotherapy which encourages detailed diagnosis of weaknesses and strengths, and rational utilization of an armamentarium of treatment intervention based upon diagnosis (1).

Is insight therapy possible with the brain damaged? Christ (7) uses the concepts of Piaget diagnostically to answer this question with children. If the brain-damaged child is functioning cognitively at the "preoperational or sensorimotor stage," insight therapy is not possible. They are in effect so self-oriented that they are unable to deal with generalizations or mobilize empathy. New situations, altered routines, are tantamount to crises for them and they require crisis management to establish predictable sequences. The need to shift and to adjust to new elements provokes rapid disorganization, but, he notes, reintegration is equally rapid with straightforward situational interpretations, instruction, support, and operant conditioning.

Brain-damaged children who function at a higher level, the "concrete and formal operational stage," are amenable to insight, he finds. They are able to see and feel outside themselves, to think hypothetically, to see situations from the point of view of others, to use deductive logic.

Insight involves the interaction of cognition and affect, and the ability of the individual brain-damaged patient to achieve and benefit from the insight depends upon that interaction. The therapist must make the determination with each patient. The nature and degree of cognitive defect influence the patient's understanding of situations, statements, interactions. Failure to react appropriately, either cognitively or emotionally, may result from failure to understand the situation. As Goldstein (10) observes, inappropriate expressions of anxiety, humor and other affects may reflect such cognitive misunderstanding. But also operating is the need to discharge tension as quickly as possible, so that the therapist must not assume that a seeming emotional over-reaction is cognitively inappropriate to the situation.

The psychotherapist tends to look for repression as one indication of conflict. He must keep in mind that faulty memory may be conflict-free, that the capacity for retention of experience in a brain-damaged person may be weak, or that once-established memory traces may have been wiped out. The interpretation "You want to forget; you are afraid to remember" may drive the patient up against an impenetrable barrier in his effort to cooperate in a task for which he is poorly equipped. Emotional re-education may be the best approach, through the offering of the therapist's personal reactions or the interpretation of the universality of many reactions. The patient by repeated discussion may be helped to see that almost everyone including the therapist would react to or feel in a given situation in a given way and so it is probable that the patient has forgotten that he, too, reacted in that way.

The therapist may find that he must modify his method of working with resistance if not his very concept of it. Brain damage often results in regression to earlier forms of behavior, necessitated because higher levels of cognition and integrative capacity are impaired. As healing takes place, many patients cling to the earlier behavioral mode, even though it is no longer necessary. Careful encouragement, support, and step-by-step hierarchical training are necessary to enable such a patient to utilize his restored capabilities. If his slow relinquishing is dealt with as resistance, the patient may feel under pressure to abandon the regressive clinging more quickly than he can tolerate. A modified concept of resistance allows the therapist to be flexible in accepting, even encouraging, interruptions of sessions for varying lengths of time to allow the patient to "try it on his own" or to have time in his schedule for an activity that otherwise he might have to forego. Provisions of sessions much shorter than the traditional length will also seem reasonable when the therapist understands that the patient is burdened with a short attention span rather than that he is being resistant.

Diagnosis of other defenses should be carefully scrutinized. Aversions need not be accompanied by decathexis in the schizoid sense, even though the patient lives in isolation; pain of loneliness and fear of rejection for cognitive inadequacy can co-exist with withdrawal. Obsessive-compulsive behavior may be more a repeated demonstration of performance competence in a small area, serving to maintain a feeling of "I can do something," than an unconscious effort to control impulses.

Denial, when severe and pervasive, is probably the most difficult of the defenses to penetrate. Therapists are correctly wary of any effort at its hasty removal, sensing its protective necessity to the patient who without the defense may be exposed to an intolerable view of himself. Denial is widely used by handicapped persons to protect their self-esteem, a use in which they are likely to be encouraged by parents eager to protect their child from pain and anxiety. If the handicapped patient is to take on the tasks and make the efforts necessary to circumvent or overcome his dysfunctions, he and his family must be helped to substitute an increasingly realistic view of his situation, capabilities, and difficulties for the more distorted picture the denial allows. Goldstein (10) warns that denial in the brain-damaged person is among his efforts to avoid the sense of catastrophe. This caution does not mean that the effort should not be made, nor that it is most likely to fail. Many such patients sense that something is wrong with their brain, as was widely expressed by Sam, the patient described at the start of this book, but have been diverted from realistic awareness by the misguided "protective" impulse of family and therapists. Recognition of a handicap and understanding of its origins and parameters are necessary to habilitation and rehabilitation efforts.

Approaching this task requires perceptiveness, courage, good judgment and skill in interpretation from the therapist, as does all psychotherapy. Confrontation carries risks of intensifying the denial and precipitating a catastrophic reaction (18). But the necessity to develop a realistic and clear view of defects is imperative, as Christ (7) states. This requires that denial be penetrated so that behavioral, emotional, and learning problems are faced, examined, clarified, related to the basic diagnosis, and to the patient's self-concept. As with all patients who use denial, the effort should not be a confrontation but a gradual focus on reality that continuously tests for the patient's ego tolerance as it proceeds. Partial interpretations should precede the ultimate one so that time is allowed for a reaction to the partial interpretation to develop and be judged. Often a patient needs only to be asked what he thinks is the cause of his difficulties for him to express and thus engage the ultimate question.

Another technique is to encourage the substitution of a more "negotiable" defense (rationalization, for example) for denial. Still another turns attention to the patient's goals rather than to insight and clarification of his emotional patterns. The patient's perception of a goal's enormity is likely to correlate positively with both degree of denial and the danger of a catastrophic reaction. Setting a series of goals, each achievable in short-range and each introduced only after the preceding one has been achieved, guards against increasing defensiveness by increasing stress.

The therapist must be undisturbed by the rationalizations of the neurological-impaired patient in his effort to conceal failures and inadequacies. These may be irritating to the unwary therapist, because many such defensive efforts will seem so blatantly obvious. Nor must the therapist be disturbed by the quick hyperirritability, the explosive anger, most often verbal, of the rapidly escalating and ebbing emotional flurries that have been likened to summer storms. The brain-damaged person may erupt into loud obscenities and in the next moment be sweetly friendly. The obscenity protects his self-esteem; the friendliness is his apology and effort to keep a friend. The therapist must be alert to any language difficulties of the brain-damaged patient, to those intrusions of aphasic barriers to easy expression and comprehension that may mimic a thought disorder or mental retardation.

Secondary gains are, of course, as likely in the recovered neurological patient as in others, and may require therapeutic work. But what the brain-damaged person is asked to do, through giving up the pleasure of passivity and special attention, must be kept within his competence. The therapist must be careful to keep his demands within the patient's competence by virtue of healing or training, or by calling upon a capacity that was never impaired. Untimely pressure upon activity or task, or even upon independence, may promote regression.

Perhaps the most pronounced change required of the psychotherapist by the brain damaged is in the amount of activity that must characterize his participation in the treatment relationship. Therapist anonymity, passivity, and insistence that the patient develop his ego strength by making his own decisions are almost certain to forbode failure with many brain-damaged patients. Seeking to resolve anxiety by a resolution of conflict through choice when the anxiety generates from failure of adaptive capacity only increases that anxiety. The psychotherapist of the brain-damaged person must not only be a diagnostician; he must be an active therapist, serving steadfastly as tutor, encourager, discourager, judge, and guide. He must be willing, especially with the younger patients, to help parents, often in direct ways, often indirectly by encouraging them to seek information from and affiliation with other parents of brain-damaged children. The therapist himself must actively keep in touch with scientific, professional, social, and legal developments in the field.

To place first things last, we should stress that the major intervention in the psychotherapy of the brain-damaged person is the nature of the therapeutic alliance. This must be positive and open from the first contact. The patient must know that the therapist is on his side, that he is constantly so through hell and high water, through failures, rages, anxieties, and depressions. The positive alliance communicates that the patient and therapist are working together for the patient's benefit. The positive therapeutic alliance helps the patient accept clarification of reality, the penetration of denial, the setting of and working toward achievable goals. The alliance imparts support and understanding; it exacts application to goals. Failure of the therapist to understand the brain-damaged person's emotional reaction is likely to precipitate a catastrophic reaction. Failure to help the patient into reconstructive efforts is likely to leave the patient mired in a sense of helplessness and futility.

The nature of the alliance with a patient is determined by consideration of the patient's cognitive assets and deficits, his emotional status, and his psychosexual developmental level. Obviously, if the patient is a child, the parents are more readily and logically incorporated into the treatment alliance. The child's progress into adolescence and adulthood must be supported by changes in the alliance that emphasize the patient's increasing need and capacity for autonomy and individuation from them. But equally patent is the clinical reality that some brain-damaged adolescents and adults will need and benefit from more protracted support and dependency.

Finally, last things last. Termination, in Christ's (7) phrasing, may well be interminable. The therapist must be willing to continue with the patient long past the point where cognitive success is achieved if emotional fragility remains. The on-going relationship may be continuous, unbroken, or it may become an irregular on-demand one in which the patient manages on his own with occasional returns to the alliance as he encounters new stresses. The willingness of the patient to use the alliance in this manner is itself solid indication that the alliance has been successful.

BIBLIOGRAPHY

1. *Bellak, L.* and *Small, L.:* Emergency Psychotherapy and Brief Psychotherapy. Second edition. New York: Grune and Stratton, 1978.
2. *Bellak, L.* (Ed.): Schizophrenia: A Review of the Syndrome. New York: Logos Press, 1958.
3. *Bellak, L.:* The psychoanalytic concept of the ego and schizophrenia. *In* L. Bellak (Ed.): Schizophrenia: A Review of the Syndrome. New York: Logos Press, 1958.
4. *Brown, B. B.:* New Mind, New Body: Bio-feedback. New York: Harper & Row, 1974.
5. *Brown, G. W.:* Suggestions for parents. J. Learning Disabilities, 2:2, 1969.
6. *Browning, R. M.* and *Stover, D. O.:* Behavior Modification in Child Treatment. Chicago: Aldine-Atherton, 1971.
7. *Christ, A. E.:* Psychotherapy of the child with true brain damage. Amer. J. Orthopsychiat., 48:3, 1978.
8. Conditioned Learning in the Brain-Damaged Child. Literature Search No. 70-17, January 1967 to March, 1970. Washington, D. C.: U.S. Dept. of Health, Education and Welfare.
9. *Dodd, F. G.:* Art therapy with a brain-damaged man. Amer. J. Art Therapy, 14:3, 1975.
10. *Goldstein, K.:* The effect of brain damage on the personality. Psychiat., 15, 1952.

11. *Goodkin, R.:* Case studies in behavioral research in rehabilitation. Percept. Motor Skills, 23, 1966.

12. *Kardiner, A.:* The Traumatic Neuroses of War. New York: Hoeber, 1941.

13. *Kraines, S. H.:* The neurophysiologic basis of neuroses. Psychosomatics, 10:5, 1969.

14. *Lazarus, R. S.:* A cognitively oriented psychologist looks at biofeedback. Amer. Psychol., May, 1975.

15. *Lempp, R.:* Psychotherapy or ortho-education of children with slight early brain damage. Acta Paedopsychiatrica, 39:7, 1973.

16. *Shaffer, D.:* Psychiatric aspects of brain injury in childhood: A review. Devel. Med. Child. Neurol., 15:2, 1973.

17. *Shelsky, I.:* The effect of disability on self concepts. Unpublished doctoral dissertation. Teachers College, Columbia University, 1957.

18. *Small, L.:* The Briefer Psychotherapies. Revised edition. New York: Brunner/ Mazel, 1979.

19. *Stabler, B., et al.:* Parents as therapist: An innovative community-based model. Prof. Psychology, Nov., 1973.

20. *Sullivan, D. S., et al.:* Reduction of behavioral deficit in organic brain damage by use of hypnosis. J. Clin. Psychol., 30:1, 1974.

21. *Swinyard, C. A., et al.:* Neurological and behavioral aspects of transcendental meditation relevant to alcoholism. Annals N. Y. Acad. Sci., 233, 1974.

III

NEUROPSYCHOLOGY AND
NEUROPSYCHODIAGNOSIS

Psychology and medicine are both described as science-professions, and indeed, their practice is derived from, closely related to, and dependent upon the research scientist. It is to the scientist that the professional practitioner looks for the upgrading of his methods for new insights and the unraveling of old mysteries.

Students of both professions are exposed to the sciences as an integral part of their training, and some few always remain scientists as they practice, using their clinical populations as their research universe. For most, the diagnostic aspect is perhaps the most closely related to the scientific heritage, demanding the rigor of thinking, the respect for alternatives, the weighing of probabilities, the precise observation and careful evaluation of data that are the hallmarks of scientific inquiry.

Neuropsychodiagnosis is the child of neuropsychology, in its turn the offspring of neurology and psychology. This section surveys these fields for the psychotherapist, delineates the relationships that have been developed between them, and describes their integration into a clinically applicable body of knowledge.

CHAPTER 14

The Brain and Behavior

We return here to the science underlying all that has been advocated in this book: Neuropsychology, the study of brain-behavior relationships. Behavior is concerned with adaptation; the brain in its role of integrating and acting upon information arriving from the various senses is the principal organ of adaptation. Ability of the brain to receive, assimilate, and organize varied inputs underlies the capacity of the higher animals for plasticity of behavior and its modification. These abilities provide the organism with the potential for variety, flexibility, and choice of response, in contrast to the narrow repertoire of lower forms of life. Birch and Belmont (1) cite Sherrington's observation that the course of evolution has not been to increase the number of sensory organs in the higher organisms but rather to bring the five major sensory modalities into closer touch with each other so that the brain became a "central clearing house of sense" (7), an organ of intersensory integration.

The complex activities of this complex organ of integration can be viewed rather simply by considering the number of tasks it is called upon to mediate, initiate, and respond to. Another simple view is to consider the number of modalities through which the brain receives information (sensory input), the methods of response of which it is capable (output), and the seemingly infinite levels of integration within the brain that intervene between the two. The permutations of these variables are incredibly large, and their full number is probably not yet appreciated. Mark (4) has calculated that a total of 42,432 data points are fundamental to an analysis of the integrity of the brain in a patient suspected of Minimal Brain Dysfunction.

The complex role of the brain in adaptive, integrated behavior became manifest through the minute observation and testing of the

323

effects of brain pathology. As in embryology or stomach physiology, for examples, knowledge of normal anatomy and functioning in the brain has been facilitated by, even dependent upon, the study of pathology; here the behavioral and psychological deficits can be associated with injuries to the brain.

Some order has been brought to this complexity by increasingly strict adherence to scientific methods: random selection of brain-damaged patients studied, increase in size of populations, standardization of observational and testing methods, and the controlled ablation of brain locales in animals by laboratory methods. Earlier studies were content to draw conclusions from isolated, so-called "pure" cases. Resounding arguments were the rule between workers who would precisely localize the anatomical seat of functions within the brain and those who held that the whole of the brain was involved in all behavior, arguing that localization of function was fantasy, not fact. These have been essentially debates between the clinician and the experimentalist, with opposing orientation.

The history of the study of aphasia is a prototype of the course of development of the field of neuropsychology, Geschwind (2) traces this course from Broca's report in 1861 that disorders of language were associated with localized lesions of the brain. Holistic explanations countered the mosaic ones. While both approaches resulted in valuable contributions, considerably more advance was made by Wernicke's advocacy of a connectionist understanding of brain function. Thus the study of the complex brain-behavior relationship has sought to associate anatomy with behavior, has pursued this search through pathology, and has created historically at least three theoretical camps: mosaicist, holistic, and connectionist.

The assumption of the mosaicist is that a behavioral function is exquisitely located or represented within the brain, and that pathology, if circumscribed, will be reflected in that function alone, producing a specific behavioral defect. Some, while still subscribing to a mosaicist position, view this assumed result as a gross underestimation of the inevitably complex effects of any brain lesion because of the multiple variables, both independent and dependent, that operate.

The holistic view denies the confinement of location and representation to specific areas of the brain; its holders argue that the entire brain participates in all functions and that the entire brain is in some way affected by an injury or lesion. Kurt Goldstein (3), a respected advocate of this view, considered that a brain lesion was always discernible in an impairment of abstract thinking.

Current theory amalgamates these views into the connectionist position that while some functions may be strongly localized—as verbal functions appear to be in the left hemisphere—connections nevertheless exist between those locations and sites in the other hemisphere, where the function is also represented, albeit not so strongly. Hence a specifically located lesion will impair one type of function more than another; a differently located lesion will more impair another type of function. A specific function may have a circumscribed representation in one hemisphere and a diffuse one in the other hemisphere. Pure syndromes—the disturbance of one isolated function—are very rare. Poeck (5) cautions: most neuropsychological syndromes are the result of interaction between two or more basic disorders, with or without one or several general disturbances. This interaction is dependent upon the anatomical location of the lesion and upon the interruption of associational pathways connecting one brain area with another.

For the neuropsychologist, the clinical syndromes they seek to correlate with anatomical locations are relatively few in number, but each is multitudinous in its aspects, shades, and combinations of manifestations. Chief among these syndromes are:

1) Language disturbances, *Aphasia*—impairment of ability to deal with verbal symbols, either numbers or words. The deficit may be specifically fluent or non-fluent. In *Fluent Aphasia* there is abundant speech, but content is irrelevant or lacking because the patient has trouble using the correct word. In *Non-Fluent Aphasia*, speech is slow, poorly articulated, and made with great effort. The terms "receptive" and "expressive" are also used to describe types of aphasic impairments.

2) Impairments of spatial orientation and capacity for constructional tasks, *Constructional Aphasia*—difficulty in placing objects in relationship to the whole. (It is important to differentiate these deficits from impairments of visual perception or manual control.)

3) Difficulty in performance of purposeful movements, *Aphaxia*—in the absence of a sensory deficit or paralysis, a difficulty in handling objects and in gesturing.

4) Impairments of sensory recognition, *Agnosias*—in the absence of a defect of the sensory organ itself, an impaired ability to recognize and identify objects through that sense organ. Visual, auditory, and haptic (touch) sensory functions are the chief

concerns, although kinesthesia, smell, and taste may also be affected. Body image constitutes an important sensory conception, a fundamental component of the "sense" of self. Agnosia of the cutaneous senses of the fingertips is an example of an isolated impairment of a body-image component. More complex examples are found through studies of phantom body parts (8). Ordinarily, the neuropsychologist is concerned with suppression of the sensory modality, but there are conditions —psychomotor epilepsy is an important example—in which excitation of the sensory modality occurs adventitiously, and hallucinations are experienced.

Other aspects of neurological syndromes are more general in their manifestations. Being less specific, they are more likely to be confused with psychogenic symptoms. They include:

1) Alterations of consciousness (experienced as depersonalization, feelings of unreality, bewilderment, confusion, and perplexity);

2) Impairment of recall (which may be distinguished between recall for recent or past events, or by the sensory modality through which the data to be recalled are or have been presented to the brain);

3) Disorders of orientations (such as orientation in space, time, and in self-location, that is, disturbances of balance and in right-left discrimination);

4) Intellectual deficits (objectively, appearing in performance on intelligence tests, which in themselves test some or many of the functions considered in this list and the one preceding);

5) Disturbance of drive (hyperactivity and apathy being the extremes of this continuum);

6) Disorders of attention (loss of vigilance; difficulty maintaining concentration or in sustaining an activity; susceptibility to distraction by intervening stimuli); and

7) Emotional disturbance (some concomitants being damage to self-esteem, depression, elation, lability of mood, sensitivity, impulsivity, and easily exacerbated anger).

These, then, are the major elements of concern to the neuropsychologist in the role of the brain in behavior. Pathology, when traceable, illuminates "normal" functions; the relationship is discernible through the effects of clearly established traumas, poisonings, febrile episodes, hemorrhagic accidents in humans, or through laboratory-controlled damage to the brain of lower animals. The behaviors have been categorized into the specific disturbances of language, spatial orientation, motor and sensory functions, and the general disturbances of consciousness, recall, orientation, intelligence, drive, attention, and emotion. Study of these leads to investigation of localization, and of dominance or lateralization within the brain. Theories and methods of neuropsychodiagnosis are based upon these explorations.

In considering the use of neuropsychodiagnosis, the clinical psychotherapist will benefit above all from Reitan's (6) caution against reliance upon univalent causal factors. The psychological deficit we observe in a patient is seldom attributable to a single cause; this fact is especially evident with children. Damage to the brain may indeed be at the causal bottom of the syndrome observed by the clinician. But intervening between causal past and clinical present, a variety of influences may have been operating, primarily a chain of consequences of the initial impairment. Brain damage produces change in behavior, capabilities, and personality. These changes affect both the self and others. Interactions with others are altered and these lead to further changes in the self.

Nowhere is ambiguity more likely than in assessing brain-behavior relationship; nowhere is there more need for consideration of alternative causes or contributing causes; nowhere is avoiding flatfooted, singleminded assumptions wiser.

BIBLIOGRAPHY

1. *Birch, H. G.* and *Belmont, I.:* Auditory-visual integration in normal and retarded readers, Amer. J. Orthopsychiat., 34, 1964.
2. *Geschwind, N.:* Problems in the anatomical understanding of the aphasias. *In* A. L. Benton (Ed.): Contributions to Clinical Neuropsychology. Chicago: Aldine, 1969.
3. *Goldstein, K.:* The effects of brain damage on the personality. Psychiat., 15, 1952.
4. Minimal Brain Dysfunction in Children: Educational, Medical and Health Related Services; Phase Two of a Three Phase Project. Washington. D. C.: U.S. Department of Health, Education and Welfare, Public Health Service Publication No. 2015, 1969.
5. *Poeck, K.:* Modern trends in neuropsychology. *In* A. L. Benton, (Ed.): Contributions to Clinical Neuropsychology. Chicago: Aldine, 1969.
6. *Reitan, R. M.:* Psychological assessment of deficits associated with brain lesions in subjects with normal and subnormal intelligence. *In* J. L. Khanna (Ed.): Brain Damage and Mental Retardation: A Psychological Evaluation. Springfield, Illinois: Charles C Thomas, 1967.
7. *Sherrington, C. S.:* Man and His Nature. Cambridge, England: Cambridge University Press, 1951.
8. *Weinstein, S.:* Neuropsychological studies of the phantom. *In* A. L. Benton, (Ed.): Contributions to Clinical Neuropsychology. Chicago: Aldine, 1969.

CHAPTER 15

Cerebral Localization and Dominance

Brain-behavior relationships have been explored through many channels, and many hypotheses have resulted. Prominent among these since the earliest phrenological proposal has been the concept of anatomical residence or location, the idea that a specific, observable behavioral function resides in and is controlled or is mediated by a more-or-less specifically proscribed part of the brain. Neurology has indeed been able to establish that the major sensory and motor functions are symmetrically arranged in the two sides of the brain, and that the motor and sensory behavior of one side of the body is localized in or controlled by the opposite or contralateral side of the brain. Pursuit of residence for higher functions in the brain led to findings of longitudinal anterior to posterior organization, with specific functions localized in the different lobes: frontal, parietal, temporal, and occipital. Extensive investigation of "localization" produced claims of more precisely defined sites where behavioral functions are believed to be organized, to reside, so to speak.

Of special interest for the psychotherapist is the activity of the limbic system within the temporal lobe. Doty (10) reports that 50 to 90 percent of patients with temporal-lobe epilepsy manifest behavior resembling that of psychotic patients without demonstrable brain lesions. The fact that epilepsy in other areas of the brain is not accompanied by similar emotional disruption allows the conclusion that the emotional disorders in temporal-lobe epilepsy are associated with the temporal-lobe, not with the epilepsy. Stimulations of and/or lesions of the hypothalamus and the limbic system within the temporal-lobe produce profound alterations of basic behavior marked by rage, fear, and distortion in reality perception. Stimulus elsewhere within the hypothalamus produces a pleasurable response.

328

Then it was observed that the same functions might be handled somewhat differently by each of the identical sites of the two sides or hemispheres of the brain: visual agnosia arising from a lesion in the left hemisphere impairs reading and writing, while a similarly located lesion in the right hemisphere is more apt to impair object recognition (27). Such observations contribute to accumulated evidence that the two cerebral hemispheres differ fundamentally in their functions, and from this evidence has developed the concept of lateral cerebral dominance.

This progression in formulation has not been smooth, nor is there consensus or harmony among theorists and clinicians. The idea of strict localization as fostered by the nineteenth-century surgeon-anthropologist Paul Broca has given way to admited differences in cerebral dominance, but conflict continues over whether the dominant functions of either hemisphere are immutably fixed or subject to a takeover by the other hemisphere when damage occurs. Two different annual meetings of the International Neuropsychological Society have heard these reflections of the conflict offered, only partly in jest: "If you don't believe in localization you should get out of neuropsychology," and "Broca is alive and well and living in Boston." The concept of dominance, although not thoroughly comprehended, still disputed, and the stimulus for such hypotheses as excitingly suggestive lines of research and excitingly obscure notions of two kinds of brains, is important to the understanding of brain-behavior relationships in man, the language-maker and the tool-maker.

The best established difference between the hemispheres is in language, for which the left hemisphere plays the predominant role. As Poeck reports, lateralization of the language function continues to play a central role in disputes between mosaicist and holist: "We speak with the left hemisphere" *versus* "We speak with the whole brain" (35). Many studies attribute visuomotor dominance to the right hemisphere. These findings promoted investigations of the hypotheses that the left hemisphere is dominant for verbal functions, the right for nonverbal functions. Greatest agreement was obtained for the first, that the left hemisphere is dominant for verbal functions. Findings more often conflict with the second hypothesis, ascribing nonverbal dominance to the right hemisphere. This chapter reviews some findings for the major activities subsumed by the terms verbal and nonverbal functions and considers some of the confusing variables.

The issue is important: reliable findings here illuminate our understanding of the development of verbal and motor processes. The neuro-psychologist needs this understanding if he is to contribute to the identification and location of brain lesions.

LATERALIZATION OF MAJOR FUNCTIONS

Standard neurological examinations emphasize the effect of a lateralized lesion upon the contralateral extremities. The functions here considered—language and constructional ability—while in some measure lateralized within the brain, have no manifest contralateral body expressions. However, evidence of the predominant lateralization of verbal and constructional functions, among others, comes from several major sources. The validity and reliability of the data coming from each source are, of course, necessarily affected by the conditions governing the situations where the data emerge.

1) Damage to brains of persons formerly normal. This damage may arise from tumors, penetrating wounds, cerebrovascular accidents, metabolic disorders, anoxia, severe febrile episodes, concussions, psychosurgery. When the damage can be identified as localized to one hemisphere or to both, or to more specific sites along the longitudinal axis of either hemisphere, an association between such localization and lateralization and the loss of specific behavioral functions may be made. But there is serious question that lesions can be so precisely defined. Not only do they vary in etiology but also in size (often overlapping one presumed site and another), in type (expanding or contracting), and in possible extension of effects. Unidentifiable inflammatory processes may radiate far beyond the central locus of the lesion; cerebral blood vessels remote from the lesion site may respond to the disease process with constriction. "Distance" effects, diaschisis, have been identified as disrupting "the functions of the anatomically intact opposite hemisphere" as well as the intact parts of the affected hemisphere (38).

2) Recent neurosurgical interventions in extremes cases. Dramatic illustrations of the functional dominance of each hemisphere and the interaction between the hemisphere have resulted from surgical procedures to sever neural pathways of the corpus callosum that connect the two hemispheres (commissurotomy), or to remove one hemisphere totally (hemispherectomy). For commissurotomized patients, stimuli of different kinds and the same tasks may be presented to each of the isolated hemispheres and the nature of their responses studied. For

the hemispherectomized patients, different types of stimuli and the same tasks are presented to the remaining hemisphere, right or left, and its response capability studied. These radical surgical procedures were developed to relieve patients with intractable epileptic seizures, tumors, or progressive mental deterioration. Prominent in their development and/or the study of their behavioral consequences have been Sperry (42), Bogen (3, 4, 5), Gazzaniga (16), Smith (39, 40), Smith and Burkland (41), Gainotti (14), and Nebes (33), among others. Compared to the numbers of patients having suffered lateralized brain damage, as in hemiplegia, for example, the number of commissurotomized patients studied is small. Moreover, the evidence increases that the remaining, so-called intact, hemisphere is likely to be damaged by the drastic surgical procedures.

3) Dichotic listening and visual field experiments. The normal anatomical arrangements can be exploited by "indirect" methods that employ dichotic listening and the selective reaction of right and left visual fields. Dichotic listening experiments are based upon the observation that each ear is more under the dominance of its opposite hemisphere. Stimulation of the right visual field proceeds more rapidly to the left hemisphere and conversely from left visual field to right hemisphere. These processes are based upon the anatomical fact of contralateral innervation of ears and visual fields. However, each ear and each visual field is also connected with its ipsilateral hemisphere.

4) Selective hemispheric anesthesia. Each hemisphere may be selectively anesthetized by barbiturate injections into the right or left carotid arteries. The "awake" and the anesthetized hemispheres are then tested for their responses to a variety of stimuli and tasks.

5) Laboratory ablation of selected sites and sides of lower animal brains. While much information is yielded by animal experiment, the controls possible in a laboratory do not assure that the damage is limited to the surgically-created lesions. Further, the justification for translating inferences acquired from a non-language-capable animal to a language-capable one is questionable. Readers interested in a review of many significant animal studies are referred to Mountcastle (31).

Language

The discussion of aphasia and dysphasia in Chapter 4 is pertinent at this point. The reader may benefit from a review of it, especially of the early discoveries of Broca and Wernicke of, respectively, an expressive and receptive language disorder, with different anatomical sites.

Most studies clearly associate verbal deficits with lesions of the left hemisphere. Lansdell observes that the extent of left temporal-lobe surgery has been correlated with certain verbal scores, as for Verbal Comprehension, which he identifies as a general verbal factor (25, 26).

Three out of four patients with left hemiplegia were found by Diller and Weinberg (9) to manifest higher verbal than performance skills; conversely, the same ratio of right hemiplegics showed higher performance than verbal skills.

Reitan's studies (37) of aphasic symptoms provide convincing evidence of their relationship to damage of the left hemisphere. Forty-seven patients with established damage of the left cerebral hemisphere were compared with 58 patients with similarly established right-side damage. Each patient was examined for the presence of specific symptoms of aphasia: naming, reading, spelling, writing, and calculating. Serious difficulties in these activities were far more frequent among the patients with leftside damage (Table 1).

TABLE 1

Percent of Left- and Right-Hemisphere Damaged Patients
Showing Aphasic Symptoms (Reitan, 37)

	left	right
dysnomia	53	0
dyslexia	47	0
spelling dyspraxia	49	7
dysgraphia	51	2
dyscalculia	55	14

This tendency to left-side lateralization of language functions was not affected by the handedness of the individual, and the aphasic difficulties of the left-side damaged patients were associated with lowered scores on the Verbal subtests of the Wechsler-Bellevue scale.

In another study by Reitan and Tarshes, cited in the same report (37), a two-part Trailmaking Test was used. The first part employed numbers only, the second part required alternation progressively between numbers and letters. Forty-four patients with left-hemisphere damage had more difficulty with the second part than with the first;

the converse was true for fifty patients with right lobe damage. Significant mean differences ($p = .001$) were obtained as predicted; the prediction was based upon the anticipation of greater difficulty for patients with left-side damage in using the additional symbolic material to make the alterations between symbolic systems—numbers and letters—required in the second part of the test.

The relationship of handedness to the lateralization of speech functions has been investigated. Of historical interest is Orton's attempt to apply the concept of cerebral dominance to the development of speech and writing. He believed that lags or deficits in language development arose from a failure to establish dominance of one hemisphere in hand use, often because of outside interference with expression of the child's early manifestation of such dominance. Reitan and Kløve report (37) that the left hemisphere was almost always dominant for speech even in left-handed persons. Some few left-handed individuals were found by them to have bilaterally represented speech centers (mixed dominance); in such persons speech and writing may develop more slowly and be more susceptible to outside interference.

The presence of so-called right-hemisphere speech—speech efficiency under the control of the right hemisphere—is demonstrated by disruption of speech when Amytal is injected into the right carotid artery. Lansdell (23) studied this phenomenon in patients in whom the age when neurological symptoms first appeared was identified in medical records. He related the phenomenon to the capacity of the right hemisphere to take over some verbal functions if damage to the left side occurs early enough in childhood or infancy.

Speech is a highly complex function, and the tendency to view it only as "verbal" behavior is an over-simplification, one that may lead to overlooking the actual impairment. In Jackson's (21) words, "speaking is not simply the utterance of words . . . speaking is 'propositionizing.'" Language is not only an external phenomenon expressed in speaking and writing but an internal one as well, expressed in thought. Involved in speech, among other processes, are voluntary expressions and automatic expressions, visual and auditory recognition and imagery. Jackson observed that a brain-damaged person may be able to utter involuntary remarks ("God bless you!" when someone sneezes) but not be able to say the same thing volitionally in response to the question, "What does one say when a person sneezes?" Jackson further observed that voluntary speech is within the domain of the left hemisphere. This, along with many corollary findings relative to the complicated process of speech, led him to the conclusion that there is no single speech center, that is, no "faculty" of speech, but many faculties residing in many parts of the brain that combine to produce that complex phenomenon, language, of which speech is one part.

Right-left confusion is sometimes interpreted as evidence of mixed cerebral dominance; while there is not always that correlation, right-left confusion is sometimes found associated with impaired language development, and often found in dyslexia, where letters of the alphabet which are mirror images of each other are reversed: b and d, p and q, m and w. It is possible, of course, that reversals and confusion of right and left may have a common cause—a lesion—rather than one being the cause of the other.

Constructional Functions

Pure constructional apraxia—difficulty in assembling parts into a whole, relating parts to each other, building and drawing—is observable in persons with adequate visual form perception and discrimination, ability to localize objects in visual space, and with no evidence of Ideomotor Apraxia (1).

Through the years, many tasks of varied complexity have been used to identify the existence of the deficit. These have included block arranging in the horizontal, block building in the vertical, three-dimensional block building, stick arranging, mosaic patterns, drawing from a model, and free or spontaneous drawings. The level of difficulty of any of these approaches may be increased to almost any degree desired: two dimensional construction may be made three dimensional; multiple figures may be required to be drawn with specific spatial and size relationships between them; or the model from which the subject makes the construction may be made increasingly an abstract representation of the desired product.

Consistency in the types of instruments used or in levels of complexity being lacking, a review of the literature tends to show considerable intraindividual variation in performance: an individual will succeed with some types of tasks but fail others. Constructional Apraxia may be a single deficit or it may encompass many discrete types of disabilities. There is reason to identify at least two separate types of constructional activity: 1) assembling tasks, sticks, and blocks; and 2) visual-graphic procedures or copying of designs.

Constructional Apraxia has been demonstrated with greater frequency in patients with lesions of the right hemisphere than in those with left-hemisphere lesions. Reitan (37) found that 64 percent of patients with right-hemisphere lesions manifested Constructional Apraxia, in contrast to 15 percent of patients with left-hemisphere damage. This ratio—better than four to one—is greater than is usually reported. According to Benton (1) right-hemisphere-damaged patients fail constructional tasks more frequently than left-side-damaged patients by a ratio of two to one, or three to one at best. Benton notes further that these ratios vary with the nature of the constructional task given to the subject and with the criterion for failure or deficit established. Usually, the more stringent the criterion of failure the greater were the differences between right and left hemisphere groups.

Benton asks whether Constructional Apraxia has true localizing significance for brain damage, or is more a reflection of "general mental impairment" with accompanying defects in attention and planful activity. If the latter is true, the evidence for localization in the right hemisphere becomes less useful. He sought to resolve this dilemma by comparing constructional ability in 35 patients with cerebral disease whose Verbal Scale I.Q. was 20 to 49 points below that to be expected for their age and education with 65 patients with cerebral disease whose Verbal I.Q. was 19 points or less below their expected I.Q. The first group were assumed to be "impaired," the latter group "unimpaired." The "impaired" group in four separate constructional tasks showed more failures (37 to 46 percent) than did the "unimpaired" group (8 to 15 percent). An equally clear relationship between Constructional Apraxia and general impairment is evident, but the relationship is not a *necessary* one since on all four tasks, the majority of the "impaired" patients did not show sufficient defect in constructional tasks to meet the rigorous criterion of Apraxia employed (performance level below that of 98 percent of control patients).

The severest degree of Constructional Apraxia was found in patients with bilateral lesions by Critchley (8), ascribing some influence to the left hemisphere in such functions.

Association of Constructional Apraxia with right-hemisphere lesions is clear, according to Costa and Vaughan (7), and is linked with consistently poor performance on perceptual-motor tasks by these patients. They suggest that the constructional deficits found in patients with right-side lesions are part of a larger pattern of visual-spatial deficits, that is, the apparent constructional deficit is actually a perceptual one.

The role of the left hemisphere in Constructional Apraxia may be explicable by the fact that certain forms of the Apraxia are dependent upon whether or not the *idea* of the construction has been clearly conveyed to the motor area (2). A recent study (34) supports this hypothesis. Difficulties in visual-constructional tasks were demonstrated by right hemiplegics. These difficulties suggested an ideational component in these tasks which may operate as a "silent" disability. Deafness, for example, is known to disrupt or impair other perceptual processes, the visual, for example (32); visual perception and ideation are both essential in construction tasks. Precise and limited localization of a manifest function probably does not exist, in the sense that most functions are not simple but complex. So with the constructional tasks as with language, many partial functions are used, involving many different parts of the brain.

The dominance of the right hemisphere for constructional praxis is not clearly established. Indeed, the verbal dominance of the left hemisphere is not without questions. What can now be said is that the verbal dominance of the left hemisphere has wider acceptance than does the constructional dominance of the right hemisphere, and that some evidence contests the purported dominance of each hemisphere.

EVIDENCE FROM PSYCHOLOGICAL TESTS

The Wechsler Intelligence Scales (the Wechsler-Bellevue, the Wechsler Adult Intelligence Scale, and the Wechsler Intelligence Scale for Children) have been used widely in efforts to test dominance and predict lateralization of brain damage (18).

The Wechsler-Bellevue Scale is reported by Reitan (37) to provide significant clues to the lateralization of brain damage. He finds that in patients with established lesions of the left hemisphere total weighted scores of the Verbal Scale are consistently less than the comparable total for the Performance Scale. Conversely, in patients with lesions of the right hemisphere the total weighted Performance-Scale score is consistently less than for the Verbal-Scale scores. This proved to be the fact also when the EEG findings were used as an indicator of lateralization of lesions. Some evidence suggests to Reitan and Kløve that the Performance Scale of the Wechsler Intelligence Tests is more sensitive to right-hemisphere damage than the Verbal Scale is to left-hemisphere lesion. In another report, Reitan (36) consolidates studies from 20 groups of patients, 19 with direct or inferential evidence of specific involvement of the left or right hemisphere, one group with diffuse cerebral damage. Rank orders of subtest mean scores were employed. Comparable groups showed consistencies in such rank order that far exceeded chance expectancies. Highly significant differences were obtained between right- and left-hemisphere-damaged groups.

Yet even such striking effects of lateralization of damage upon Verbal and Performance scores are attenuated and even possibly obliterated by the influence of the age of the patient, his educational level, duration of the lesion, and location and type of the lesion. For example, patients with tumors and vascular lesions intrinsic to the brain tend to demonstrate the greatest differences between Verbal and Performances scores, the most clearcut psychological-test evidence of lateralization of cerebral damage. More marked Verbal-Performance differences are found with the more posteriorly located lesions, that is in the posterior temporal-parietal area. A much less clearcut relationship is found in patients suffering traumas. No consistent relationship is obtained in patients with extrinsic tumors, those affecting the meningeal tissue surrounding the brain.

Very similar results are reported by Fields and Whitmyre (13), who were able to relate impaired integrity of the left hemisphere to deficits in verbal functioning on the Wechsler Adult Intelligence Scale and performance deficits to right hemisphere disorders. While their statistical analysis supported these statements, the actual differences were somewhat attenuated, the investigators believe, by the fact that more than half of their patients had lesions of long standing, although unilateral, and that patients with extrinsic cerebral lesions (meningiomas) were included in their study population. The investigators suggest that cerebral plasticity may account for the attenuation of differences in Verbal-Performance with chronicity, perhaps because with the passage of time after the acute phase of a lesion there is some compensation and some recovery of function. (Chapter 18 discusses recoverability from brain injuries.)

In a factor-analytic study of the usefulness of the Wechsler-Bellevue to identify side of temporal-lobe surgery Lansdell (26) obtained a relationship between the Verbal-Comprehension factor and the *extent* of tissue removed from the left temporal lobe; the factor did not distinguish the *side* of the operation. Some rather confusing results were obtained by Cohen (6) for the other two factors identified in the Wechsler scales—Perceptual Organization and Freedom from Distractibility. However, he found that the scores of the four subtests making up the Verbal factor when compared with the scores of the other seven subtests provided a simple illustration of the differential effects of left-side and right-side lesions.

Failure of the Verbal-Performance discrepancy to appear among either aphasic and nonaphasic patients with left-hemisphere or dominant-hemisphere damage is reported by Smith (40). Among patients with left-hemisphere tumors, one in three produced lower Verbal than Performance scores. He thus was not able to substantiate reports of differential effects of acute lateralized lesions, but rather produced evidence that appears to refute such differential effects. He suggests that much research is invalidated by important methodological difficulties in precise definition and differentiation of the effects of brain lesions combined with the relative insensitivity of the Wechsler tests and subtests to specific defects associated with circumscribed lesions. Smith concludes that while Wechsler Verbal-Performance discrepancies may expose a variety of expressive and receptive aphasias, additional tests, more various and more sensitive, must be used, both to define these impairments more precisely and to test functions not tapped by the Wechsler subtests.

Efforts at more precise site identification and more sensitive psychological instrumentation have occupied Lansdell for some years. He studied (24) the effect of temporal-lobe ablations upon two deficits —vocabulary and visual closure. From a group of patients who had undergone therapeutic temporal-lobe removals he excluded those for whom there was evidence of right-hemisphere dominance for speech and writing or reasonable presumption of diffuse cerebral damage. To forestall the possibility that a verbal deficit following left-temporal ablation might be due to the usual auditory mode of testing (as in the Wechsler scale), a paper and pencil test was used. Clearcut lateralization effects were obtained: lower vocabulary scores correlated with left-hemisphere surgery, lower closure scores with right-side surgery. The extent of tissue removal was positively and significantly related to vocabulary deficit when the surgery was on the left-side; extent of right-side surgery was negatively related to closure deficit. Lansdell suggests that the vocabulary function may be more localized on the left and that closure representation on the right may have multiple sites, some of which (as in the nearby right parietal lobe) function despite damage to the right temporal lobe. He considers as interesting but less feasible a difference in functional organization in which closure efficiency involves a pattern of connections in the right hemisphere, while verbal efficiency is related to volume of intact temporal tissue of the left side. Other investigators, notably Heilbrun (20) and Meier and French (29), have also failed to confirm Reitan's reports.

Exploring the issue further, Landsdell (25) used the Differential Aptitude Test (DAT), which measures aptitudes in verbal reasoning numerical ability, abstract reasoning, space relations, mechanical reasoning, clerical speed, and sentence usage, with two groups of patients who had undergone temporal-lobe surgery. One group was tested more than four years after surgery, the other within a mean of seven days after. Of the eight DAT tests, only Verbal Reasoning scores were significantly related to the side (left, as was expected) from which tissue had been removed. Apart from this, Abstract Reasoning scores were generally and symmetrically, both right and left sides, related to extent of temporal-lobe tissue removal. The findings are, of course, supportive of Kurt Goldstein's concept of abstract thinking as a diffuse, non-lateralized cerebral function. Thus some functions, e.g., verbal reasoning, appear to be strongly lateralized and asymmetrical and others, e.g., abstract reasoning, are generalized and symmetrical.

The factors which appear to influence test findings in support of these statements include: the general plasticity or equipotentiality of brain tissue (there is some evidence that the dominant hemisphere is relatively more plastic); the age at which injury takes place (the earlier age is associated with greater plasticity); the diffuse or localized brain representation of the function; the location of the lesion (subcortical lesions tend to have more diffuse effects than cortical ones); the area of brain tissue affected by the lesion. Lesions of the meninges extrinsic to the cortex tend to show less clear lateralizing effects; lesions located more posteriorly tend to have more clearcut effects.

Subtle (perhaps equivocal is a better word) sex differences are also reported. Men with right-side ablations produced a lower mean score on nonverbal Wechsler subtests than did men with left-side operations. This was in the direction generally expected. But the converse was true among women: those with left-side removals had a lower mean score than did those with right-side operations. Lansdell (26) suggests that these sex-linked differences may represent either a difference of localization in the brain, or differences in both the types and amounts of training the sexes receive culturally.

As stressed in Chapter 11, the Wechsler scales are not "pure." The Verbal scale includes tasks requiring attention and memory as well as verbal material, and the Performance scale includes considerable verbal material as in the nomic aspects of Picture Completion. Kløve (22) emphasizes that diagnostic reliance cannot be placed solely in the Wechsler-Bellevue Scales, that they must be understood as adjuncts in the assessment of lateralized dysfunctions.

THE EFFECTS OF COMMISSUROTOMY
AND HEMISPHERECTOMY

The vast and complicated literature on this subject is beyond the scope of this writer and this book, except for the following review of some major findings. Bogen (3, 4, 5) reports an intensive study of the effects of commissurotomy in eight right-handed patients and hemispherectomy in two patients in whom he sought to correlate his findings with other observations of lateralized dysfunctions. Following commissurotomy he reports that there is impairment of writing ability with the left hand (under the dominance of the right hemisphere) and impairment of the copying ability of geometric figures for the right hand (under the dominance of the left hemisphere). The dysgraphia was restricted to the left hand; although some of these patients were mute, they could write adequately with the right hand. The left hand dysgraphia, therefore, was the result of some defect of the right hemisphere. While this would seem to establish that the right hemisphere had been cut off from the language centers of the left hemisphere, Bogen was not content with this disconnection hypothesis, because he could also demonstrate language functions in the right hemisphere: the right hemisphere could recognize words: although mute and unable to write, these patients could tactilely identify in a bagful of objects with their left hand whatever object was named. He proposed that the agraphia of the left hand resulted from an "inhibition" between intact gnostic centers and intact effector centers in the right hemisphere as a result of differential pre-operative development in the two hemispheres. His hypothesis implies that as a specific function becomes more active in one hemisphere it is increasingly inhibited in the other hemisphere. Finally, his hypothesis postulates that when a hemisphere is released from this inhibition, as would be the case in commissurotomy, it gradually becomes able to develop a function that had been "suppressed rather than lost."

Bogen's hypothesis finds corroboration in the neuropsychological studies of hemispherectomized patients by Smith (39, 41). Smith is continuing studies of the initial and later effects of right and left hemispherectomies in both children and adults, using a standard neuropsychological test battery. They support the hypothesis that a single hemisphere, which may be either the right or the left, is sufficient for the development of normal language and intellectual ability. Campbell, *et al.* (5a) have reported some recent findings with commissurotomized patients that indicate that the left hemisphere may compensate for some nonlanguage deficits after damage to the right hemisphere.

Bogen also addresses himself to the right hemisphere and its dominant functions. He identifies its superior ability to copy, for spatial gnosia, recognition of faces, and musical ability (30). He suggests that the concept of cerebral dominance has obscured the fact that we actually have two brains, each of about the same size, weight and metabolic activity, each with the same potential for functional capacity. As the left hemisphere developed its superior language capability, the right hemisphere experienced an inhibition, not a loss, of its language capability, and instead developed an appositional mode of function and thought.

Bogen's postulations also receive support from data correlating handedness and aphasia. Eisenson (11) has reviewed this problem. Aphasia is usually associated with damage to the left hemisphere, regardless of the handedness of the person. Yet aphasia following damage to the right hemisphere is found in up to 10 percent of right-handed persons. The incidence is somewhat higher among left-handed patients suffering right hemisphere damage. These distributions indicate that left-hemispheric dominance occurs more frequently than does right handedness, and that right-hemispheric dominance occurs much less frequently than does left handedness. In general, functional asymmetry —hand, ear, eye and foot preference—is greater in the right-handed than the left-handed, among whom the asymmetry is less strong and less consistent. In the truly ambidextrous (a very small proportion of the population) an active bilateral language representation is postulated.

Gazzaniga (15) finds that the long and continuing study of commissurotomies has produced one of the "clearest" syndromes seen in clinical neurology: impairment of *information* processing between various centers of the brain. The dominant hemisphere, in this view, is the site of this central processing. If dominance is not established there is no central point to which cognitive data are channeled to be appraised and reacted to. The lack of such a center causes confusion, which may produce some of the symptoms observed in minimal brain dysfunction. He cites studies that indicate that the right hemisphere is superior to the left in some word-classifying activities, but not in their semantics, so that transmission of information between the hemispheres is important.

This view of interlocking rather than separate functional organization of the two hemispheres is widely-held. Luria (28) proposes that the integrated activity of both hemispheres governs psychological activity, although the specific contribution of each may be at a different level. Hécaen (19) postulates a gradient of interhemispheric integration, greatest at subcortical levels, least at the higher cortical levels. These reflections return us to the work and theories of the connectionist.

CONTRIBUTIONS OF THE CONNECTIONIST APPROACH

Many symptoms do not indicate a dysfunction of circumscribed, specifically localized areas of the cerebral cortex. Rather they point to the interruption of association fibers which connect cortical areas within the same hemisphere, and the interruption of pathways which connect corresponding areas of the two hemispheres.

Important findings in this area have evolved from the pioneering work of Geschwind (17), who identified some of the syndromes associated with disconnection of association pathways. The concept of contralaterality is that each hemisphere sends motor commands to the appendages of the opposite side, and in turn receives somatosensory data chiefly from that opposite side of the body. As indicated, these sensory data or signals are sent also to the ipsilateral hemisphere, on the same side from which the signals arise. This has been demonstrated by conditioning experiments: an animal trained to perform a task with his right forelimb, largely affecting the motor area of the left hemisphere of his brain, then indicates on testing that some learning had taken place in the motor area of the right hemisphere as well.

Studies of commissural connections surveyed by Ettlinger and Blakemore (12) demonstrate the plasticity of the mammalian brain in the organization of behavior. The two hemispheres of the brain are connected with each other in two ways: 1) haphazard connections of nerve fibers take place between the two hemispheres at many levels, in many directions, and are intermingled with nerve cells; 2) organized connections occur in which fibers are gathered together into a bundle, excluding all nerve cells, and traverse between the two hemispheres, connecting each with the other. Such an organized collection of fibers is called a commissure.

Nerve fibers from each eye usually are connected to both the left and right hemisphere, not only to the ipsilateral hemisphere. Cutting of the interhemispheric connection results in temporal field blindness in each eye, so that the left part of the left eye is blind, as is the right part of the right eye. In similar fashion, each ear is connected to both cerebral hemispheres. But the fibers do not cross in a single bundle; they transverse the midline at many levels, so that auditory input from one ear cannot be entirely limited to a single hemisphere. A limited degree of ipsilateral connection for the limbs has been demonstrated. The limbs project somatosensory inflows largely into the contralateral hemisphere. In effect, therefore, ipsilateral projection is pronounced in vision, considerable in audition, and minor in tactile transmission.

Some experiments in auditory perception highlight this functional asymmetry. The left hemisphere was found to play a leading role in the perception and analysis of verbal stimuli. The right hemisphere was found superior in the perception of nonverbal stimuli, such as melodies and noises. Auditory asymmetry is particularly pronounced when the stimulus consists of syllables composed of both vowels and consonants, and is far less pronounced when the stimulus consists of vowels only. In left-handed individuals, the functional asymmetry of the two hemispheres for auditory perception is less clearcut and there is pronounced equipotentiality of the two halves of the brain.

Similar experiments have been conducted with visual recognition. In visual perception, the right half-field of each eye is projected to the left striate area; the left half-field of each eye is projected to the right striate area. Since both striate cortices are connected by associational pathways, the signals are not confined to the respective hemispheres. The right half-field was found to be superior for letters, words, and for concrete objects which are readily verbalized. The left half-field is superior in the recognition of meaningless figures and similar nonverbal visual patterns.

Geschwind (17) describes some of the possible effects of lesions in the area of the temporo-parieto-occipital congruence—the area in which data in two sensory modalities are associated. As one example: given a lesion in Wernicke's area of the brain—the area of auditory association—a word may be received here, but no response will be arousable in the area, so that response elsewhere in the brain also will not be arousable. The word therefore will not be understood, nor will the person be able to repeat it. Furthermore, the victim of such a lesion will be unable to describe what he sees, since stimuli from the visual cortex will not arrive at Broca's area. He will be unable to comprehend written language, as the visually perceived word will not be able to arouse its corollary form.

Geschwind reports similar observations of the effects upon speech of lesions in Broca's area in which the victim continues to understand both written and spoken language but is unable to speak properly.

These effects are comprehensible when the pathway by which visual stimuli arouse auditory associations is depicted: from visual cortex to visual association area of the cortex to angular gyrus to the auditory-association cortex (Wernicke's area). Broca's area—the motor association region—mediates the transposition of perceived sound into a motor response.

Given this anatomical-functional arrangement, the pathway by which a visually perceived object is named is this: the visual cortex is stimulated, the stimulus goes to the visual-association cortex, then to the angular gyrus which arouses the name of the object in Wernicke's area, and then through the arcuate fasciculus into the motor association area (Broca's area) where the motor pattern associated with the sound form is aroused, then to the motor cortex and finally downward to emerge as speech.

Knowledge of the anatomical-functional model permits predictions about the effects of lesions, as were described above. However, Geschwind observes certain difficulties. Some of these effects are not readily explicable by the model, for example, why Wernicke's Aphasia is fluent, and Broca's Aphasia is non-fluent. Some syndromes exist which are not predicated by the model; patients with Broca's Aphasias have little trouble in naming, Wernicke's Aphasias have considered anomia. Also the former have great difficulty in sentence construction, while the latter are likely to form well-constructed sentences that lack specific words. Also, despite a seemingly sufficient lesion, cases are observed in which predicted deficits do not appear. Even with these difficulties, Geschwind favors the conclusion that the localization of anatomical-functional model is the most efficient in explaining known information, predicting new phenomena, designing experiments, and in accommodating improvements checkable by both observation and experiment.

These findings derived from the connectionist approach highlight the limitations of any single psychological test of cerebral function to identify the existence of brain damage, then lateralize it, and ultimately localize it. A lesion may be so located that its effect upon a pathway is not detectable. Thus a lesion that may affect comprehension of written language may not be detectable by the subtests of the Wechsler scales, where most of the instructions and questions are spoken. Awareness of these limitations does, however, enable the psychologist to take steps to overcome them to the extent that our instruments are so alterable.

The significance of commissural connections is seen by Ettlinger and Blakemore (12) to illustrate the plasticity of the brain: "Under certain conditions the subcortical commissures acquire the capacity to take over some of the functions normally sustained by the four brain commissures, or the ipsilateral projection system can attain greater functional importance, or cortical systems in an isolated hemisphere come to function in a way previously not possible."

A reasonable conclusion according to Poeck (35) is that some functions have a bilateral cerebral representation, but that it is asymmetrical, so that one hemisphere is more dominant with a particular function than is the other hemisphere. Thus, the nondominant hemisphere is involved in psychological activity, but this does not mean that the left hemisphere does not play the leading role. Poeck believes that the evidence suggests that there is a differential functional organization of the human brain in which "each hemisphere plays its part in a particular field and makes a separate contribution to human experience and behavior."

OVERVIEW

So goes the theoretical discussion and debate. The same data may be interpreted in different ways. The differences may arise primarily because the experiments have been restricted to anatomical features and do not incorporate biochemical physiological variables. The role of neurotransmitters, for example, has only recently begun to receive research attention. The coordination of three variables, in this case the anatomical, the physiological, and the behavioral, will be no easy matter, as multiple-variable research into the etiology of schizophrenia, for one example, demonstrates.

For the present, functional asymmetry is demonstrable, albeit with enough inconsistency to suggest that cerebral dominance has developed from an original equipotentiality of the two hemispheres, a suggestion supported by case study evidence that the non-dominant hemisphere may acquire language and intellectual functions, that cerebral dominance is reversible.

Finally, dominance does not appear to be complete or absolute. Many functions have been demonstrated to require the interaction of the two hemispheres for their complete operation even though "dominated" by a single hemisphere.

Within the bounds of these caveats these are some of the functions most often, but not always "dominated" by each of the hemispheres:

Left	*Right*
Language:	Visual and tactile
speech	recording and processing
reading	of spatial data, the
writing	recognition of forms
comprehension	and shapes.
expression	Directional orientation
Verbal ideation	Perspective
Verbal symbols written	Copying and drawing
on the skin	Constructional activities
Muscular control of	Musical ability
speech for both	
contra- and	
ipsilateral sides	

BIBLIOGRAPHY

1. *Benton, A. L.:* Constructional apraxia: Some unanswered questions. *In* A. L. Benton (Ed.): Contributions to Clinical Neuropsychology. Chicago: Aldine, 1969.
2. *Ben-Yishay, Y., et al.:* Similarities and differences in block design performance between older normal and brain-injured persons: A task analysis. J. Abnorm. Psychol., 78:1, 1971.
3. *Bogen, J. E.:* The other side of the brain; I: Dysgraphia and dyscopia following cerebral commissurotomy. Bull. Los Angeles Neurol. Soc., 34:2, 1969.
4. *Bogen, J. E.:* The other side of the brain; II: An appositional mind. Bull. Los Angeles Neurol. Soc., 34:3, 1969.
5. *Bogen, J. E.* and *Bogen, G. M.:* The other side of the brain; III: The corpus callosum and creativity. Bull. Los Angeles Neurol. Soc., 34:4, 1969.
5a. *Campbell, Jr., A. L., et al.:* Neuropsychological test functions in long-term postoperative studies of patients with commissurotomy. Presented at annual meeting of the International Neuropsychological Society, February, 1979.
6. *Cohen, J.:* The factor-analytically based rationale for the Wechsler Adult Intelligence Scale. J. Consult. Psychol., 21, 1957.

7. *Costa, L. D.* and *Vaughan, Jr., H. G.:* Performance of patients with lateralized lesions; I. Verbal and Perceptual Tests. J. Nerv. Ment. Dis., 134, 1962.
8. *Critchley, M.:* The Parietal Lobes. London: Arnold, 1953.
9. *Diller, L.* and *Weinberg, J.:* Learning in hemiplegia. Presented at the annual convention, Amer. Psychol. Assoc., 1962.
10. *Doty, R. W.:* Limbic System. In A. M. Freedman and H. I. Kaplan (Eds.): Human Behavior: Biological, Psychological and Sociological. New York: Atheneum, 1972.
11. *Eisenson, J.* Adult Aphasia. New York: Appleton-Century-Crofts, 1973.
12. *Ettlinger, G.* and *Blakemore, G. B.:* The behavioral effects of commissural section. In A. L. Benton (Ed.): Contributions to Clinical Neuropsychology. Chicago: Aldine, 1969.
13. *Fields, F. R.* and *Whitmyre, J. W.:* Verbal and performance relationships with respect to laterality of cerebral involvement. Dis. Nerv. Sys., 30:3, 1969.
14. *Gainotti, G.:* Studies on the functional organization of the minor hemisphere. Int. J. Ment. Health, 1:3, 1972.
15. *Gazzaniga, M. S.:* Brain theory and minimal brain dysfunction. Annals N. Y. Acad. Sci., 205, 1973.
16. *Gazzaniga, M. S.:* The Bisected Brain. New York: Appleton-Century-Crofts, 1970.
17. *Geschwind, N.:* Problems in the anatomical understanding of the aphasias. In A. L. Benton (Ed.): Contributions to Clinical Neuropsychology. Chicago: Aldine, 1969.
18. *Guertin, W. H., et al.:* Research with the Wechsler Intelligence Scale for Adults: 1960-1965, Psychol. Bull., 66, 1966.
19. *Hécaen, H.:* Functional hemispheric asymmetry and behavior. Soc. Serv. Info., 12:6, 1973.
20. *Heilbrun, A. B.:* Psychological test performance as a function of lateral localization of cerebral lesions. J. Comp. Physiol. Psychol., 49, 1956.
21. *Jackson, J. H.:* On the nature of the duality of the brain. In J. Taylor (Ed.): Selected Writing of John Hughlings Jackson. New York: Basic Books, 1958.
22. *Kløve, H.:* Validation studies in adult clinical neuropsychology. In R. M. Reitan and L. A. Davison (Eds.): Clinical Neuropsychology: Current Status and Application. New York: John Wiley, 1974.
23. *Landsell, H.:* Verbal and nonverbal factors in right-hemisphere speech: Relation to early neurological history. J. Comp. Physiol. Psychol., 69:4, 1969.
24. *Landsell, H.:* Effect of extent of temporal lobe ablation on two lateralized deficits. Physiol. and Behav., 5, 1968.
25. *Landsell, H.:* Evidence for a symmetrical hemispheric contribution to an intellectual function. Proc. 76th Annual Convention, Amer. Psychol. Assoc., 1968.
26. *Landsell, H.:* The use of factor scores from the Wechsler-Bellevue Scale of Intelligence in assessing patients with temporal lobe removals. Cortex, 4, 1968.
27. *Lezak, M. D.:* Neuropsychological Assessment. New York: Oxford University Press, 1976.
28. *Luria, A. R.* and *Simernitskaya, E. G.:* Interhemispheric relations and the functions of the minor hemisphere. Neuropsychologia, 15:1, 1977.
29. *Meier, M. J.* and *French, L. A.:* Longitudinal assessment of intellectual functioning following unilateral temporal lobectomy. J. Clin. Psychol., 22, 1966.
30. *Milner, B.:* Laterality effects in audition. In V. B. Mountcastle (Ed.): Interhemispheric Relations and Cerebral Dominance. Baltimore, Md.: The Johns Hopkins Press, 1962.

31. *Mountcastle, V. B.* (Ed.): Interhemispheric Relations and Cerebral Dominance. Baltimore, Md.: The Johns Hopkins Press, 1962.
32. *Myklebust, H. G.* and *Brutten, M.:* A study of the visual perceptions of deaf children. Acta Oto-Laryngologica. Supplement 105, 1953.
33. *Nebes, R. D.:* Hemispheric specialization in commissurotomized man. Psychol. Bull., 81:1, 1974.
34. *Nielsen, J .M.:* Agnosia, Apraxia, Aphasia: Their Value in Cerebral Localization. New York: Hafner, 1962.
35. *Poeck, K.:* Modern trends in neuropsychology. *In* A. L. Benton (Ed.): Contributions to Clinical Neuropsychology. Chicago: Aldine, 1969.
36. *Reitan, R. M.:* Problems and prospects in identifying the effects of brain lesions with psychological tests. Sinai Hospital J., 14:1, 1968.
37. *Reitan, R. M.:* The effects of brain lesions on adaptive abilities in human beings. Indianapolis, Indiana: Indiana University Medical Center, Mimeo, 1959.
38. *Smith, A.:* Neuropsychological testing in neurological disorders. *In* W. J. Friedlander (Ed.): Advances in Neurology. New York: Raven Press, 1975.
39. *Smith, A.:* Dominant and nondominant hemispherectomy. *In* W. L. Smith (Ed.): Drugs, Development and Cerebral Function. Springfield: Charles C. Thomas, 1972.
40. *Smith, A.:* Verbal and nonverbal test performances of patients with "acute" lateralized brain lesions (tumors). J. Nerv. Ment. Dis., 141:5, 1966.
41. *Smith, A.* and *Burkland, C. W.:* Dominant hemispherectomy. Science, 153, 1966.
42. *Sperry, R. W.:* Some general aspects of interhemispheric integrations. *In* V. B. Mountcastle (Ed.): Interhemispheric Relations and Cerebral Dominance. Baltimore, Md.: Johns Hopkins Press, 1962.

CHAPTER 16

Criterion Problems

Many problems impair confidence in neuropsychological diagnosis. Some relate specifically to the research efforts of neuropsychology in the determination of brain-behavior relationships by studying the effects of lesions, as surveyed in Chapter 15. Some are more specific to the clinical goals of neuropsychodiagnosis, and relate directly to the use of behavioral tests to assess and localize possible brain damage. Most of the problems affect both disciplines.

The populations available to the two disciplines for study are different, as are their conditions. The neuropsychologist may study animals under conditions which permit control of the introduction and manipulation of variables, as in split-brain experiments. Or he may investigate the behavioral effects of known neurological damage in human subjects, sometimes generally established, as in the hemiplegic consequences of a cerebral vascular accident, sometimes more precisely established, as in brain-surgery cases where the site, the amount and the geometry of tissue removed are determined with precision and photographically recorded. The neuropsychologist will also have available identifying and diagnostic data from many neurological tests and instruments. With animal subjects, autopsy and histological study are always possible; with human surgery patients these validating procedures are frequently impossible. With animal subjects, before-and-after objective behavioral comparisons are always available. These are rarely possible with human subjects; brain-surgery patients have already suffered damage before the surgical procedure, so that the pre-lesion status can only rarely be established in precise terms. Observations upon animals are largely confined to sensory and motor processes; with human subjects language and other cognitive processes can be studied in addition to these.

349

In contrast, the neuropsychodiagnostician observes only human subjects in whom a brain lesion is usually suspected rather than known. The psychodiagnostician sees persons in whom emotional problems are the primary reason for diagnostic observation, where any neuropsychodiagnostic concern that may arise becomes a matter of checking out differential probabilities. Some neurological tests are available, but, as we will see, the full range is seldom deployable. Autopsy and histological studies are rare at best. Earlier behavioral assessments from tests may be available if the patient has a preceding history of emotional problems, but usually the tests then employed were not sensitive to brain-behavior impairment, or reflective of the entire range of brain functioning.

Both disciplines try to answer these questions: 1) Is there brain damage? 2) If so, where is it located? 3) If so, can the behavioral manifestations observed be ascribed to the lesion? 4) Can the symptomatic behavior be modified?

While the neuropsychologist's "harder," more precise data are obviously more likely to establish confidence in his answers than are the data of the neuropsychodiagnostician, he too has problems of criterion similar in kind if not degree to those that plague the diagnostician. These basic criterion problems are: 1) difficulties in establishing a neurological diagnosis, and 2) uncertainty in ascribing behavioral manifestations as the exclusive effect of a brain lesion.

ADEQUACY OF THE NEUROLOGICAL DIAGNOSIS

Nearly ideal criteria can prevail in animal studies; the site of ablation in the brain is planned and carefully executed; behavioral changes are measured; histological evidence is available; and the precision of the techniques minimizes the need for large study populations. The neurological diagnosis is exact. Yet the validity of the criterion for precise localization is still subject to question. While the path of a scalpel may be exquisitely guided with microsurgical techniques, the molecular effects of the incision upon the intact tissue adjacent to the incision are unknown, nor is the extended effect upon more remote tissue establishable. Histological study will not reveal whether such molecular effect has taken place nor how extensive it may be. A symptom may be due less to a lesion than to disorganization of the physiology of the rest of the brain. Interaction among nerve cells apparently takes place in ways more subtle than gross anatomy reveals.

Recent findings indicate that nerve cells transmit more than electrical impulses to their neighbors. Damaging one nerve cell may cause adjacent cells to shrink. Chemical passage has been traced from the eye to the visual cortex.

The history, approached from a developmental viewpoint, may shed some light upon the difficulties that medical diagnoses sometimes encounter in determining whether, where, and to what extent there has been an injury to the brain. This attitude of exploration is discussed by Kennedy and Ramirez (5). They note that impairment of function and behavior may be absent, even in the presence of extreme malconfiguration of the brain, as in hydrocephalus, and that if the remaining hemisphere is healthy after a diseased hemisphere has been removed, behavior and mental function are not seriously affected. On the other hand, extensive injury to the immature brain of the neonate may not be recognized until years later when its effects appear as skill deficits, behavioral problems, or seizure disorders; or a limited injury may so affect surrounding tissue that behavior and function are much affected. In short, the physiological effects of an injury may be more extensive than the anatomical limits at first suggest.

Difficulties in obtaining conformance to ideal criteria for neurological diagnosis are inherent in work with human subjects. A population known to be brain-damaged is often far from homogeneous in crucial variables: etiology, age at injury, nature of injury, site and extent of the lesion, elapsed time since injury, age at the time of observation, sex, and a host of pre-injury factors among which are intelligence, education, training, and lateral preferences for hand, eye, ear, and foot.

Defining a lesion, particularly, is a basic necessity that more often than not eludes even reasonably accurate neurological diagnosis. Smith (12, 13) comments that in many neuropsychological studies dependent upon neurological diagnosis, there is a "lack of precision in definition of the cardinal variable in most studies—namely, the lesion." The behavioral effects of a lesion, he reminds us, in addition to the factors above, vary according to: 1) pathophysiological effects on both adjacent and remote cerebral structures and on the entire brain; and 2) the momentum of the lesion—an eruptive lesion, as in a stroke, destroys nerve cells and tracts, and produces aphasia, while a slowly developing tumor at the same site does not. Tumors, notes Joynt (3), most commonly are glial in origin, inserting themselves between nerve cells and tract, leaving the function intact.

Frequently, neurological findings fail to corroborate psychological-behavioral findings, and vice-versa. The view is often encountered that a correct diagnosis is determined by the neurological data, that these establish positive and negative findings, and that any incongruence with behavioral indices is the fault of the behavioral methods. This attitude probably had its origin in the belief that neurology is a "hard" science, psychology a "soft" one. Tests performed upon the body, the use of instruments or electricity, x-rays, kymographic recordings, are often regarded as superior in validity to observation and measurement of behavior. This hard-nosed attitude may be soft-headed. It ignores the frequency, for example, with which normal EEG tracings have been found to be associated with diseased brain tissue. A similar phenomenon is the not infrequent autopsy finding that any tissue damage is lacking in a person who had displayed pronounced neurological disability.

Neurodiagnostic procedures now available vary markedly in their predictive ability; paradoxically, the greatest accuracy among them is associated with greater risks of pain, injury, or death. A hierarchy of increasing accuracy among neurological diagnostic techniques is suggested by Russell, et al. (11): 1) the standard physical neurological examination is the least accurate; then follow in order 2) procedures requiring special equipment, the EEG, and brain scan; 3) tests requiring minor surgical procedures; the pneumoencephalograph and the angiogram; 4) brain surgery permitting direct observation of the brain; 5) autopsy, with unlimited direct observation and crude sectioning of the brain; and finally most revealing of all; 6) histological study of brain tissue.

Reviewing the use of the EEG in psychological disorders attributable to brain damage, Kennard (4) in 1953 cited general inability to associate the two indices—behavior and EEG pattern. At that time she attributed the failure to the immature state of EEG-pattern classification and variations in psychological criteria associated with different schools of treatment. But 20 years later these difficulties remained little mitigated (18).

ADEQUACY OF THE PSYCHOLOGICAL DIAGNOSIS

Psychological and behavioral test procedures suffer at least as much as neurological procedures from ambiguity of criteria. Neuropsychological tests assay "functions": sensory, motor, cognitive, and the rest.

Luria (6) stresses the need for clarification of what constitutes a function. And indeed, when many tests used in the neuropsychological diagnosis are examined critically, they are seen to overlap, to combine elements of distinctly different functions. Uncontrolled variables are the nemesis of much research in this field. According to Meier (7), they may not be readily apparent in the experimental setting, they may confound each other, and they may obscure both criteria and behavioral measures.

Dependent upon the neurological diagnosis for a first discriminative base, the construction of a psychological test begins with subjects with established brain damage, although the many variables that determine a lesion may be imprecisely established. Successful discrimination in this first stage of research all too often is followed by sharp drops in predictive validity when the test is then used in efforts to discriminate the brain-damaged from non-brain-damaged patients in an unselected population, or when it is asked to separate patients with neurological diagnoses from those with severe psychiatric ones, for example, schizophrenia. The test may be inadequate, or undetected brain damage may be present in the so-called non-brain-damaged populations. Indeed, the very assumption that a psychiatric population is not a neurological one as well would appear to be unwarranted until the subjects have been examined carefully in depth for "soft" as well as "hard" signs of neurological pathology before they are grouped.

Research populations may be contaminated unwittingly by factors of "field-dependence" and "field-independence," in Witkin's terms (19). Many psychological tests used in the effort to identify brain damage require ability to separate figure from ground or field. Research may show that these factors should be controlled in comparisons of presumably brain-damaged and non-brain-damaged populations.

In the examination of a single patient, the diagnostician is dealing with the smallest possible population. In discrimination studies with groups of patients, the multiple variables operating require sifting through an enormous population to get even a small sample. Preceding levels of functioning of the subject usually are not available, neurological diagnostic work-ups on both brain-damaged and non-brain-damaged patients are not equal in scope, nor it is feasible usually that they be so. Equally lacking in uniformity are the neuropsychodiagnostic instruments used. Poeck (8) cautions, for example, that an adequate description of the speech difficulties of an aphasic patient would require a broad spectrum of performance testing. Were researchers and diagnosticians to establish a uniform battery of tests, some clarification might be achieved in time.

A special difficulty is encountered in the effort to separate psychological-behavioral problems from neurological ones. This difficulty obscures the differential diagnosis of schizophrenia and brain damage to an embarrassing degree. Tumors of the brain—especially in the areas of the frontal and temporal lobes—are often accompanied by and frequently preceded by severe psychopathology which masks the diagnostic picture until signs indicating intracranial pressure become manifest.

A consistent series of failures in efforts to discriminate between schizophrenic patients and brain-damaged ones is reported by Watson (14, 15, 16). In his studies, the Bender-Gestalt, the Graham-Kendall Memory for Designs, the Reitan-Halstead Battery, and the WAIS appeared to be non-discriminating. He reported significant differences only for the Benton Visual Retention Test, but these only to a degree that caused him to advise that this test be used cautiously in settings that serve both brain-damaged and schizophrenic patients.

Watson's work appears to be based upon an assumption that probably is not warranted until it is clearly established: that a patient diagnosed as schizophrenic is not also brain-damaged. While he is careful in one study (15) to identify those patients among his schizophrenic subjects who had had lobotomies, there is no indication that he searched the histories for data suggestive or implicative of brain injury, fevers, traumas, or birth difficulties.

Perhaps the greater difficulties in evaluating a full history of an adult schizophrenic patient for neurological implications explain why there appears to be somewhat more consensus that neuropathology is also present in large numbers of schizophrenic children. In one study (17), abnormal EEG's were obtained for only 10 percent of neurotic children, but in 59 percent of children diagnosed as autistic or symbiotic schizophrenics. Ritvo, et al. (10) argue convincingly that children with established and probable neuropathology must be eliminated from studies of EEG readings in childhood psychosis. Their chief point, however, is that the organic dysfunction that contributes to similar disturbance in both brain-damaged and schizophrenic children is too subtle to be detected by existing investigative procedures.

The difficulty of separating brain-damaged from emotionally-disturbed children on the basis of patterns of intellectual ability was encountered by Bortner and Birch (2). Their subjects were 131 emotionally disturbed children and 116 brain-damaged children, ranging in age from seven to eleven years. Apart from I.Q. level and certain patterns of factorial organization, they found that the intellectual patterning in these two groups of children were markedly alike. Emotionally disturbed children tended to be superior in the I.Q. level as as a whole, in Verbal I.Q., Performance I.Q., Full Scale I.Q., and on subtest scores. When the I.Q. level was controlled, these differences disappeared. Discrepancies in Verbal-Performance scores were insignificant at all grade ages in the emotionally disturbed group, contrary to the generally held opinion that verbal abilities lag behind performance abilities in emotionally disturbed children. As a counterpart, it was established that Verbal-Performance I.Q. discrepancies were not significant among the brain-damaged children, thereby contesting the corollary opinion that performance scores tend to be lower than verbal scores in brain-damaged children.

In a related way, it was indicated that individual subtest scores could not be correlated with either diagnostic group. Neither group was distinguished by an especially verbal or non-verbal disability. However, both groups evidenced disability in attention and concentration (Arithmetic, Digit Span, Coding). The authors were compelled to suspect that the manner in which children are assigned or designated as emotionally disturbed or brain-damaged was responsible for the findings. *Children designated as emotionally disturbed, may in fact be brain-damaged; conversely, a brain-damaged child may manifest emotional disturbance.* Considerable evidence points to overlap between emotional disorders, mental subnormality, and brain damage.

It is difficult to separate brain-damaged populations from normal ones as well. Reitan (9) reminds us that almost all of the conditions thought to be associated with cerebral damage in children—hyperactivity, impulsivity, learning disorders—are found in "perfectly normal children."

Schizophrenia in both children and adults is a complex, multiple phenomena. Efforts to sharpen diagnostic inferences among populations of schizophrenics on the basis of the process-reactive dichotomy have not been too fruitful. Bellak's (1) conceptualization of schizophrenia as a syndrome of variable ego function deficiencies resulting from multiple possible etiologies stresses the rigor required to isolate and hold constant the many related variables.

INCREASING CONFIDENCE IN DIAGNOSIS

More congruence between neurological and behavioral criteria would be within reach if certain emphases develop in the practices of both neurology and psychology. Diagnosis would become more reliable if:

1) Greater credence were given to the so-called "soft," equivocal neurological signs;

2) EEG procedures were always extensive and always included needle electrodes, nasopharyngeal leads, sleep readings, photo-stimulation and hyperventilation;

3) psychological tests were "purified" as to the function tested, by eliminating overlap and combination;

4) psychological test batteries were expanded and refined to make them more reflective of and sensitive to the wide range of brain-behavior relationships;

5) histories were invariably pursued for data significant of neurological as well as psychological implications;

6) neuropsychologists and neuropsychodiagnosticians agreed upon a uniform test battery and upon procedures for accepting innovative additions to that battery as they are developed;

7) psychological, psychiatric, and neurological data were systematically collected from control groups as well as patient groups;

8) double-blind evaluation of all data was made routine;

9) both initial and long-term studies of patients were also made routine.

Meanwhile, all professional workers responsible for the welfare of patients must realize the enormity of the criterion problem. We all need increased respect for the contributions of disciplines other than our own, and more humility about our own current limitations.

If neuropsychological and neurological methods produce congruent data, confidence in diagnosis of pathology is increased. However, even if they concur that the patient shows *no evidence* of brain damage, there still remains the possibility that the patient is suffering a neurological impairment that none of the investigative procedures has been sensitive enough to detect. Even if one discipline reports brain damage and the others do not, the likelihood of brain damage is not necessarily diminished; that patient's impairments may be so subtle as to escape the discipline that finds nothing. A lesion may be "silent," unresponsive to the exploration of one method, or to all, or perhaps more responsive to one than to others. In general, confidence in diagnosis mounts with increase in the number of similar judgments derived independently from different and/or related investigative procedures. This increasing probability is what the clinical neuropsychodiagnostician must pursue in the one-to-one professional relationship with a single patient.

BIBLIOGRAPHY

1. *Bellak, L.:* The psychoanalytic concept of the ego and schizophrenia. *In* L. Bellak and P. K. Benedict (Eds.): Schizophrenia: A Review of the Syndrome. New York: Logos Press, 1958.
2. *Bortner, M.* and *Birch, H. G.:* Patterns of intellectual ability in emotionally disturbed and brain-damaged children. J. Spec. Ed., 3:4, 1969.
3. *Joynt, R. J.:* Language disturbances in cerebrovascular disease. *In* A. L. Benton (Ed.): Behavioral Change in Cerebrovascular Disease. New York: Harper and Row, 1970.
4. *Kennard, M. A.:* The electroencephalogram in psychological disorders: A review. Psychosom. Med., 15, 1953.
5. *Kennedy, C.* and *Ramirez, L. S.:* Brain damage as a cause of behavior disturbance in children. *In* H. G. Birch (Ed.): Brain Damage in Children. Baltimore, Md.: Williams and Wilkins, 1964.
6. *Luria, A. R.:* Higher Cortical Functions in Man. New York: Basic Books, 1966.
7. *Meier, M. J.:* Objective behavioral assessment in diagnosis and prediction. *In* A. L. Benton (Ed.): Behavioral Change in Cerebrovascular Disease. New York: Harper and Row, 1970.
8. *Poeck, K.:* Modern trends in neuropsychology. *In* A. L. Benton (Ed.): Contributions to Clinical Neuropsychology. Chicago: Aldine, 1969.
9. *Reitan, R. M.:* Psychological effects of cerebral lesions in children of early school age. Mimeo., 1970.
10. *Ritvo, E. R., et al.:* Correlation of psychiatric diagnoses and EEG findings: A double-blind study of 184 hospitalized children. Amer. J. Psychiat., 126:7, 1970.
11. *Russell, E. W., et al.:* Assessment of Brain Damage. New York: Wiley-Interscience, 1970.
12. *Smith, A.:* Practice and principles of clinical neuropsychology. The Int. Neuropsych. Soc. Bull., March, 1979.
13. *Smith, A.:* Appraising the neuropsychological literature. The Int. Neuropsych. Soc. Bull., August, 1978.
14. *Watson, C. G.:* The separation of NP hospital organics from schizophrenics with three visual motor screening tests. J. Clin. Psychol., 24:4, 1968.
15. *Watson, C. G., et al.:* Differentiation of organics from schizophrenics at two chronicity levels by use of the Reitan-Halstead Organic Test Battery. J. Consult. Clin. Psychol., 32:6, 1968.
16. *Watson, C. G.:* Intratest scatter in hospitalized brain-damaged and schizophrenic patients. J. Consult. Psychol., 29:6, 1965.

17. *Webb, W. W., et al.:* The sequelae of acute bacterial meningitis: A possible clue to early school problems. J. Spec. Ed., 2:4, 1968.
18. *White, P. T., et al.:* EEG abnormalities in early childhood schizophrenia: A double blind study of psychiatrically disturbed and normal children during Promazine sedation. Amer. J. Psychiat., 120, 1964.
19. *Witkin, H. A., et al.:* Personality Through Perception. New York: Harper and Bros., 1954.

CHAPTER 17

Neurodiagnostic Approaches

This chapter considers two major approaches to neurodiagnosis, the neurological and the psychological, as they bear upon equivocal conditions.

NEUROLOGICAL DIAGNOSTIC TECHNIQUES

Standard neurological diagnostic techniques include a routine physical examination, a mental status examination, special tests, and instrumental and surgical procedures.

The Routine Neurological Examination

The routine neurological examination (9) consists of:

1) estimates of general cerebral function—intellectual, emotional, and social behavior, memory;
2) tests of motor and sensory functions—muscle tone and strength, gait, involuntary movements, performances of rapid alternating movements, cortical and discriminatory sensations;
3) tests of cerebellar functions—such as finger to nose, path pointing, heel to knee, coordination;
4) tests of reflexes, including the deep reflexes;
5) tests of cranial-nerve functions—eye muscles, visual fields, audition, balance, and speech production.

The usual examination does not include assessment of perceptual-motor functions, constructional praxis, abstract thinking, or body-image concept, nor other higher level subtle cerebral functions.

Some neurologists, depending upon training and orientation, in-

359

clude measures of cognitive functioning. Although I have not formally surveyed practices in neurological examinations, my personal experience in obtaining neurological consultation for my patients, as well as my observations from the literature, indicates that the usual emphasis is upon assessment of the subcortical areas and lower cortical functions of the central nervous system, and that the usual examination is of infrequent value in illuminating cognitive and behavioral functions.

A recent publication (36) stresses the mental-status examination in neurology as a corollary to the physical exploration. It presents a comprehensive and detailed procedure for the examination of cortical functions: levels of consciousness, appearance, mood and social behavior, language, memory, constructional ability, spatial comprehension, information, abstract thinking, arithmetic, ideomotor and ideational praxia, right/left orientation, visual gnosia, and geographical orientation. The approach both borrows much from and lends much to neuropsychology, which is treated rather cursorily. The approach presented is unlike most neuropsychology practice in being unstandardized, and similar in requiring much time. The authors seek to reassure student neurologists that once they have mastered the lengthy procedure it can be truncated. In practice one generally finds that outside of the teaching hospital, the neurological exploration of higher cortical functions is rather superficial.

The practice of neurology concentrates upon the definite, upon clinically recognizable manifestations of dysfunction; it has recognized the existence of "soft" or equivocal signs, but these, even when they signal the possibility of motor or sensory dysfunction, are seldom credited. This emphasis upon hard signs and subcortical functions, coupled with rather cursory survey of cognitive functions, limits the value of the standard neurological examination in the detection of equivocal conditions (19, 23, 25), a primary concern of this book. Submicroscopic lesions may cause primary or only soft signs on both neurological and psychological tests, states Gross (15), and the neurological examination as now constituted cannot rule out disease at the microscopic or molecular levels. Another major problem in neurology, as throughout much of medicine, is the possible multiple causation of a single symptom, as Drachman and Hart (11) have demonstrated in dizziness. Moreover, Reitan (29) has shown that severe organic brain pathology is not necessarily correlated with clearcut neurological indices. A population of 26 patients with diffuse cerebral damage from cerebrovascular disease showed minimal positive finding on neurological examination. The EEG's of 35 percent were entirely normal, and contrast studies on 13 patients failed to find a lesion. Further, Benton and Joynt (3) observe that often changes in behavior after cerebrovascular accidents are hard to recognize. The changes may be inconspicuous, for example, in speed of reaction, or in time taken to make decisions in complex situations, or short-term memory. These may be brought out only by careful comparisons with peers, or preferably with the person's own preceding performance level, if available.

Nonetheless, current instruction in neurology, and hence neurological practice, emphasizes precise relationship between lesion and behavior. The certainties are highlighted, while the areas of ambiguity and even frank ignorance are underplayed. Usually the patients who present ambiguous disorders or those not understood are referred for treatment to psychiatry, a profession no better equipped than neurology to diagnose and treat such ambiguous conditions.

However, the presence of soft or equivocal signs does not always mean that hard signs are absent, and these must be sought diligently in difficult cases, as well as in more obvious ones. The neurological examination remains important in equivocal conditions, to probe for possible brain pathology of a progressive nature requiring intervention, or non-progressive pathology that might benefit from a protracted treatment regimen. Even in this determination, however, the examination is only a starting point for what may have to be an extended, elaborate, sometimes painful and dangerous process of diagnosis. In itself, the standard, routine neurological examination is limited in its capacity to diagnose all orders of cortical lesions.

Special Instrument Tests

Diagnotic acumen now has at its service new and significant neurological procedures using special instrumentation. In recent years, the brain scan and computerized axial tomography have emerged as useful devices. Electroencephalography has been widely used for about four decades; validity of its results as a criterion of brain damage and its location is still the subject of controversy.

The Electroencephalograph (EEG)

The EEG test measures and records the frequency and voltages of oscillating potentials originating in brain-tissue activity. Classically, leads, i.e., electrodes, are placed upon the scalp. Recently, needle electrodes have been placed under the scalp. Less frequently, deep electrodes ase placed directly into the brain tissue itself. Since the variables—frequency and voltage—vary with regions of the brain, the aim is to deploy the electrodes so as to capture as much as possible of the brain's electrical activity. The surface area of the brain available for EEG scrutiny has been increased by the recent development of naso-pharyngeal leads. These are electrodes placed relatively close to the inferior and medial surfaces of the temporal lobes. The leads are inserted through the nostrils, and advanced along the septum into the naso-pharynx (2). Only about one-third of the brain is at present directly available to electroencephalography.

Electrical activity varies with state of consciousness and with sensory stimulation. Thus readings may be taken while the patient is sedated or stimulated (as by flashing lights) for comparison with those obtained during a waking-resting state.

Within limits, normal patterns of the recorded EEG tracings for rate, regularity, amplitude, and configuration of waves have been established. These are related to the age of the subject, his resting state (that is, his relative metabolic equilibrium), and freedom from known or suspected central-nervous-system pathology. Experience indicates that within these parameters even a "normal" adult population will produce abnormal EEG records in five to 15 percent of the subjects.

Normal patterns for children have also been established; these are more varied and less stable than those obtained for adults. The patterns change in a fairly predictable process from birth to adolescence; thereafter the changes are more gradual. Some evidence indicates that a young brain which produces abnormal EEG readings may mature into an adult brain with dominantly normal rhythms, although this does not mean pathology is no longer present.

The validity of the EEG as a criterion of brain pathology is in considerable doubt. The consensus is that positive readings may be accepted; negative readings are less reliable, in light of the frequency of normal readings found to be associated with pathological brain tissues (8). This evidence indicates that the EEG alone is not a clear-cut diagnostic tool (14).

While they often correlate with a diagnosis of brain pathology derived from clinical history and behavior patterns, EEG tracings—reflecting electrical activity of the brain—are apparently influenced by factors other than brain pathology which in many ways have similar effects. Factors of age, metabolic states, levels of consciousness, and sensory excitement have already been mentioned. Thought disturbances and other psychopathology have been related to abnormal EEG characteristics (17, 18), with an incidence much higher than in a normal population. Here, of course, which factor is causal is not clearly established. No particular abnormal EEG patterns have been associated with psychological problems alone. A 14-and-6 per second positive spiking pattern has been found with some psychological problems, but such a spiking pattern may also be associated with a seizure disorder (23).

Part of the difficulty may arise because of the limited area of the brain read by EEG electrodes. Since only about one-third of the brain is ordinarily scrutinized by them, this limitation may account for reports of seizures observed after normal readings were recorded, or of frontal-lobe tumors diagnosed only after a patient had spent years in a psychiatric hospital, or of normal readings obtained from patients found to have deeply situated tumors.

The EEG taps only the outer shell and a small portion of the under and medial surface of the cerebrum, only the outer centimeter or so. The electrodes employed, although very small, are large in comparison with the size of brain cells, so that the tracings produced are summations of the activity of groups of cells, not of a single cell.

Still another difficulty is that the EEG is extremely sensitive to stimuli unrelated to the processes that are being studied. The observer must be trained to rule out the effects of coughing, blinking, and sneezing, for examples.

A basic difficulty with the EEG has been reading the recorded tracings accurately. In the early days of EEG use, the electroencephaloger scanned the tracings visually so that the technique and ultimate diagnosis were only as good as his specific skill and experience. Later, careful but time-consuming measurements were made by hand with rulers and calipers of the length, height, and shape of the tracings. The frequency of each variable was then counted by hand. It is now possible to do all of this by computer. The technique allows the banding together of some spectral components and the eliminating of others, a data-reducing device. Another new approach involves evoking nerve-cell electrical activity by appropriate stimulation and averaging the results to arrive at the average evoked potential (12). Monroe (24) employs an activating drug, alphachlorose, to increase the sensitivity of scalp recordings and to discriminate behavior arising from epilepsy, for example, from that of so-called motivational disorders.

The electrodes used in EEG studies may contribute to confusing artifacts. They may create asymmetrical readings because they are unequally spaced, or two electrodes may be accidentally connected by perspiration or the electrode paste employed, or the electrodes may be in poor contact with the scalp (6).

Efforts to improve the validity of the EEG have brought suggestions that needle electrodes and naso-pharyngeal leads be universally employed, that sleep readings always be an essential component of the EEG examination, that repeated or serial tracings be obtained, and that double-blind interpretations be standard in order to minimize bias. As one example, perceptual inconstancy is a neuropathological condition contributing to childhood psychosis, according to Ritvo, *et al.* (31), that appears in EEG readings *only* during varying states of consciousness and when "telemetered monitoring for spectral and discriminant analysis" is employed.

Despite criterion difficulties, much reliance continues to be placed in the EEG. A nationwide review of the diagnostic process for Minimal Brain Dysfunction finds the EEG "widely and erroneously regarded as the *sine qua non* for the identification of Minimal Brain Dysfunction" (23). This important publication of the Federal government states that no EEG pattern of abnormality can be associated diagnostically with "diffuse brain damage, minimal brain dysfunction or in behavior disorders of any kind."

Rid of the myth of infallibility, the EEG, like so many other diagnostic procedures, has its valued role. The procedure could be more helpful in cases where seizures are suspected but cannot be established, in behavior abnormalities of paroxysmal nature, in possible seizure-equivalent states, and where there is a suggestion of global or focal neurological dysfunction. In these instances, confidence in EEG find-of multiple EEG techniques is increased where application of multiple EEG techniques is thorough, even exhaustive, and includes tracings recorded during wakefulness, hyperventilation, intermittent photic stimulation, sleep, serial tracings, hour-long recordings, repeating the procedure another day at a different time, use of needle electrodes and naso-pharyngeal leads, activating drugs, and special montage for detecting 14-and-6 per second positive spiking. Its best role, however, is always in association with corollary procedures: the history, the neurological and neuropsychological examinations, and other neurological procedures; in itself the EEG is not *the* diagnostic tool. And, again, while a positive EEG usually is diagnostically significant, a negative one need not be. This seeming paradox is not without parallel among medical diagnostic procedures: generations who lived in dread of veneral diseases knew that a positive Wasserman most likely was valid, a negative one often enough was not.

The Brain Scan and the C.A.T.

In recent years a technique of brain scanning has been found a useful device. It requires the injection of a small amount of radioactive material, and is said to be without harm to the patient, exposing him to less radiation than a chest x-ray. Tinterov (38) emphasizes its diagnostic value early in the examination of patients with convulsive disorders and psychiatric conditions that may mask intracranial pathology. In some specific clinical incidents it is preferable, he states, to the lumbar-puncture technique, described below. Again, he cautions "a negative scan is of no value. . . ."

A more sophisticated technique has emerged recently: computerized axial tomography (C.A.T.). In this procedure a large number of x-ray pictures are taken simultaneously and collated by computer. The technique allows a large number of serial reading along any body axis, the equivalent of histological sections but of tissue *in situ*.

Tests Requiring Minor or Major Surgery

In the *lumbar puncture* procedure, a hollow needle is inserted between lumbar vertebrae into the fluid surrounding the spinal cord; fluid is withdrawn and analyzed for its chemistry, for blood and tumor cells, as evidences of histopathology.

In a related procedure, the *pneumoencephalogram,* spinal fluid is replaced with air or other contrast material; the air reaches the spaces surrounding the brain and the ventricles of the brain, more clearly delineating their shapes; x-rays then are taken. *Angiography* is the x-ray examination of the brain's vascular system after injection into the blood stream of radiopaque material.

The *Wada test* utilizes the injection of amytal into the carotid arteries, allowing the selective anesthetization of each cerebral hemisphere and thereby facilitating the lateralization of a lesion.

Brain surgery and *biopsy* permit more direct examination, the former of the gross anatomy of the brain and the manifest extent of visible lesions, the latter of small portions of suspect brain tissue removed for histological study.

Diagnosis Through Therapy

Sometimes in the absence of trustworthy diagnostic evidence of any kind, except for behavioral manifestations, a patient improves when trial courses of medication are introduced. This often happens in children suspected of Minimal Brain Dysfunction who demonstrate the paradoxical effect of stimulant drugs by becoming less hyperactive and better able to sustain concentration. Another example of a *post facto* therapeutic diagnosis is found in those instances when phenomena, unidentifiable by EEG but suspected to be seizure equivalents, are mitigated by anticonvulsant medication.

Improving Neurodiagnosis

Most of the procedures identified above were believed by Poeck (27) to be too crude to accomplish precise localization, although continued refinement of radioactive scanning was expected to lend more precision to neurodiagnosis. The C.A.T. (computerized axial tomography) scan is one current fulfillment of his prediction. Developments in the studies of evoked cortical responses (10) are promising. Unlike the EEG, these procedures use a controllable stimulus, e.g., light. Computers separate the brain's responses to this stimulus from the rest of the brain's usual electrical activity. These responses to light have been found to be highly complex, and possibly to consist of components from different cortical areas. An intriguing brain activity identified in this research, the meaning of which is still being investigated, is the emergence of a slow negative-rising wave when an event or stimulus is being anticipated.

Continued exploration of the diagnostic import of equivocal signs through longitudinal age studies can be expected also to improve neurodiagnosis over the long term. These should chart the development and course of normal functions, the appearance and fate of impairments, and their effect upon functioning at all ages. The differentiation of psychotic from brain-damaged children probably will improve only when equivocal signs are better understood, better described, and more widely accepted as having meaning. The future should bring refinement of microanatomical, molecular, chemical, electrical, and x-ray scanning procedures that will improve criteria for the definition and classification of equivocal signs. These signs should be identified in historical data, behavioral patterns, and psychological-test patterns, as well as in sensorimotor functions, language, and learning behavior. Wider use of extant age norms such as the Gesell scales (13) and development of newer scales, standardized for all types of signs, could result in significant clarification. Promising among these is the classification and description of very early neurological signs that may evolve in later years as neuropathology; Dargassies (7) has been studying such signs in the first year of life. The standard neurological examination typically is not concerned with aspects of maturation and development. Yet many of these functions involved in learning, for example, particularly in reading, could be scrutinized. Improved age norms for cortical functions in the preschool child might facilitate early identification of a child who will later manifest learning difficulties, and make possible early therapeutic intervention or special teaching.

Refinement and standardization of these equivocal signs should increase the diagnostician's ability to separate signs strongly suggestive of serious brain pathology from those suggestive of minimal brain dysfunction, so that the valuable role of the standard neurological testing procedures may be more discriminately applied.

PSYCHOLOGICAL PROCEDURES

As we have seen, psychological testing techniques have a role in establishing brain damage, identifying the function(s) affected if it exists, and identifying the nature and degree of the impairment, as well as the possible location of the lesion. In this section, the major psychological methods for inferring brain damage are described, along with the approaches of some outstanding neuropsychodiagnosticians.

Methods for Inferring Brain Damage

A critical review of psychological methods for inferring the existence of cerebral damage is presented by Reitan (30).

1) *Level of performance.* Central-tendency measures of variability are established for single tests for groups with known cerebral damage and without it. The performance level of either an individual or a group of subjects then may be compared with a normative standard. Reitan finds data of this kind difficult to apply. Level of performance

on psychological tests is known to be affected by many variables other than brain damage: genetic factors, cultural deprivation, educational disabilities, the presence of severe emotional conditions such as psychosis, and the normal aging process. Therefore, a psychological-test score departing from the normative standard may do so for many reasons other than brain damage. The functioning level of the patient prior to his presumed injury or impairment is not usually known; if originally he were of superior ability, he may have sustained a pronounced loss but still be functioning within the average range of individuals whose norms contributed to the criteria for the non-brain-damaged characterization.

The deficits resulting from cerebral damage may vary considerably with the passage of time, even though the essential neurological diagnosis remains the same. Reitan concludes that a definite possibility of obtaining so-called false-positive results with any instrument that yields "scaled, continuous score distributions" of psychological abilities is inescapable.

2) *Qualitative deficiencies in psychological-test performances.* Goldstein (14) has contended that the abstract function is different and distinct in nature from concrete behavior and that there is no gradual transition from one to the other. He held that the distinct difference between the two vitiates the meaning of the quantitative results of test data where the same test is administered to both non-brain-damaged and brain-damaged subjects, because in his view the results fundamentally are not comparable. Reitan contests this opinion. Using graded subtests of the Halstead Category Test, Reitan demonstrated that while normal and brain-damaged subjects made significantly different numbers of errors on tests measuring abstract functions, there was no such significant difference between the groups in either absolute or proportional improvement from one subtest to the other. Reitan concludes that the effects of cerebral lesions represent quantitative deviations from normal levels, rather than sharp qualitative differences. Clinically, I have been impressed by sustained capacity for abstract reasoning, as measured by intelligence scales such as the Wechsler, along with pronounced impairment in other areas such as verbal conceptualization.

3) *Pathognomic signs of cerebral damage.* A familiar instance of the use of one or several behaviors as evidence of pathology is found in Piotrowski's (26) Rorschach signs, for example, his Impotence and Perplexity signs. These are signs of specific deficiencies, said to be more

commonly associated with brain damage than with any other type of impairing condition. Yet their application to the identification of brain damage is difficult. They are dependent upon subjective observation by the examiner, hence are not easily replicated by other examiners. They produce rather high numbers of false negatives; that is, many persons with clearly established cerebral deficits fail to produce evidence of signs. They are of value in alerting the examiner to the possibility of cerebral damage and as supplements to other measures which yield more quantitative results.

4) *Pre-damage versus post-damage comparisons.* This method of investigation is rarely possible, since test data prior to traumatic episodes or critical disease eruptions are seldom available for sufficient members of a population to be of value. Exceptions are those cases in which seizures are reported for the first time *after* examination. In question, however, is the reliability of the report that the seizure observed was indeed the first.

5) *Differential score comparisons.* This method, dating back to the work of Babcock in 1930 (1) presumes that some functions are easily and adversely affected by cerebral damage, while others are more resistive. Wechsler's *Hold-Don't Hold* tests are an example. Reitan cites inherent sampling difficulties as responsible for the poor data obtained with this approach. He demonstrated that the Block Design subtest —held to be the subtest of the Wechsler-Bellevue battery most sensitive to brain damage—was of great value in identifying patients with right-cerebral lesions, but relatively inefficient in identifying patients with limited left-cerebral hemispheric damage. He finds the subtest a useful instrument in comparing the integrity of the two cerebral hemispheres, and considerably less useful in a general determination of whether or not cerebral damage is present.

The differential-score method does not address the problem of identifying *general* versus *specific* deficits resulting from cerebral lesions. It does not take into account the effects upon psychological-test results of variations in brain damage, such as location, type, momentum, or duration of lesion. Its assumption, which baldly is that "a given brain lesion in any individual will manifest its psychological effect in the same way," ignores the complexity of the brain-behavior relationship.

6) *Statistical methods.* Multivariate statistical analysis is sometimes employed. A comparison is made between two groups of subjects: a non-brain-damaged group and a brain-damaged group; or a group with left-hemispheric lesions and another with right-hemispheric le-

sions. A single weighted score resulting from the discriminant function is obtained for each subject, along with an optimum least-squares separation between the scores for each group. The point of minimal overlap between the groups is established from the distribution of summed weighted scores, so that an individual's weighted score will place him in a particular group depending upon whether if falls above or below this overlap point.

Reitan's criticism here is not with the statistical method but rather with the identification of the groups of subjects. This objection takes us back to that persistent haunting problem in neuropsychological diagnosis: the problem of the criterion. Individual variation within the group characterized as brain-damaged is so great that generalizations about such a group are usually not permissible. Even success in differentiating right- and left-hemisphere damage from diffuse cerebral damage is only a first step in the discrimination process.

7) *Comparison of results from the two sides of the body.* This is an intra-individual comparative method, and thus is free of many of the problems inherent in other methods of inference. It is derived from the classical physical neurological examination which compares the right with the left side of the body. The method requires that the extent of difference in a given performance be established for the two sides of the body, as for example, in finger-tapping speed or strength of grip. Validity of interpretation depends upon using a number of different tests of such lateralized performance at different times during the examination period, so that if the patients shows consistent impairment on one side as compared with the other, the operation of transient fluctuations of attention and effort may be minimized in the assessment. Again, the variety of possible causal factors must be kept in mind. Reitan cautions that impairment of strength or of finger-tapping speed could be the result of muscle strain, a joint injury, or injury to the peripheral nerve, rather than to some central damage. Therefore, he adds tests of right and left sensory-perceptual and complex performance tasks to his investigative armamentarium.

A major disadvantage is that some of the tests will not show differential results if there has been nearly equal damage in both lobes of the brain. Reitan finds the method promising, however, because he has observed pronounced differences between right and left performances in many subjects, including mental retardates, in whom no neurological evidence suggested involvement of only one of the cerebral hemisphere.

A major advantage of the method is its relative freedom from the effects of conscious resistance, deliberate simulation of impairment, or the effects of emotional problems. Conceivably, however, a classical hysteria affecting one side of the body might produce false-positive results with the method.

Reason, Reitan concludes, dictates that the special strength of each method be appreciated and that the methods be combined for their synergistic enhancement of each other.

Some Individual Neuropsychodiagnostic Approaches

Differences of approach are apparent in the procedures, techniques, and emphases developed by certain innovative neuropsychodiagnosticians who have made their clinical styles and orientations quite clear in their writings. These examples of style are valuable to the student and to the developing clinician, who may find that identification with one or another facilitates his own emerging approach. Only some of the outstanding workers are reviewed below, those whose contributions epitomize the major historical trends in neuropsychology. The contributions of many other outstanding scientists and professionals are described elsewhere in this volume.

The "nose" of the astute diagnostician is a hallowed concept among clinicians; indeed, some insist that the best instrument for organicity is an astute clinician so equipped. This emphasis stresses the process "within" the clinician, the rapid concatenation of observation, evaluation, and judgment, the on-the-spot selection of tests in response to observation, even the instant invention of tests to assess a specific function in an individual patient. It is not that standardized tests are not deployed, but that their deployment is not formalized, and that it is the clinician who is the primary test instrument via his observation of "how" the patient performs, not what he scores. Luria's approach, an exemplary demonstration of this clinical style, is made abundantly clear in his writings.

As detailed below, another approach places the test instrument in the foreground of the clinical examination and gives the scores obtained by its use prominence in the ultimate judgment. Some investigators still pursue a single test instrument that will sort out the brain-damaged from all others in statistically significant ratios. More promising is the use of a battery designed to test a variety of brain functions. The battery is presented uniformly to all patients in a manner that has been standardized. Validation of each test in the battery is pursued in statistical analysis. New tests are invented to meet perceived needs to fill in and round out the battery; their invention and application follow the dicta for validation and standardization. Halstead and Reitan are noteworthy for this mode of rigorous development and testing of tests as instruments of clinical diagnosis. A recent extension of their approach has been the development of a "key" method of neuropsychodiagnosis, in which the reliance upon the test as "clinician" is pronounced. One should not presume, however, that the Halstead-Reitan tradition does not call upon clinical acumen or devalues it. The clinician in this tradition operates with the test battery to assure that the fullest range of observations is made in every case, and that none are overlooked. His clinical style may be proscribed; his clinical acumen is not limited but rather is buttressed.

Nonetheless, the test-battery approach can lead to de-emphasis of the human being as test instrument, especially in the "key" method and in the paper-and-pencil computer method (23) when technicians rather than clinicians administer tests constructed by the systems analyst in conjunction with the clinician. The initial shock to one's clinical convictions may be mitigated if one keeps in mind the possibilities for coping with enormous numbers of data points and thus their potential for great social usefulness. For example, screening millions of young children to detect those with possible cerebral deficits for early intervention and special training becomes feasible with these methods.

Halstead's Pioneering Work

Seeking to identify and measure the dimensions of what he called "biological intelligence," Halstead developed 27 different tests of intellectual functioning, with the aim of distinguishing the brain-damaged from the non-brain-damaged person. These tests contributed to the final Halstead Battery of Neuropsychological Tests. In 1947, Halstead published (16) a description of his tests and a factorial analysis derived from their application to 237 control and experimental subjects with various types of brain lesions.

From this analysis Halstead identified four factors in "biological intelligence": 1) A central integrated field factor, representing the organized experience of the individual; it is the "familiar" against which the "new" is experienced. 2) A factor of abstraction, the basic capacity to characterize according to criteria; this involves comprehension of basic essential similarities and differences. 3) A power factor, which regulates the forces of affective drives and permits the operation of the ego in its differentiation functions. 4) A directional factor, the process whereby the reality of the experience is determined on the sensory side and the "final common pathway" is determined on the motor side.

Measuring Halstead's contribution is difficult; one may easily be unjust because of limited capacity for description. Essentially, he emphasized 1) that brain functions are such that the effects of a lesion in one location are different from those that would result from a lesion in another location, and 2) that a lesion can be detected only by use of a combination of neuropsychological tests that tap as many brain functions as possible. His signal contribution is undiminished by the fact that some later research has not corroborated his particular battery or his hypotheses of localization. Whether the failure on occasion to obtain corroboration rests in Halstead's battery or in the design and execution of the research is not relevant at this point. What is important is that his work stimulated development and improvement of neuropsychological test batteries and has been the vehicle through which much knowledge of brain function has been obtained.

His neuropsychodiagnostic battery remains his monument, despite the challenges. He reduced his original battery of 27 tests to 10, selected for their statistically demonstrated ability to separate brain-damaged from non-brain-damaged subjects. These 10 he used to compute what he called the Impairment Index: if a subject scored within the brain-damaged range on any five of the 10 tests, his Index score was considered to identify him as brain-damaged. Halstead also set a pattern for cooperation in diagnostic research between neurologist, neurosurgeon, and neuropsychologist, no mean accomplishment, and a standard to which we should all repair.

Reitan's Contributions

Reitan worked with Halstead. He developed his own modifications of Halstead's approach and added his own procedures. His work is guided by the view that the complexity of the brain calls for recognition of the major strength of any specific method and its exploitation in the assessment process. Since a cerebral lesion may impair one or more of many types of functions, a broad spectrum of psychological tasks testing various functions is required in the composition of a neurological test battery. Tests selected for use, regardless of which function they are presumed to measure, should as much as possible have demonstrated in control studies that they validly reflect impairments of the integrity of the brain.

Reitan in his work at the Neuropsychological Laboratory at the University of Indianapolis, and at the University of Washington in Seattle since 1971 extended the Halstead Battery to include tests of a wider range of behavioral functions. These apply first to 1) simple motor functions; 2) sensorimotor functions; and 3) psychomotor problem-solving procedures. These test relatively simple levels of functioning. However, Reitan emphasizes sensorimotor comparison of the two sides of the body, so that the individual provides his own basis of comparison to lateralize a dysfunction if it is present. Higher-level tasks in Reitan's battery include: 4) measurements of symbolic and communicational aspects of language; 5) manipulatory tasks, requiring ability to deal effectively with visual-spatial relations; 6) abstract and concept-formation ability; and 7) general intelligence. His battery thus examines for aphasia, apraxia, and various sensoriperceptual deficits.

Reitan has contributed significantly to the ability of the neuropsychologist to lateralize and localize brain lesions. He brought special sensitivity and acumen to the development of test methods, and to the illumination of existing ones as neuropsychodiagnostic instruments. This has been true especially of his application of the Wechsler Scales, consigned previously to disuse by the inadequacies of the *Hold-Don't Hold* measures. Although his claims that the scales are definitively able to discriminate between left and right hemispheric damage are seriously contested, he brought them back to respected employment as a preliminary neuropsychological battery in the hands of a general psychodiagnostician, and as part of the larger armamentarium of the wider-ranging neuropsychodiagnostician.

The Neuropsychological "Key" Approach

In biological classification systems, *keys* were developed to facilitate placing a specimen within a system using the organism's characteristics. The characteristics of a specimen are checked against a series of descriptive statements in the key. These statements are usually dichotomous, comparable to the basic "go, no-go" method of computers. If the specimen's characteristics are congruent with the first statement, the key is pursued according to the directions attendant to that statement; if not, the key is followed to the next alternate statement, and so on. In this way, the group for which the key has been constructed is separated into smaller and smaller units of classification.

Russell, *et al.* (32) have adopted some of the more modern concepts of biological classification by the key method to the discrimination of brain-damaged and non-brain-damaged individuals. Earlier biological keys were based upon a rigorous black-and-white method whereby a specific characteristic or number of characteristics defined the subgroup. This "monothetic" method was derived from the assumption in evolution theory that the animal or plant groups most like each other in key characteristics were developed from a common ancestor more recently than had those groups less alike. The progression along the evolutionary tree was thought to be logical and rigid.

In contrast, and more readily applicable to neuropsychodiagnosis, the "polythetic" arrangement places together organisms which have the greatest number of similar characteristics, but no single characteristic is either necessary or sufficient in itself to identify an organism as a member of a group. In essence, this is the way in which the Halstead Impairment Index operated in diagnosing brain damage if the subject scored in the brain-damaged range on any five of the ten tests in the battery.

The definition of a polythetic group is extremely important for neuropsychodiagnosis because it can reflect the complexity and variability in the brain-behavior relationship: a group is defined by a set of characteristics; each characteristic is found in large numbers of the group members; each member of the group possesses a large, but unspecified, number of the group characteristics; and no single characteristic is necessarily found in every member of the group.

Russell, *et al.* employ 41 test scores in their method. The scores are derived from some of Halstead's tests, an Aphasia examination, some of Reitan's contributions, and the WAIS. Twelve of the 41 scores are averaged to obtain an Impairment rating. Rating scales are applied to tests where they will increase quantification and objectivity. Scores are derived for sensorimotor functions of both sides of the body and for the visual fields.

Two major keys were constructed. 1) The *Localization Key* first seeks to determine the presence or absence of brain damage, then lateralization or diffuseness if brain damage is present, and finally the degree of lateralization, strong or weak, if lateralization has been established. 2) The *Process Key* attempts to discriminate between acute, congenital, and static brain-damaged conditions.

This approach is essentially an actuarial one. Among their validation studies, the authors compare the ability of their key to predict neurological criteria with a "sophisticated clinical approach"—the neuropsychological report. Little difference was found between the two methods, and they suggest that if these findings receive continued corroboration, the actuarial approach's greater economy will give it a marked advantage over the clinical inferential procedure.

A computer program was developed for ordering obtained data through the keys. In practice, the keys are fairly complicated because the traditional binary form of "go, no-go" did not always serve. For example, diagnosis of left-hemisphere involvement requires combinations of as many as 13 different indices. This procedure is part of the contemporary trend toward using systems-analysis techniques to order large collections of data and make decisions. A variation of the method has been developed by Mark for the diagnosis of Minimal Brain Dysfunction; it is described in Chapter 2.

Research psychiatrists and psychologists are also beginning to apply systems analysis to the study of complicated diagnostic problems. Their potentiality for bringing some order into the diagnosis and therapy of syndromes with multiple etiological and therapeutic possibilities, for example schizophrenia and school phobias (4), is intriguing.

Luria's Clinical-Analytic Method

Luria, the distinguished Soviet neuropsychologist, insisted that the fact that a patient solved a test problem is not the important datum in neuropsychodiagnosis, but rather *how* the patient solved it. In a 1966 publication in English (21), Luria judged "psychometric" tests (Binet, Terman, Wechsler) as having limited ability to determine the qualitative features of a cerebral dysfunction.

He saw four essential features in neuropsychological examination:

1) The investigation must be based first upon comprehension of the *possible* types of disturbance that may be caused by a given brain lesion and that may be brought to light during the examination of the patient. The neuropsychologist must know all the syndromes and behavioral disturbances caused by lesions in different locations in the

brain. His investigation must be directed toward exploring for the existence of any of these syndromes. His essential requirement is a range of pilot tests sufficiently wide to screen for the great variety of disturbances that may arise from different types of brain lesions, variously located. Even a preliminary investigation, therefore, must include tests which evaluate auditory, optic, and kinesthetic processes, and motor behavior.

2) An identified impairment must then be analyzed qualitatively to determine whether the deficit is in a relatively elementary mental activity or results from a disturbance of a more complex level of activity. The investigation must further try to determine whether the observed deficit is the primary consequence of a specific aspect of the functional system under investigation or a secondary result of a more primary deficit. The value of the neuropsychological examination is its ability to make such a qualitative analysis and to state its effect upon the entire range of the patient's mental activity.

3) Therefore, the neuropsychological examination must further include tests of integrated activity which examine complex forms of behavior, among them repetitive and spontaneous speech, writing, reading, ability to comprehend textual material, and solution of problems.

In sum, the neuropsychological investigation in Luria's view should be less whether or not a particular problem is solved and more with the way in which it is solved, that is, with "a careful qualitative analysis of the patient's activity, of the difficulties experienced, and of the mistakes made."

Luria recommends that the neuropsychological investigation begin with administration of preliminary tests which are relatively standardized and which aim to generally evaluate various aspects of mental activity and process. In addition to being relatively standardized, these preliminary tests of Luria's first stage must be able to determine the state of what Luria calls the brain's "individual analyzers": optic, auditory, kinesthetic, and motor. The psychologist must be able to describe the various levels of mental processes: direct sensory reaction, mnestic organization of activity, and complex mediated operations. Tests must be graded in complexity and difficulty, and adjustable according to the patient's level prior to his illness, lesion, or disease. Naturally, they must be congruent with the person's cultural background. A large number of these tests are needed, all of short duration because of the fatigability of many brain-damaged patients, to permit identification of as many impairments as possible as well as those functions which reveal no impairment. Undue fatigue in a patient is in itself a meaningful clinical datum suggestive of organicity when resistance, passivity, regression, hunger, and lack of sleep, among other possible causes, are ruled out.

The second stage of Luria's procedure entails more minute and specific exploration of those mental processes in which impairments had been detected by the preliminary testing. This stage is almost strictly individualized. It is developed from the data obtained in the preliminary stage and throughout accommodates itself to the data which successively emerge during the course of the second stage itself. Far more complex and addressing more complicated data, the second stage requires great flexibility in its administration and conduct. The investigator here attempts to verify the intact functions, to determine what remaining form of abilities, analysis, and synthesis the patient is using to circumvent his impairment, to solve problems, and conduct mental activity by mobilizing those "analyzers" which have survived and by moving the attempt at solution to a higher level.

The last stage of Luria's neuropsychological investigation is the making of an ultimate diagnosis or conclusion. Here he describes as fully as possible the basic impairment, how it is manifested in and influences various forms of mental activity in the patient, and the possible organic factors which could underlie such an impairment.

Luria begins with standardized procedures as the basis for neuropsychological examination, then moves into a highly individualized, qualitative exploration, culminating in the diagnosis. All diagnosis requires experience; Luria's qualitative emphasis additionally demands flexibility. The neuropsychological investigator cannot rely solely upon standardized administration of a test or task, but must be able to modify its presentation if he is to discover the factors that make performance difficult for the subject and those used to compensate for difficulties. Luria's dicta of flexibility and qualitative analysis are not totally absent from the orientation of some American neuropsychologists. Burgemeister (5) discussed the need for flexibility in the selection of tests and the order of their deployment "as the patient's diagnosis *emerges*," in her telling phrase. Her recommendations concur with Luria's admonition that the neuropsychologist attends constantly to the evidences of disturbances revealed *as* tasks are required of the patient. Variation in fatigue levels on different tasks, the inhibitory

effect of an irrelevant stimulus upon one activity but not another, response to a change of pace or an increase in complexity, all become significant diagnostic data. Lezak (20) also advises flexibility in selecting tests for the individual patient. Acknowledging that standardized test batteries are invaluable in research, she believes that when they are applied in individual examinations "most patients undergo more testing than is necessary" but, paradoxically, not enough to answer the questions raised by their specific problems.

LEVELS OF CERTAINTY IN NEUROPSYCHODIAGNOSIS

Types of neurological-psychological inquiry, each presenting criteria with a different degree of certainty, number at least three.

1) The neuropsychologist as the experimental investigator working with animals enjoys the most certainty. In laboratory conditions of his own design and control, he usually selects a single process of input, output, or integration, and creates the presumably precise lesion in animals necessary to study the process. His attention is focused upon a single process to the exclusion of others. His tests of behavior have been carefully tailored to the process he is studying.

2) The neuropsychodiagnostician, either clinician or researcher, works with human subjects to investigate known or suspected cases of brain lesion. If the lesion is known, he anticipates specific impairments and assesses these as well as others. If the lesion is unknown, he must first determine the brain-behavior relationship that merits more concentrated study, and so, in Luria's concept (21), he makes a preliminary general investigation of the patient's mental processes, identifies those that appear to have altered in a crucial way, and explores them further. He must also be aware of causal factors other than brain damage: muscle weakness, end-organ impairment, peripheral nerve damage, and cultural, developmental, genetic, and psychodynamic contributants. His data are so complex that he can enjoy far less confidence in his findings than the experimental investigator with animals.

3) The psychodiagnostician sees patients for assessment of emotional-behavioral problems. His investigation is heavily biased in the direction of psychogenic causality. But he too should maintain a routine alertness to the possibility that brain damage is either the etiology of the emotional problem he is exploring, or a contributant to it. He should be acquainted with or reminded of the capacity of his customary test instruments to suggest the behavioral effects of a brain lesion

—their sensitivity to brain-behavior relationship—and be prepared to extend his investigation somewhat if the routine procedures produce data suggestive of brain damage. After this, he requires the same consultative skills as the neuropsychodiagnostician and the neurologist. Obviously, the neurodiagnostic criteria are most clouded for the psychodiagnostician.

CREDITABILITY OF NEUROPSYCHODIAGNOSIS

Sometimes diagnosis is abandoned because too much is demanded of its tools. Conditions necessary before a psychological test may be considered an effective diagnostic tool have been advanced by Theaman (37): 1) the patient's behavior must be altered by the condition being diagnosed; 2) this behavioral change must be measureable by the psychological test being used; 3) the change must be the same for all cases in which the condition is the same; 4) the behavioral change must be unique for the condition being studied; 5) the change must be large enough to be discernible from the normal variability anticipated in the area of behavior being tested. These admirably rigorous standards of validity and reliability are unlikely to be survived by any single psychological test instrument currently available.

Validity and reliability are both extremely important and extremely elusive. Validity turns on the ubiquitous criterion problem. Reliability technically hangs on the degree of concurrence between independent investigators using the same procedures, that is, the concurrence between measurements made at different times, either by the same investigator or different ones using the same procedures. But in clinical practice, the word reliability retains the meaning it has in general use: how dependable is the diagnostic impression of the individual clinician? How much faith can he put in it? The faith the neuropsychologist places in his diagnosis may contribute to the neurosurgeon's decision to use surgery, and if so, where. The psychodiagnostician has often to decide whether or not his diagnosis is a firm basis for exposing the patient to the anxiety and the possible or probable pain of a neurological consultation. The well known phenomena of false positives and false negatives in diagnostic testing of all types prevent reliance upon any single test finding when the fate of an individual is at stake, even though the test has been corroborated by hard neurological findings in, say, 75 percent of a study population. Repetition of test procedures may ameliorate concern about reliability somewhat, but is not always fully feasible in neuropsychodiagnosis. Many areas must be explored, many tests must be administered, and fatigue may mount while motivation drops.

In clinical practice, too, the qualitative approach is to be emphasized. The appropriate flexibility requires varying conditions of investigation from one time to another, from one patient to another. Luria (21) suggests that reliability of the clinical diagnosis is derived from "syndrome analysis": results obtained by different methods in the investigative procedure are compared; if each method points to a common type of disability, even though in a different way, credibility of the diagnosis is increased.

As with equality in some societies, where "all are equal but some are more equal than others," creditability, reliability, for the clinician is indeed variable, a fact that is especially pertinent in evaluating equivocal signs. Here a combination of congruent signs may leave him in doubt of a diagnosis because despite their congruence they still do not develop enough conviction, even synergistically, in him. In contrast, a single sign may be so clear, so convincing, that creditability can be accepted by the clinician despite the weakness or absence of parallel signs. These, then, are the essential sources of creditability in clinical diagnosis: 1) signs lending strength to each other; and 2) the clarity and convincingness of a single sign. Signs that augment each other may be derived from different tools or tasks in the same method of investigation, or from different but complementary methods of investigation: thus a test finding may accumulate creditability from other test findings, observation of the patient's behavior in the waiting room, details of his history like an accident or a febrile episode, from the patient's physician, or from the electroencephalogram. Reliance upon the single, clear sign increases with clinical experience, against which the clinician may "candle" the present diagnostic problem, and draw upon his conscious and preconscious memory of similar clinical patterns and their outcomes.

A MODEL FOR THE NEUROPSYCHODIAGNOSTIC PROCESS

Reitan's advice—to exploit the value in *all* tested methods—is convincing. It is realistic about the limitations inherent in any method, about the numerous independent variables, often undetectable, the complexity of brain-behavior relationship, about the variable effects of variously located lesions. It accepts the ambiguity surrounding criteria, the factors influencing recoverability. It emphasizes concern with and responsibility for individual human welfare.

Reitan's advice was directed toward the use of testing techniques, but it also provides a fundamental guideline for a model of diagnosis incorporating all methods of observation—history, behavioral scrutiny, neuropsychological test, and neurological examination techniques. Such a model would muster all of them in a directed scrutiny of brain-behavior functions both broad and deep. This concept visualizes the diagnostic process as the exploration for factors that gradually quantify the probability of the presence of a lesion, and close in as much as possible upon its location and nature. The neurological examination here is the last stage in the process, because of the alarm it may cause the patient, and the pain and potential danger sometimes required. Thus history taking, behavioral observation, and the neuropsychological examination would precede it, but the order of these three is not important. Indeed, the diagnostician may shift back and forth from one to another as data acquired suggest that some behavior be elicited and studied, or the possibility of a past event be explored, or that a function be measured and compared with other functions. However, usual clinical procedure roughly follows a course that begins with the patient's complaint and present status, then moves to a history to establish antecedents and a baseline for comparing present functioning, and finally initiates special testing and inquiry.

This model derives from the multivariate concept of brain damage and its effects rather than the unitary. The view that brain damage is a unitary phenomenon was inherent in Goldstein's hypothesis that capacity for abstraction is impaired in brain damage of whatever location, so that a single test of abstract ability if graded from the simplest to a sufficiently complex level of abstract reasoning should detect brain damage wherever it may be localized. Satz (33), however, now finds that non-verbal perceptual tasks of more complex level are affected by a brain lesion irrespective of its location or laterality. A number of different functions are apparently necessary for unimpaired performance in a complex task, so that a lesion affecting any one of the functions is likely to affect performance of the complex task itself.

Both types of lesion effects appear to operate: 1) a common end result irrespective of locus; and 2) very specific results characteristic of lesions in specifically defined locations. Research in pursuit of validation for each of the concepts produced ingeniously designed instruments and tests—imbedded figures, rotated and substitution block tasks, background interference procedures. Percentage ability to separate brain-damaged from non-brain-damaged groups, inelegantly termed the "hit rate," has improved. The clinician responsible for the individual patient, however, must use all available methods to improve as far as humanly possible the probabilities for accuracy of diagnosis in an individual case. A neuropsychological testing procedure therefore will encompass all significant sensory modalities, motor functions, manipulative and visuo-spatial tasks, concept formation, language and communication skills, alertness and memory, and, in addition, probe each of these at increasing levels of difficulty and complexity with requirements for intersensory integration, introduction of unfamiliar requirements in visuo-motor tasks, comparison of the two sides of the body, and bilateral simultaneous sensory stimulation. In a similar fashion, the neuropsychodiagnostician will use all those other methods that improve the creditability of findings—history, behavioral observation, and neurological examination. Lack of agreement between methods should not lead to rejection of either of the methods producing the contradictory finding but rather promote continued diligent exploration to improve understanding of the patient's puzzling condition.

TRAINING IN NEUROPSYCHOLOGY FOR THE PSYCHODIAGNOSTICIAN

Ideally, the psychodiagnostician to equip himself in neuropsychology would spend a post-doctoral year in one of the neuropsychological centers attached to hospitals and universities which have proliferated in the past several decades in all parts of the country. More realistically, an informal arrangement can sometimes be made by the practicing psychologist for a brief period of testing experience with brain-damaged patients in one of these centers. Some centers or their personnel acting individually offer workshops in neuropsychological procedures. These are advertised by direct mail brochures or announcements in professional publications such as the *Monitor* of the American Psychological Association (APA). Excellent workshops have been routinely provided at annual conventions by the Clinical Division of the APA. Symposia and paper presentations at conventions of APA, International Neuropsychological Society, Association for Children and Adults with Learning Disabilities, Orton Society, and American Orthopsychiatric Association often address issues of specific interest to individual psychodiagnosticians. The bulletins, newsletters, and journals of these organizations do the same.

Some recent publications are helpful. A compact and cogent chapter-long summary of the role of neuropsychological testing in neurological disorders is presented by Smith (34). His approach is cautious; he cites the lack of precision in tests and batteries, arising from the effect of diaschisis, for example, and discusses the significant subjects of redundancy and cost-efficiency in the selection of tests. He also reviews a small and useful battery of tests.

A volume by Lezak (20) published in 1976 offers the most comprehensive extant effort at a text in neuropsychology; it presents basic concepts, the structure of the brain in relation to behavior, and many neuropsychological procedures and tests.

McFie (22) in a small book emphasizes localization of behavior in the brain, using a small battery of tests familiar to clinical psychologists, with heavy reliance on subtests of the Wechsler scales.

Another volume edited by Smith and Philippus (35) is informative although scattered and somewhat confusing in organization. It stresses the matter of localization, with papers by proponents on both sides of the issue.

Davison's introduction to the volume edited by Reitan and Davison (28) relates neuropsychology and psychiatry and differentiates neuropsychology from clinical psychology.

Neuropsychological Tests

Psychological tests for the detection of brain damage have become numerous, too numerous to be described here. The therapist-diagnostician may want to extend his investigation of the brain-behavior relationship beyond the range of the interview and the standard psychological testing techniques described in Part II. Many of the neurological tests and tests batteries in current use are described by Lezak (20), Reitan and Davidson (28) and by Smith (34).

BIBLIOGRAPHY

1. *Babcock, H.:* An experiment in the measurement of mental deterioration. Arch. Psychol., 18, 1930.
2. *Bach-y-Rita, G., et al.:* An improved naso-pharyngeal lead. Electroencephalography Clin. Neurophysiol., 16, 1969.
3. *Benton, A. L.* and *Joynt, R. J.:* Conclusions and indications for future inves-

tigative work. Presentation 21. *In* A. L. Benton (Ed.): Behavioral Change in Cerebrovascular Disease. New York: Harper and Row, 1970.

4. *Bolman, W. M.:* Systems theory, psychiatry and school phobia. Amer. J. Psychiat., 127:1, 1970.

5. *Burgemeister, B.:* Psychological Techniques in Neurological Diagnosis. New York: Hoeber Medical Division, Harper-Row, 1962.

6. *Clenny, S.:* Problem record of the month. Amer. J. EEG Technol., 10:3, 1970.

7. *Dargassies, S. St.-A.:* Neurodevelopmental symptoms during the first year of life. Develop. Med. Child Neurol., 14, 1972.

8. *Deutsch, C. P.* and *Schumer, F.:* Brain Damaged Children. New York: Brunner/Mazel, 1970.

9. *DiLeo, J. H.:* Early identification of minimal cerebral dysfunction. Acad. Therapy, 5:3, 1970.

10. *Donchin, E.* and *Lindsley, D. B.* (Eds.): Average Evoked Potential: Methods, Results and Evaluation. Washington: National Aeronautics and Space Administration, 1969.

11. *Drachman, D. A.* and *Hart, C. W.:* An approach to the dizzy patient. Neurology, 22:4, 1972.

12. *Ferriss, G. S.:* Evoked responses and their clinical application. Amer. J. EEG Technol., 10:1, 1970.

13. *Gesell, A., et al.:* Gesell Developmental Schedules. New York: Psychological Corporation, 1949.

14. *Goldstein, K.:* Human Nature. Cambridge, Mass.: Harvard University Press, 1940.

15. *Gross, M. D.:* Violence associated with organic brain disease. *In* J. Fawcett (Ed.): Dynamics of Violence. Chicago: American Medical Association, 1971.

16. *Halstead, W. C.:* Brain and Intelligence. Chicago: University of Chicago Press, 1947.

17. *Kennard, M. A.:* The electroencephalogram in psychological disorders: A review. Psychosom. Med., 15, 1953.

18. *Kennard, M. A.:* The characteristics of thought disturbances as related to electroencephalographic findings in children and adolescents. Amer. J. Psychiat., 115, 1959.

19. *Kennard, M.:* Value of equivocal signs in neurological diagnosis. Neurology, 10, 1960.

20. *Lezak, M. D.:* Neuropsychological Assessment. New York: Oxford University Press, 1976.

21. *Luria, A. R.:* Higher Cortical Functions in Man. New York: Basic Books, 1966.

22. *McFie, J.:* Assessment of Organic Intellectual Impairment. London: Academic Press, 1975.

23. Minimal Brain Dysfunction in Children: Educational, Medical and Health Related Services: Phase Two of a Three Phase Project. Washington, D. C.: U.S. Dept. of Health, Education and Welfare, Public Health Service Education No. 2015, 1969.

24. *Monroe, R. R.:* Episodic Behavioral Disorders. Cambridge, Mass.: Harvard University Press, 1970.

25. *Mora, G., et al.:* Psychiatric syndromes and neurological findings as related to academic underachievement—implications for education and treatment. Mimeo, undated.

26. *Piotrowski, Z.:* The Rorschach ink-blot method in organic disturbance of the central nervous system. J. Nerv. Ment. Dis., 86, 1937.

27. *Poeck, K.:* Modern trends in neuropsychology. *In* A. L. Benton (Ed.): Contributions to Clinical Neuropsychology. Chicago: Aldine, 1969.

28. *Reitan, R. M.* and *Davison, L. A.* (Eds.): Clinical Neuropsychology: Current Status and Applications. Washington, D. C.: V. H. Winston and Sons, 1974.
29. *Reitan, R. M.:* Objective behavioral assessment in diagnosis and prediction. Presentation 15. *In* A. L. Benton (Ed.): Behavioral Change in Cerebrovascular Disease. New York: Harper and Row, 1970.
30. *Reitan, R. M.:* Psychological assessment of deficits associated with brain lesions in subjects with normal and subnormal intelligence. *In* J. L. Khanna (Ed.): Brain Damage and Mental Retardation: A Psychological Evaluation. Springfield, Illinois: Charles C Thomas, 1967.
31. *Ritvo, E. R., et al.:* Correlation of psychiatric diagnosis and EEG findings: Double blind study of 184 hospitalized children. Amer. J. Psychiat., 126:7, 1970.
32. *Russell, E. W., et al.:* Assessment of Brain Damage. New York: Wiley-Interscience, 1970.
33. *Satz, P.:* A block rotation task: The application of multivariate and decision theory analysis for the prediction of organic brain disorder. Psychol. Monog., 80:21, 1966.
34. *Smith, A.:* Neuropsychological testing in neurological disorders. *In* W. J. Friedlander (Ed.): Advances in Neurology, Vol. 7. New York: Raven, 1975.
35. *Smith, W. L.* and *Philippus, M. J.* (Eds.): Neuropsychological Testing in Organic Brain Dysfunction. Springfield, Illinois: Charles C Thomas, 1969.
36. *Strub, R. L.* and *Black, F. W.:* The Mental Status Examination in Neurology. Philadelphia, Penn.: F. A. Davis, 1977.
37. *Theaman, M.:* The performance of post-traumatics, post-traumatic epileptics, and idiopathic epileptics on psychological tests. Doctoral dissertation, New York University, School of Education, 1950.
38. *Tinterov, L. A.:* Brain scan in suspected intracranial arteriovenous malformation: Report of a case. Dis. Nerv. Syst., 30:7, 1969.

CHAPTER 18

Brain Injury and Recoverability

The brain, encased in bone, surrounded by meningeal tissue, and floating in fluid, is nonetheless vulnerable to many vicissitudes. Defective fetal development can result in structural malformation. Diseases of unknown etiology can afflict it, for example, narcolepsy and epilepsy. The brain is subject to demyelinating diseases (multiple sclerosis), diseases of metabolism affecting blood, nerve tissue and bone, toxic diseases caused by bacteria (diptheria), degenerative diseases, which may be hereditary, and to infections of the brain and the meninges specifically, such as abscesses, poliomyelitis, encephalitis, syphilis. The brain can be damaged by tumors, vascular lesions or accidents and traumas. It can be attacked chemically by such metallic compounds as lead, and by organic compounds like alcohol and the barbiturates. The effects of these insults were described in the preceding chapters on brain behavior and cerebral lateralization. Here we will consider how much function can be recovered after injury has been suffered and impairment has appeared.

Some effects are clearly irreversible, given the inability of neurons to regenerate themselves. Deficits of function caused by fetal structural defects are one example. A massive injury may obliterate all or most of the representations of a function, or a function may be so finely localized that a confined injury to the precise site will result in deficit. Also, interruption of a pathway at a critical point may prevent takeover or seriously impair retraining.

This irreversibility is the most dismal aspect of the prospects for brain-injured persons. LeVere (15), for one, emphasizes that recovery depends upon the nature and amount of tissue that is spared in any insult to the brain. Dawson (5) in a review of the literature finds

387

little support for a holistic view of the brain that would derive from evidence that recovery of a lost function comes about through the redundant representation of that function in the brain or from a multiplicity or overlapping of control by anatomically different neural centers.

Still, a considerable body of experience lends more optimism to the prognosis. Evidence is mounting that neural modification in response to the organism's experience does take place, that while no new neurons are created after a very early age, dendrites do proliferate in response to experience and training (19). Experiments with both young and adult animals yield persuasive evidence that changes in the CNS occur with changes in internal and external environments. The old concept of implacable irreversibility is being replaced; neuronal structure is seen to be more plastic than previously believed. Neurons receive numerous new connections from other neurons; combining and re-combining goes on (9, 12). Horn, *et al.* (13) report that new dendrite connections are more numerous in rats living in an environment rich with play activities than in rats living in a "deprived" environment. This is true even when the rats in the play environment are blind. The recent extension of investigation into biochemical influences on the brain has demonstrated chemical control of dendritic and glial cell growth (16), suggesting a chemical view of the brain instead of a purely anatomical one. The number of neurotransmitters identified has increased and their role in brain-behavior extended. They are now seen to have a role in the capacity of some of the brain to reform itself, to correct disconnections resulting from injury.

Studies of humans also provide evidence supporting the concept of plasticity. Seizure disorders may disappear, for example, even without treatment, usually with a gradual decrease in frequency and intensity of seizure episodes.

Duration of coma following serious head injury appears to be inversely related to degree of eventual recovery of motor and intellectual abilities, although some intellectual deficit remains probable (2).

The age when injury is sustained clearly influences the outcome. Gallagher's experience in tutoring brain-injured children is described by Reitan (20). Significantly greater improvement was observed in children eight to ten than in those ten to twelve years of age. Moreover, improvement was greater in verbal than in non-verbal skills. The capacity of the right hemisphere to assume language functions if the person is young enough when the left side is damaged is another aspect of the effect of age upon prognosis (6). Studies have been reported by Rosner (21) in which a majority of eight children who had left hemispherectomies for intractable seizures regained speech or developed it *de novo*. It would appear that the earlier the right hemisphere is called upon to assume verbal skills, the more likely is there to be normal or near-normal development of verbal processes. Of course, the right hemisphere must be intact if it is to assume substitute functions, and it cannot be automatically assumed that it escapes harm during the surgery.

Some clinicians would argue that the age variable in recoverability cannot be stated unequivocally. They would contend that the same lesion in two people of different ages may affect the older person less adversely than the younger one because the brain of the older person has enjoyed more years of stable integration, as contrasted, say, with the person who sustained a lesion at birth. However, the argument depends upon demonstration that two lesions are at least similar, the problems of exact neurological diagnosis being what they are.

Recovery and development of function following hemispherectomy have been extensively followed by Smith and his colleagues; they report "before" and "after" neuropsychological data in cases of both right and left hemispherectomies. A five-and-one-half-year-old boy after left-hemispherectomy developed superior language and intellectual abilities (23). A six-year-old boy demonstrated rapid and continued improvement in cerebral function, with gains of 30 points in Verbal I.Q. and 38 points in Performance I.Q. after right-hemispherectomy. These were associated with gains in performance on the Hooper's Visual Organization Test, the Raven's Progressive Matrices, the Peabody Picture Vocabulary Test, the Memory for Unrelated Sentences Test, and the Purdue Pegboard (22).

Partial cerebral plasticity, the potentiality of one hemisphere to assume functions predominantly those of the other hemisphere, is postulated by Fields and Whitmyre (7) to account for the diminution and sometimes disappearance of Verbal-Performance disparities associated with lateralized brain damage.

Over-optimism about cerebral compensation is unwarranted nonetheless. Damage to the immature brain may have more serious consequence for the subsequent development of higher functions than will damage to the mature brain in which those functions have already been established. A symposium (24) of knowledgeable workers in the field concluded that much uncertainty remains about the factors that influence recovery and that current hypotheses about recovery factors are attended by conflicting evidence. Nonetheless, recovery occurs and further efforts to comprehend its determinants are clearly justified.

The nature of the initial lesion influences what may be expected in the future course. If of a nonprogressive nature, the functional limitation is definable as of the time of observation, and the degree of reversibility may be estimated from all of the clinical facts. When the lesion is progressive in nature, the effects, of course, are less predictable. An acute lesion of nonprogressive nature tends to produce more impairment than does a static chronic condition. Thus Fitzhugh, et al. (8) found that patients with static lesions produce performances superior to those of patients with acute lesions on the Wechsler-Bellevue and on eight tests of the Halstead battery.

Promise of ability to *predict* improvement in the cerebrovascular-accident patient by the level of behavior-test performance soon after injury is held forth in work by Meier and Resch (17). Predictors were selected from the Proteus mazes, the Trailmaking Test, the Sequin-Goddard Form Board, and a Visual-Space test. These were evaluated against ratings of change in objective neurological signs over a seven-to-ten-day period of hospitalization. The extent of change in neurological signs was linearly related to the level of test performance on the second day of hospitalization.

The degrees-of-intertest (WAIS) variability was found to be inversely related to time elapsed since onset of the injury by Watson (25), who finds that differentiation of brain-damaged from schizophrenic patients by psychological tests is less clear if the brain damage is a chronic condition. EEG data (20) suggest that in nonproliferating, nondegenerative disorders that are likely with time to become static there is progressive diminution of the impairment.

The preinjury personality and constitution are important prognostic variables. The similarity of post-traumatic symptoms to pre-traumatic neurotic ones is observed by Burgemeister (3). Patients who were markedly neurotic before injury are more likely to display post-traumatic behavioral complications. Some workers believe, she reports, that the pretraumatic personality has more effect upon post-traumatic behavior than do the sequelae of the trauma.

Genetic constitution, experience, and training before injury are cited by Rosner (21) as influencing the pace and scope of recovery.

A significant component of prognosis for any individual who has suffered brain damage is the alteration in that person's "dynamic field" produced by his impairment. This factor might be called his "recovery environment." Klebanoff, et al. (14) recommend analysis of the specific demands upon the patient—social, familial, personal—to permit development of educational and psychotherapeutic techniques to help the patient to meet those demands better, even altering the environment if necessary, to bring its demands to a reasonable level.

The essential fact to be explained to important persons around a brain-injured individual may be that his ability for abstract thinking has been limited, perhaps beyond restoration. They must understand that improvement will result only from retraining—the development of substitute functions through the intact residue. Even when learned, a new behavior may soon be extinguished in the brain-damaged person unless reinforced (20), so that the environment may require modification to assure this reinforcement. Complete plasticity—hence complete recoverability—does not appear to be the good fortune of either the growing or the adult brain. K. Goldstein's (10) observation of irreversibility of abstract deficit and dependence upon remaining concrete behavior for improved performance is well-known, though now sometimes contested.

Some degrees of improvement or recovery of function are frequently possible. Increasing the flow of blood to the brain where it has been blocked and reduced is associated with improved performances in objective measures by S. G. Goldstein, et al. (11). The authors explored the subjective report of patients who felt themselves to be "smarter" than they had been for years after carotid endarterectomy (removal of plaque from a stenotic or occluded carotid artery by extracranial surgery). The improvement was partial, however, and the patients' performances were still similar to those of persons with stroke impairments.

Vigorous and persistent rehabilitation efforts with victims of cerebrovascular accidents at centers such as the Rusk Institute of Rehabilitation Medicine in New York City (1) have demonstrated that deficits in the capacity for abstraction can be modified, in contradiction of K. Goldstein's dictum. Their programs are reported also to have succeeded in helping these patients relearn the ability to focus on important points, to shift focus when necessary, to ignore the given in order to search for a higher level meaning, to maintain sets and to scan.

Recovery with intensive training in cases of severe aphasia is reported. Davies and Grunwell (4) caution, however, that the improvement in such cases occurs only in those specific areas to which the re-learning is directed.

Biofeedback techniques are said to facilitate recovery. Mostofsky (18) finds support in behavioral techniques for the hypotheses that 1) physiological change takes place through learning activity so that 2) physiological change can be taught as a therapeutic procedure.

Assessment of the prognostic probabilities is thus possible only through data gleaned about many variables: age at injury, nature and extent of the lesion, redundancy of representation of the function in the cortex, the preinjury personality and constitution, resolution of personal demands of and upon the patient, the opportunity for appropriate retraining, and enlightened reception by the recovery environment. Interacting with these variables are those of cerebral plasticity, changes with the maturational process, and the recovery function of extended time lapse. Continuing improvements up to seven years after serious brain injuries have been reported for both motor and intellectual abilities (2). To all of these must be added the nature, degree, consistency, and persistence of training or re-training, and the age at which training is introduced. If a prenatal or perinatal injury is detected at birth or soon after, and special training is instituted, the likelihood for development of functional competence is greater than if the injury is deducted *post hoc,* years later. This is illustrated by the experience with children with cerebral palsy, where greater gains in motor skills, more quickly achieved, are correlated with early training, and in turn with higher intelligence quotients.

The rewarding consequences of careful diagnostic evaluation followed by early, consistent, phase-oriented support and instruction emphasize the potentiality for some improvement in almost all cases. A major variable in all instances is the basic features of the patient's personality that combine into the determination to exercise and extend every increment of improvement any of the other variables provide. The importance of this motivating drive frequently makes psychotherapy a determining factor in recoverability.

BIBLIOGRAPHY

1. *Ben-Yishay, Y., et al.:* Prediction of rehabilitation outcome from psychometric parameters in left hemiplegics. J. Consult. Clin. Psychol., 34:3, 1970.
2. *Brink, J. D., et al.:* Recovery of motor and intellectual function in children sustaining severe head injuries. Devel. Med. Child Neurol., 12:5, 1970.
3. *Burgemeister, B. B.:* Psychological Techniques in Neurological Diagnosis. New York: Hoeber Med. Div., Harper-Row, 1967.

4. *Davies, C. L.* and *Grunwell, P.:* A new approach to the treatment of severe dysphasia: A case study. Brit. J. Disorders Commun., 10:2, 1975.
5. *Dawson, R. G.:* Recovery of function: Implications for theories of brain function. Behavior. Biol. 8:4, April 1973.
6. *Fedio, P.* and *Mirsky, A. F.:* Selective intellectual deficits in children with temporal lobe or centrencephalic epilepsy. Neuropsychologia, 7:4, 1969.
7. *Fields, F. R.* and *Whitmyre, J. M.:* Verbal and performance relationships with respect to laterality of cerebral involvement. Dis. Nerv. Syst., 30:3, 1969.
8. *Fitzhugh, K. B., et al.:* Psychological deficits in relation to acuteness of brain dysfunction. J. Consult. Psychol., 25:1, 1961.
9. Functional recovery after lesions. Neurosciences Res. Prog. Bull., 12:2, 1973.
10. *Goldstein, K.:* The effect of brain damage on the personality. Psychiat., 15, 1952.
11. *Goldstein, S. G., et al.:* Neuropsychological changes associated with carotid endarterectomy. Cortex, 6:3, 1970.
12. *Haydu, G. G.:* Experience said to modify cerebral neuronal structure. Reported anon. Frontiers of Psychiatry, 2:11, 1972.
13. *Horn, G., et al.:* Experience and plasticity in the central nervous system. Science, 181, August 1973.
14. *Klebanoff, S. G., et al.:* Psychological consequences of brain lesions and ablations. Psychol. Bull., 51:1, 1954.
15. *LeVere, T. E.:* Neural stability, sparing, and behavioral recovery following brain damage. Psychological Rev., 82:5, 1975.
16. *Lynch, G., et al.:* The response of the dentate gyrus to partial diaffrenation. *In* M. Santini (Ed.): Golgi Centennial Symposium Proceedings. New York: Raven Press, 1973.
17. *Meier, M. J.* and *Resch, J. A.:* Behavioral prediction of short-term neurologic change following acute onset of cerebrovascular symptoms. Mayo Clinic Proc., 1967.
18. *Mostofsky, D. I.:* Teaching the nervous system. N.Y.U. Educ. Quart., 6:3, 1975.
19. *Pribram, K. H.:* Languages of the Brain: Experimental Paradoxes and Principles in Neuropsychology. Englewood Cliffs, N. J.: Prentice-Hall, 1971.
20. *Reitan, R. M.:* Psychological deficit. Ann. Rev. Psychol., 13, 1962.
21. *Rosner, B. S.:* Brain functions. Ann. Rev. Psychol. 21, 1970.
22. *Smith, A., et al.:* Neuropsychological studies of a six-year-old boy with right hemispherectomy. Presented at the Annual Convention of the American Psychological Association, 1978.
23. *Smith, A.* and *Sugar, O.:* Development of above normal language and intelligence 21 years after left hemispherectomy. Neurol., 25:9, 1975.
24. *Stein, D. G., et al.:* Plasticity and Recovery of Function in the Central Nervous System. New York: Academic Press, 1974.
25. *Watson, C. G.:* WAIS profile patterns of hospitalized brain-damaged and schizophrenic patients. J. Clin. Psychol., 21:3, 1965.

Index

Abdominal epilepsy, 93. *See also* Epilepsy
Abenson, M. H., 190, 204n.
Abscesses, 387
Abuzzahah, Sr., F. S., 246, 247, 256n.
Acalculias, 39, 145, 239
Acoustic agnosia, 144. *See also* Agnosia
Acting-out behavior, 60, 63, 64, 66, 93, 100
Action syndromes, 313
Adams, J., 296, 304n.
Aggression, 230
Agnosia, 39, 143, 239, 275, 325, 326
Agrammatism, 141, 144
Agraphesthesia, 6, 10
Agraphia, 144, 239, 240
Alcohol:
  cerebral dysfunction of, 17
  intoxication from, 237
  and seizures, 96, 114
Alexia, 144, 195
Allen, R. P., 68, 89n.
Alphachorolose, 94
Alvarez, W. C., 95, 103, 134n., 135n.
Ambar, 113
American Orthopsychiatric Association, 383-84
American Psychological Association (APA), 383
Amnesia, 94
  and psychosis, 185
  retrograde, 18
Amniocentesis, 218
Amniotic sac, 218
Amobarbital, 246
Amphetamines, 17, 53, 70, 96, 237, 277
Analgesics, 15
Analytic-inferential-deductive method, 265

Anemia and infant brain damage, 15
Anesthesias, 15, 331
Angiography, 22, 352, 365
Anhedonia, 38
Anisocoria, 7
Anomia, 143, 144, 224
Anoxia, 95, 140, 181, 217, 254
  and asphyxiation, 13-15
  and brain functions, 330
  and neurological disorder, vii
  and poverty, 19
  and retardation, 17
  and structural defect, 31
Anterior aphasia, 141. *See also* Aphasia
Anticonvulsive medication, xxxi, 107, 251
Antidepressants, tricyclic, xxxi, 96, 237
Antipsychotic drugs and pregnancy, 16
Anxiety, xxxi, 254, 260, 261, 307, 308, 311, 312, 317
  denial of, 315
  and depression, 229
  and diagnosis, 264
  and epilepsy, 103, 124-26
  free-floating, 276
  and MBD, 38, 39
  and neurosis, 83
  and psychosis, 168, 170, 175, 189, 193
  and retardation, 224
  and seizures, 108, 109
  and separation, 59-60
  and therapy, 59-60, 63, 65
  tolerance of, 64, 82
  and word-finding, 144
Apgar, F., 12, 24n.
Aphasia, 39, 140-48, 169, 170, 200, 202,

395